D0229440

052363

MEN'S HEALTH

HEALTH LIBRARY

MEN'S HEALTH

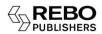

REBO
PUBLISHERS

© 2006 Ars Medica, Grupo ArsXXI, Barcelona, Spain
© 2006 Rebo Publishers

Concept and project manager: Jordi Vigué
Editor of original version: Myriam Cañas
Corrections: Ramon Aymerich
Medical advice: Dr. Gonçal Folch
Photography: Capsa Màgica Studio
Illustrations: Ana Journade, Roger Tallada, David Navarrot, Daniel Martínez
Image processing: Rosa Rigau
Graphic design: Celia Valero
Layout: Glòria Badia, Yasmín Sancho, Marta Ribón, Claudia Martínez, Martín Riveiro, Manuel Guirado
Editorial coordination: Miquel Ridola

Layout: AdAm Studio, Prague, The Czech Republic
Typesetting and pre-press services: AdAm Studio, Prague, The Czech Republic
Translation: Guy Shipton for First Edition Translations Ltd, Cambridge, UK
Editing: David Price for First Edition Translations Ltd, Cambridge, UK
Proofreading: Sarah Dunham, Jeffrey Rubinoff

ISBN 13: 978-90-366-1905-9
ISBN 10: 90-366-1905-X

C O N T E N T S

infancy and childhood

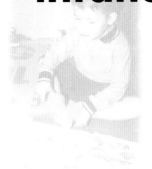

Infancy is the first stage in a human being's life. In this phase, the external appearance of males and females is very similar, their genitalia being the sole external factor that sets them apart. Characteristics of this stage include growth and the progress that a baby undergoes in terms of awareness of its own body and everything around it.

Babies: the first year of life

Increase in the baby's size and weight

Babies lose a little weight in the first few days of life, but shortly afterward they show regular gains, managing to double their weight by the age of five months. Once they have reached six months, babies grow in a slower, more irregular fashion and, by the age of one, will weigh three times more than they did at birth.

Babies also experience significant growth during their first 12 months of life, although it is in the first six months that they grow most rapidly. At one year old, a baby will be 50 percent larger than when it was born.

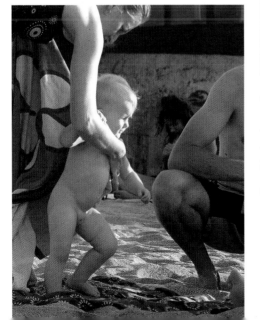

Baby achievements

- Smiles
- Can turn himself around
- Can sit up by himself
- Babbles in his first attempt at speech
- Plays at hiding and then shows himself again
- Appearance of the first teeth
- Manages to stand up
- Walks with assistance, holds onto furniture or something else for support
- Says "Mama" and "Dada"
- Is able to drink from a cup
- Understands "no," and stops whatever he is doing as a result

The cranial perimeter

A baby's cranium is not yet fully fused together, which enables the perimeter of the cranium to increase in size in step with the growth of the brain. In the first six months of life, the cranial perimeter tends to increase in size by more than 2/5 inch a month; afterward, it grows rather more slowly at approximately 1/5 inch each month. From the age of one onward, the head grows gradually and in proportion to the rest of the body.

7

RECOMMENDED IMMUNIZATION BY AGE OF 2			
Vaccine	Prevented disease	Doses	Immunization schedule
Hepatitis B	Hepatitis B	3	At birth, then at 1–2 and 6–23 months
DTaP	Diphtheria	4	At 2, 4, 6, and 15–23 months
	Tetanus		
	Pertussis (whooping cough)		
Hib vaccine	Meningitis from Haemophilus influenzae	3	At 2, 4, and 12–17 months
MPSV4	Meningitis from meningococcus C	1	At age 2–10 years
Inactivated polio virus	Poliomyelitis	3	At 2, 4, and 6–23 months
MMR vaccine	Measles	1	At 12–17 months
	Mumps		
	Rubella (German measles)		

Toddlers: from age 1 to 3

A child will have progressed greatly during the first year (in terms of size, weight, etc.) compared to when newborn, and will have achieved many things (perception of himself and others, recognition of people closest to him, understanding many things said to him, etc.). It is at this stage that he starts to move from one place to another and control his body using a wide and varied range of movement.

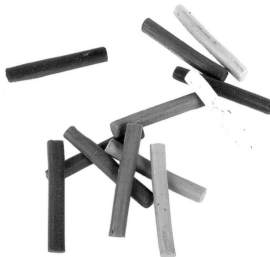

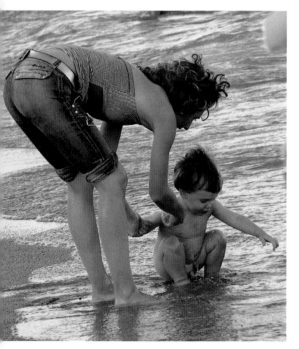

Preschoolers: from age 3 to 6

Increasing weight

Increases in weight become more regular during this stage at roughly the rate of 4 ½–5 ½ lbs a year. This growth means that the child loses the typical chubbiness associated with babies.

Increasing height

The child continues to grow rapidly up until the age of three. Thus by the age of two, he may have grown about 5 inches and by the age of three by 3–3½ inches more. From between three and five, growth becomes more regular, and he will usually gain around 3 inches a year.

▪ Toddler achievements

- Walks
- Can jump clumsily
- Can distinguish between males and females
- Uses a few words and understands simple instructions
- Can run, turn round in circles, and walk backward
- Can eat unassisted and use a knife and fork
- Can refer to everyday objects and indicate parts of the body
- Can go up and down stairs
- Imitates other people's speech, repeats words
- Starts to pedal
- Recognizes and classifies colors
- Starts to make line drawings
- Begins to dress himself
- Learns to share toys

- Begins to throw, kick, and play with a ball
- Can keep his balance briefly on one foot
- Can climb frames in children's playgrounds
- Can turn door handles and faucets
- By the age of three, has developed a preference for using one hand or the other
- Has good control over his thumbs and fingers
- Begins to have control over needing to go to the bathroom

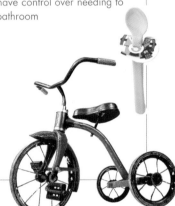

▪ Preschooler achievements

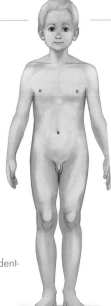

- Rides a tricycle well
- Can draw a circle
- Can make line drawings of faces with two to three features
- Can keep his balance on one leg
- Can run, turn round in circles, and walk backward
- Can catch a bouncing ball
- Can refer to everyday objects and indicate parts of the body
- Understands concepts of size
- Enjoys rhymes and word games
- Can jump
- Enjoys doing most things independently and without help

- Has better balance and is able to start riding a bicycle
- Understands concepts of time
- Starts to recognize written words and gains the ability to read
- Starts to go to school

upper teeth	primary teeth	secondary teeth
central incisor	8–12 months	7–8 years
lateral incisor	9–13 months	8–9 years
canine	16–22 months	11–12 years
first premolar	–	10–11 years
second premolar	–	10–12 years
first molar	13–19 months	6–7 years
second molar	25–33 months	12–13 years
wisdom tooth	–	17–21 years

lower teeth	primary teeth	secondary teeth
wisdom tooth	–	17–21 years
second molar	23–31 months	11–13 years
first molar	14–18 months	6–7 years
second premolar	–	11–12 years
first premolar	–	10–12 years
canine	17–23 months	9–10 years
lateral incisor	10–16 months	7–8 years
central incisor	6–10 months	6–7 years

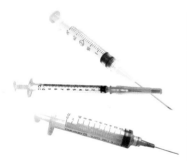

RECOMMENDED IMMUNIZATION BETWEEN AGES 3 AND 6 YEARS			
Vaccine	Prevented disease	Doses	Immunization schedule
DTaP	Diphtheria	1	At age 4–6
	Tetanus		
	Pertussis		
Inactivated polio virus (IPV)	Poliomyelitis	1	At age 4–6
	MMR vaccine		
	Measles		

The Oedipus complex

Children are capable of telling sexes apart (and, therefore, the type of emotional relationship that exists between their parents) from the age of three.

- The mother, who is the most important person for the child, loves not only him, but also has a very special and simulta-neously very different relationship with the child's father. This situation creates feelings of jealousy in the child and the desire to separate his mother and father, so enabling him to take his father's place. Between the ages of three and five, it is quite usual to see boys showing an exagger-ated preference for their mothers: this ranges from caresses and cuddling all the way to creating a scene when sepa-rated from mom, including demands that only mom is allowed to wash them at bathtime, or give them something to eat, or help dress them. Furthermore, physical displays of affection between a boy's parents can engender intense

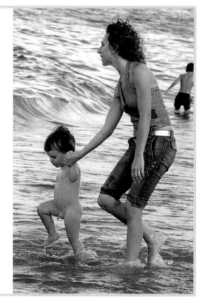

feelings of jealousy in him, giving rise to tantrums, as well as attempts to separate them. Most of the time, little notice is taken of this type of behavior and it is interpreted simply as childish silliness—a display of attachment and affection toward the mother. However, a boy genuinely suffers in this situation. As the object of his attention fixates on his mother, so his father is gradually transformed into a rival. This behavior is referred to as the Oedipus complex, and it marks the first major sexual event in a boy's life. The term was coined by Sigmund Freud, the father of psychoanalysis, and was based on the Ancient Greek story of *Oedipus Rex*, which relates the tragedy of a young man who, attempting to escape the oracle's premonitions, ends up fulfilling them by killing his father and marrying his mother.

Elementary school: from age 6 to 11

Achievements of a child at elementary school

- Can already understand and carry out a series of instructions by the age of 6
- Starts to get to grips with team sports (soccer, basketball, etc.)
- Permanent teeth take the place of milk teeth
- Develops significant routines for daily activities
- Has greater skill in reading and writing
- Friendships and social recognition start to become important

RECOMMENDED IMMUNIZATION BETWEEN AGES 11 TO 16			
Vaccine	**Prevented disease**	**Doses**	**Immunization schedule**
Td	Diphtheria	1	At age 13–16
	Tetanus		
Hepatitis B	Hepatitis B	3	monthly and with a 6-month gap after the first
MMR vaccine	Measles	1	At age 11
	Mumps		
	Rubella (German measles)		

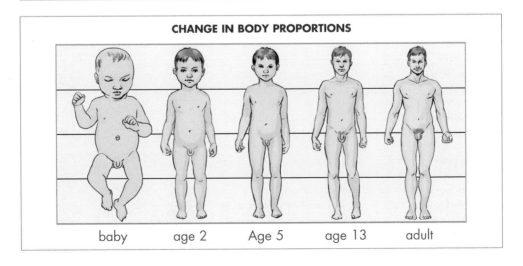

CHANGE IN BODY PROPORTIONS

baby   age 2   Age 5   age 13   adult

◾ Increases in size and weight

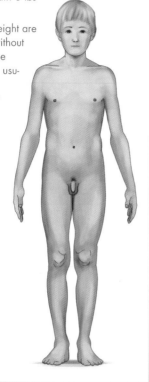

- During this period before adolescence, boys' growth is stable and without abrupt changes. As far as weight is concerned, they usually gain 6 lbs 8 oz a year.

- Increases in height are also regular without great leaps, the rate of growth usually being approximately 2–2½ inches each year.

	BOYS	
Age	Average weight in lbs	Average height in feet & inches
1st month	9 lbs 6 oz	21.7 inches
2nd month	11 lbs 1 oz	22.4 inches
3th month	12 lbs 11 oz	24.0 inches
4th month	14 lbs 0 oz	24.4 inches
5th month	15 lbs 5 oz	24.8 inches
6th month	16 lbs 11 oz	25.2 inches
7th month	17 lbs 10 oz	26.0 inches
8th month	18 lbs 10 oz	26.8 inches
9th month	19 lbs 10 oz	27.2 inches
10th month	20 lbs 10 oz	28.0 inches
11th month	21 lbs 5 oz	28.7 inches
12th month	21 lbs 10 oz	29.5 inches
18th month	24 lbs 3 oz	31.9 inches
2nd year	26 lbs 5 oz	2 feet 9 inches
3rd year	30 lbs 12 oz	3 feet 1 inch
4th year	35 lbs 7 oz	3 feet 3 inches
5th year	39 lbs 12 oz	3 feet 6 inches
6th year	43 lbs 15 oz	3 feet 8 inches
7th year	48 lbs 9 oz	3 feet 11 inches
8th year	52 lbs 0 oz	4 feet 0 inches
9th year	58 lbs 4 oz	4 feet 3 inches
10th year	63 lbs 6 oz	4 feet 4 inches

Sexuality

- Generally speaking, boys aged 7 already have an understanding of the basic anatomical differences between the sexes and, display a certain reticence and shyness about showing their bodies. This shyness is behavior learnt from the way that their parents behave in this respect; but at the same time, the child's natural curiosity comes to light in games that facilitate sexual exploration. Homosexual play between boys, as well as heterosexual play with girls, forms part of normal development at this age.

puberty

Adolescence is the stage in life between the ages of 10 and 19. It is at this time that very specific physical, psychological, and social changes take place. Puberty refers solely to the physical changes that indicate the process of sexual maturity that is in progress. Puberty generally begins in adolescence, although in some cases it can make its appearance before that age.

At age 12

Main characteristics

There is variance in facial features as the jaw and nose grow.

The voice becomes gruffer: at first, boys may find it hard to produce the right sounds, or they may make croaking noises; if so, this condition soon corrects itself.

Normally, between 60 and 70 percent of boys undergoing puberty experience development of fatty nodules below the skin around their nipples. In rare instances, these nodules can measure more than ¾–1¼ inches in diameter; at first, they may be painful, but they are not an abnormality and disappear by themselves one or two years later.

The first change seen in boys, and the one that signals the onset of puberty, is an increase in size of the testicles. In infancy, the testicles have a volume of less than 0.1 fluid oz and a diameter of ¾ inch or less. The action of gonadotropin-releasing hormones causes the testicles to grow in size and produce the specifically masculine hormone called testosterone and develop spermatozoa. Testosterone and a hormone derived from it called dihydrotestosterone are what cause the physical changes characteristic of this phase. The testicles, together with activity in other glands, begin to produce other substances, which create seminal fluid; its buildup and expulsion from the body constitute an ejaculation. A boy's first ejaculation is the sign that body and sex organs have started to develop.

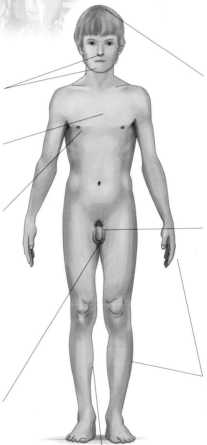

It is during puberty that the growth *spurt* occurs: the period when boys start to grow rapidly. This occurs relatively late in males and begins once the other signs of puberty have already started. It commences between the ages of 11 and 16, lasting approximately 3 years. Adolescents grow between 7 and 10 inches during this period, although they may continue growing more slowly for a few years afterward.

Shortly after the testes have started to increase in size, dark wiry hair begins to appear in the pubic region; later, this hair extends to other areas of the body, such as the armpits, the face, the chest, and limbs. Not long after, the penis increases in length and girth; this usually commences around age 11 and ends at about age 16.

Gradual growth occurs with initial enlargement of the hands and feet, followed by the arms and legs, and finally the torso and chest. Skeletal growth precedes muscular development, which causes an imbalance in the body's proportions.

Muscle mass and consequently strength start to increase at the same time as the limbs begin to lengthen, which can occur quickly enough to give rise to uncoordinated movement, making boys appear somewhat clumsy. Lethargy can accompany this clumsiness. Moreover, boys become distracted, narcissistic, and rebellious.

■ Puberty

The term "puberty" comes from the Latin word *pubes*, meaning "hair." The Romans considered body hair to be the first sign of virility in boys, and, in fact, the appearance of pubic hair is today considered to be a medical criterion for establishing the onset of puberty.

Very rapid changes take place during puberty, particularly in the body. Mental and psychological changes take more time than physical ones, and for that reason adolescent males can show a developmental imbalance between their mind and body. This imbalance results in conflicts and the typical problems of adolescence. In many cases the adolescent still sees himself as a boy, while his body is turning into that of an adult.

At age 15

Main characteristics

The skin becomes much firmer and more resistant; the most obvious changes in adolescents are eruptions of blackheads, which precede the appearance of acne. This is the result of increased activity in the sebaceous glands.

Armpit hair usually appears in adolescent males two years after pubic hair. Facial hair appears later still, firstly on the upper lip, next on the cheeks, and finally on the chin.

Hormonal changes also cause increased activity in the sweat glands, which secrete a denser fluid, causing a significant change in body odor.

As the process of puberty continues, the development of the genitals becomes greater, erections become more frequent, and the first nocturnal emissions occur.

The penis develops as well, eventually measuring between 4½ and 6½ inches when erect. The amount of pubic hair increases. At first, it assumes a triangular shape, similar to the growth pattern in females. Toward the end of puberty, it forms more of a rhomboid shape with an upper line of hair running to the navel.

In the last stage of puberty—three or four years after it first began—the adolescent is nearing young adulthood, and is very close to his final, full height. The speed of growth begins to decelerate. The genitals will have reached full development. The testicles have a volume of 0.7–0.8 fluid oz, measuring 2–2½ inches in diameter, and are contained in the scrotal sac; one testicle is often more descended than the other and their size differs slightly. The appearance of the scrotum also changes, with the skin becoming rougher and darker in coloration.

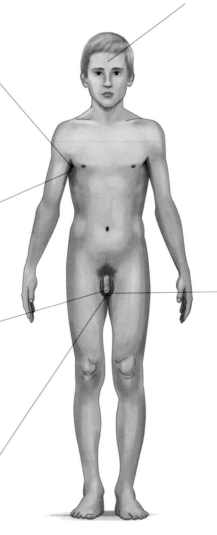

■ Precocious puberty

"Precocious puberty" denotes the development of secondary sexual characteristics in males before the age of 9. Not only do these sexual characteristics appear, but at the same time so does the growth spurt, which causes young people affected by this to seem taller than normal for a while. However, this rapid and premature development can result in young people failing to keep growing in later years. For that reason, they can end up being shorter in stature than their peers.

Precocious puberty is usually produced by a premature activation of the hormonal system. In the majority of female cases, the causes of this premature activity are unknown and do not reveal an underlying medical problem. Although precocious puberty is less common among boys, they require more careful examination. For example, growth of the testicles, penis, or pubic hair before the age of 9 can be a symptom of a hypothalamic tumor, infections (meningitis or encephalitis) or some type of trauma.

As a result of skeletal and muscular growth, weight gain is accompanied by a corresponding gain in physical strength.

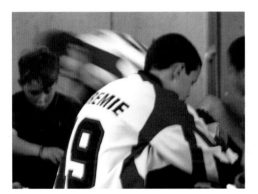

■ Delayed puberty

When the normal timeline for the development of secondary sexual characteristics is late, it is referred to as "delayed puberty." Differences vary greatly from individual to individual, but delayed puberty is usually diagnosed when a 14-year-old boy does not show the features typical for his age. The causes may be genetic, hormonal, or related to chronic illness.

Sperm production

The occurrence of ejaculations, either as the result of masturbation or during nocturnal emissions, happens around the age of 12–13—usually, two years after the testicles start to enlarge and one year after the penis starts to grow. On the first occasion, an adolescent will ejaculate a clear, slightly sticky fluid that contains few spermatozoa. Generally speaking, and despite being able to ejaculate, adolescents do not usually produce normal (adult) levels of sperm until the age of 16.

Nevertheless, from the onset of puberty an adolescent boy is still able to produce more than enough spermatozoa to cause a pregnancy and thus become a father.

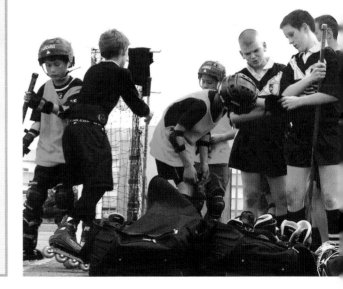

The Tanner stages

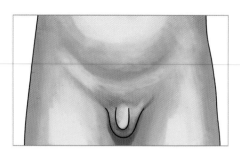

GRADE I

Also referred to as prepubescent. There is no pubic
hair, and the testicles, scrotum, and penis all have
infantile characteristics.

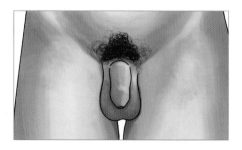

GRADE II

The penis does not alter in size; however, the scrotum
and testicles do enlarge. The scrotum's skin reddens
and becomes slacker. There is a slight growth of pubic
hair at the base of the penis. This is either long and
silky, or slightly wiry.

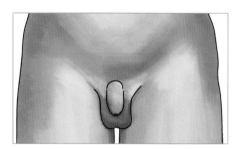

GRADE III

This phase is characterized by an increase in the
length and girth of the penis, and by the enlargement
of the testicles and scrotum. Hair is more abundant,
darker, coarser, and more wiry in the pubic area.

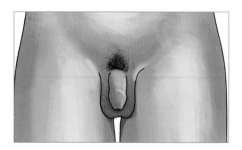

GRADE IV

Penile development continues: increase in diameter
and development of the glans. The testicles also grow,
and the scrotum becomes darker in color. Pubic hair
is similar to that in the adult but covers only a small
area without reaching the thighs or the navel.

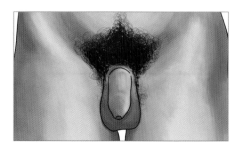

GRADE V

The testicles and penis are fully developed and reach
adult proportions. Pubic hair covers the whole pubic
area, extending to the thighs and navel.

Hormonal changes during male puberty

Puberty is a unique hormonal phenomenon that is not fully understood.

Between the ages of 6 and 8, the adrenal glands located above each of the kidneys begin to increase their secretion of androgens, such as DHEA (dehydroepiandrosterone), which the body uses as the raw material for manufacturing other steroids.

These androgens prepare the hair follicles for growing pubic hair and also cause the skin to thicken and become oilier. They also stimulate the sweat and sebaceous glands, causing a change in body odor—a characteristic feature of puberty.

Another major change concerns the sex hormones. The hypothalamus controls the endocrine system and is connected to the pituitary gland. In adult males and in women of child-bearing age, constant pulses of the hormone GnRH (gonadotropin-releasing hormone) direct the pituitary gland to secrete its hormones.

In turn, these hormones act on the ovaries and testicles to produce ovulations and sperm, as well as estrogen and testosterone.

These hormones have a significant influence on both behavior as well as the body shape of adolescents, who are slowly but surely transformed into sexually active adults.

GnRH remains inactive during childhood. Puberty commences only once this hormone is activated, but precisely how the GnRH hormone is activated is still unknown, although recent studies show that the GPR54 gene and the KiSS-1 peptide are central to the onset of puberty.

In adolescent males, the luteinizing hormone secreted by the pituitary gland stimulates the testicles to produce testosterone.

The body alters once estrogen and testosterone start to appear, changing from childhood to adolescence.

In males, testosterone sculpts the body by increasing muscle mass and gives rise to other features, including the appearance of body hair and beard growth.

TIMELINE OF CHANGES DURING MALE PUBERTY	
Age 11	Enlargement of the scrotum and testicles
Age 12	Time of maximum growth
Age 12	Growth of the penis
Age 13	Growth of pubic hair
Age 14	Growth of armpit hair
Age 14	Change in voice depth
Age 15	Growth of facial hair

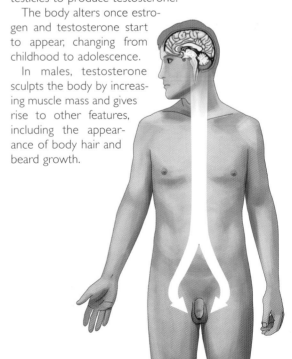

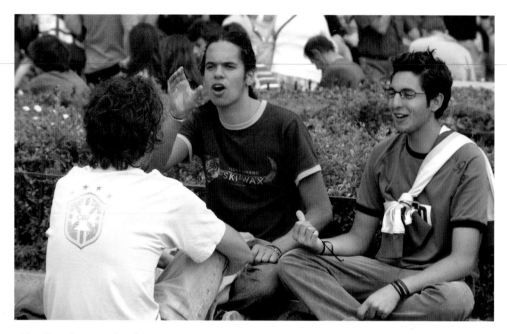

▪ The hypothalamus

- The hypothalamus is responsible for releasing the hormone that secretes gonadotropin (GnRH).

- The production of gonadotropins stimulates the pituitary gland, which produces the luteinizing hormone (LH) and the follicle-stimulant hormone (FSH).

- These hormones are responsible for stimulating the testicles to produce both the hormone testosterone and spermatozoa.

- The pituitary gland controls the production of testosterone and its level in the blood.

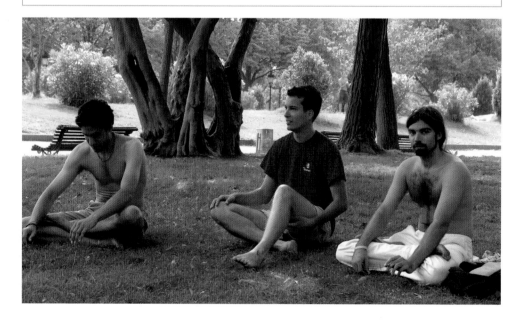

adolescence and teenagers

Adolescence is a process in the human lifecycle without fixed time limits—a transition stage. Adolescence commences with puberty. In other words, it begins with relatively rapid, physiological changes that culminate in full sexual maturity and thus the capacity to reproduce and have sexual relationships. However, adolescence cannot be reduced to these changes alone, because it is further characterized by significant psychological and social transformations.

Teenager traits

Teenagers are at that stage in life in which they desire more independence from their parents as they start to feel more adult and capable of making their own decisions. In some families, this fact is considered to be normal and logical; in others, it can give rise to conflict, as the teenager rebels against attempts by the parents to assert control and impose obedience on their teenage son or daughter. The more that teenagers distance themselves from their parents in the search for their own identities, the more importance they attach to a group of friends or buddies, as this peer group becomes a refuge in which to try out new ideas and compare their physical and mental growth with that of others.

It is a stage when teenagers begin, bit by bit, to discover their own identities, and this allows them to form bonds with others of a more lasting nature: the process of seeking out a partner has commenced.

Teenagers are typically egocentric, but at around the age of 16 to 17, they become capable of understanding that the world does not revolve solely around them and that others have worries of their own as well.

In early adolescence, a group of friends usually consists of members of the same sex who form gangs, cliques, or clubs in which they try to behave and dress in similar ways, share

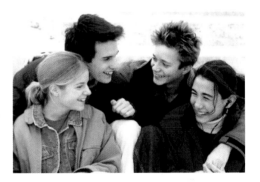

The more that teenagers distance themselves from their parents in the search for their own identities, the more importance they attach to a group of friends or buddies.

secret codes or rituals, and take part in the same activities. As teenagers approach the final stage of adolescence, their circle of friends expands to include members of the opposite sex.

Mid- to late adolescence is characterized by the need to establish a sexual identity, as well as accommodating to one's own body and sexual feelings. Through friendships, first dates, and experimentation, adolescents learn to express and comprehend sexual intimacy gradually and comfortably, in a way that does not undermine their identity. Adolescents without the opportunity to have such experiences can have difficulty with intimate relationships when adult.

Great changes in thought patterns also occur during adolescence. These derive from the growth and development of the brain as the result of hormonal variations and the accumulation of experience at a social and educational level.

Unlike children, adolescents can develop abstract ideas and concepts on matters such as morality, religion or infatuation. Teenagers see the world from a far more idealistic point of view and fight for what they believe is right and just.

Emotions

Studies have revealed that four out of every ten teenagers experience a phase of feeling so unhappy that they cry and want to get away from it all, even to the point of running away. At some stage during the course of adolescence, one in every five teenagers will think life is no longer worth living.

These common feelings can produce a state of depression that may not be obvious to others. Overeating, drowsiness, and excessive concern about physical appearance can also be signs of unease or emotional dissatisfaction. More obvious signs may take the form of phobias and panic attacks. Furthermore, teenagers who are used to being ignored by other members of their family or by friends will not usually want to discuss their problems.

Frequent problems in adolescence

Sexual issues

The dramatic physical changes during this stage can be a source of concern for some adolescents, especially for those who are shy and do not like to ask questions on the subject. At the other extreme, these concerns can manifest themselves in teenagers showing off excessively—in terms of their sexual prowess as well as their experiences. More than half of

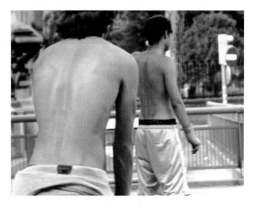

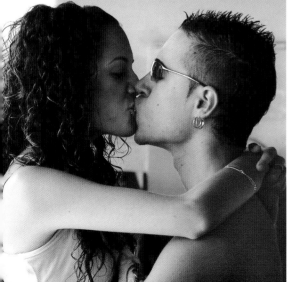

all adolescent boys have their first full sexual experience before the age of 16 or 17, girls by 17 or 18. Those who start having sexual relations early are exposed to a greater risk of unwanted pregnancy and health problems, as well as to the risks posed by HIV, the virus which can lead to AIDS. Moreover, a teenage boy may be unsure of his sexual orientation and wonder whether or not he is homosexual. Unconditional support, straightforward reference material, and reliable information on the various types of sexuality are of great value at this stage of life, whether this comes from his parents, high school, family physician, or

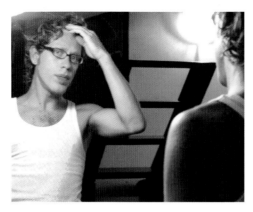

some areas, adolescents can take seriously to heart any restriction of their growing sense of freedom and capacity to make their own decisions. Disagreements are commonplace, because adolescents fight hard to forge their independence. Although all of this is pretty normal, the situation can reach the point at which parents lose control and can no longer keep track of their children or be aware of what is going on in their lives.

family guidance center. The majority of adolescents are relatively careful about their choice of partner. Sexual promiscuity and frequent, unsafe, unprotected sex are usually signs of underlying emotional problems, although this can also reflect an extreme lifestyle.

Drugs, tobacco, and alcohol

Most adolescents do not use illegal drugs or sniff glue, and most of those who do will go no further than occasional experimentation. Despite the publicity surrounding the subject of drugs, it is alcohol that most frequently causes problems in adolescents.

Behavioral issues

Adolescents and parents usually complain in equal measure about each other's behavior. Typically, parents feel that they have lost some measure of control or influence over their children. For their part, while still wanting their parents to provide clarity, rules, and limits in

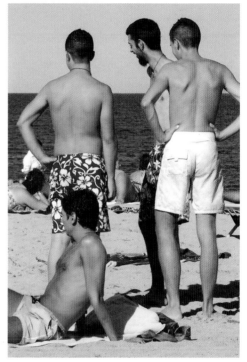

Eating

Being overweight is a frequent cause of unhappiness in teenagers. If they are criticized or laughed at because of their physical appearance, they can become upset and depressed, and this sets a vicious circle of behavior in motion. They do little and eat for comfort, but this succeeds only in aggravating the issue concerning their physical appearance. Diets can make the situation even worse. Fat or skinny, the most important thing is that they feel happy about themselves. Despite the fact that many teenagers go on diets—particularly teenage girls—only a few develop food-related conditions such as bulimia or anorexia nervosa. However, it is adolescents with low self-esteem who are most likely to suffer from bulimia and anorexia, particularly if they feel under pressure or anxious, or if they have had a weight problem in childhood.

Male urogenital organs

The male urogenital organs consist of a series of organs that, sharing a common embryological origin, can be classified separately according to their urinary or genital functions, although these functions sometimes overlap. The reproductive organs consist of the gonads and a series of tubes for transporting spermatozoa, as well as the organs used for copulation.

vas deferens
This is the continuation of the epididymis. It measures some 20 inches in length and conducts spermatozoa from the testicles to the ejaculatory ducts. At the end of its course, it dilates to form a slight bulge—the ampulla of the vas deferens—where the spermatozoa are stored. Each ampulla is linked to a seminal vesicle.

urinary bladder
A bag-shaped organ into which both ureters empty and in which urine is stored before being expelled from the body.

prostate gland
A gland located below the bladder and encircling the urethra. It does not play any role in the erectile function of the penis, but it is important in protecting and lubricating the spermatozoa.

seminal vesicle
This is an accessory gland to the male genital organs and is located to the rear of the bladder. It consists of a blind tube that coils around itself. During ejaculation, these vesicles secrete a fluid rich in fructose —the principal component of semen.

symphysis pubis
The joint created by the union of the pubic bones (pubis, ischium, and ilium) forming the lower limit of the pelvic cavity.

bulbourethral or Cowper's glands
The size of a pea, these glands are located underneath the prostate and are paired either side of the urethra. They are responsible for the minor fluid secretion produced in the penis when a man becomes sexually aroused. Although this secretion cannot be described officially as semen, it does sometimes carry spermatozoa in it and thus can cause pregnancy even when there is no ejaculation.

urethra
The duct through which urine and semen is expelled. It extends from the urinary bladder to the end of the penis. It measures 6½–7¾ inches.

penis
A cylindrical structure that can be divided into three sections: the base of the penis—not visible and formed by the part of the corpora cavernosa (two tubular structures) that is joined to the pelvic bone like an anchor; the shaft or body, which is the most visible part between the base and the glans; and the glans penis, which is the smooth, rounded extremity of the penis and also its most sensitive area.

ejaculatory duct
Formed by the joining of the vas deferens with the seminal vesicle, the duct passes through the prostate, where it joins the urethra.

glans penis
A cone-shaped bulge at the end of the penis.

scrotum
This is the external sac that contains and protects the testicles and is composed of somewhat wrinkled skin, usually darker in complexion than the rest of the body. It becomes covered with pubic hair during puberty.

epididymis
This is a long, narrow tube some 19 feet in length and coiled tightly around itself to form one mass fitting around the back of the testicle. Its function is to store the testicle's secretions, which are propelled toward the vas deferens and urethra during ejaculation.

testicle (testis)
The two testicles are responsible for producing spermatozoa and secreting testosterone. These ovoid sex glands are contained inside the scrotum. They measure 2 inches in length, 1¼ inches in width, and 1 inch in thickness. The interior of the testicle is formed by tiny lobes, each of which houses the seminiferous tubules—ducts that produce spermatozoa. The seminiferous tubules are separated by cells responsible for producing male hormones.

Spermatozoa

Spermatozoa (sperm cells) are the male sex cells capable of fertilizing an egg and they contribute half of the chromosomes or genetic information that go toward creating a new being. A sperm cell is mobile, and its function is to transport the DNA from its nucleus and unite it with the DNA in the egg (ovum), thus producing fertilization. A mature sperm cell is composed of two parts: the head and the tail. The head contains the nucleus and, therefore, the genetic traits that the father will transmit to his descendents. The head is capped with a protuberance called the acrosome, which contains the enzymes necessary for penetrating the egg. The tail, or flagellum, gives the sperm mobility and allows it to travel. A sperm measures 0.05 mm and can be seen only with the aid of a microscope. It can reach a speed of 7 inches an hour and can take an average of two hours to reach the egg.

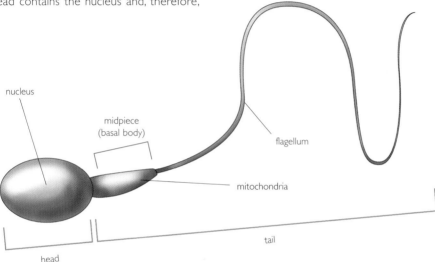

nucleus

midpiece
(basal body)

flagellum

mitochondria

head

tail

▗▘ Seminal fluid

Also referred to as "semen" or "sperm," this is a whitish, viscous fluid with a characteristic odor and is expelled at the time of ejaculation. Seminal fluid is a complex mixture composed of spermatozoa—which represent only a small fraction of the volume ejaculated —and secretions from the testicles and epididymis, secretions from the prostate, and fluid from the seminal vesicles. The latter represents approximately two-thirds of the total volume, while most of the rest of the fluid is from the prostate gland. The volume of ejaculated sperm—normally between 2 and 5 milliliters) —depends on the secretion of male hormones. The number of sperm varies between 25 and 300 million per milliliter. If a man ejaculates twice on the same day, the quantity of sperm in the second ejaculation may be reduced. This also applies to an ejaculation on the day afterward.

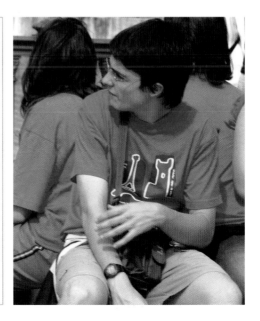

Phases of male sexual function

Spermatogenesis

- The unbroken line shows the concentration of testosterone in the blood over the course of a man's lifetime. The broken line shows the production of sperm during the different phases of his life.

Spermatogonia

MITOSIS

Primary spermatocyte

- The sex hormones set to work even as the embryo is developing in the womb. Because of its genetic code, the fetus produces testosterone, which is responsible for stimulating the development of the reproductive organs. The sex hormones are dormant during childhood. In puberty, however, the body undergoes a genuine hormonal revolution. Testosterone production increases, causing the physical changes typically associated with puberty (growth of body hair, increase in body size, changes to the skin and to the voice, etc.). Testosterone levels are maintained until old age, when they start to diminish, but do not disappear altogether. Due to their continued production of testosterone, men have the ability to produce sperm throughout their entire lives.

MEIOSIS

haploid secondary spermatocytes

- Two distinct processes occur during spermatogenesis—the process that creates the male gametes, which are developed in the testicles. The first of these processes is called meiotic division in which the number of chromosomes is reduced, and the genetic material is reordered (recombined). The second process—referred to as spermiogenesis— produces the most significant structural changes, the compaction of the chromatins, the appearance of the acrosome, and the development of the flagellum.

Differentiation and maturation

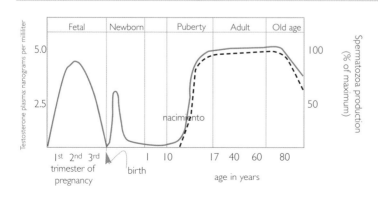

Testosterone plasma: nanograms per milliliter

| Fetal | Newborn | Puberty | Adult | Old age |

5.0

nacimiento

2.5

1st 2nd 3rd
trimester of
pregnancy

birth

1   10   17 40 60   80

age in years

Spermatozoa production
(% of maximum)

100

50

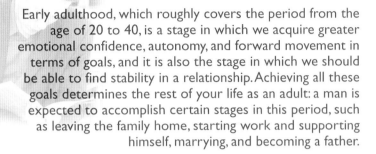

adulthood

Early adulthood, which roughly covers the period from the age of 20 to 40, is a stage in which we acquire greater emotional confidence, autonomy, and forward movement in terms of goals, and it is also the stage in which we should be able to find stability in a relationship. Achieving all these goals determines the rest of your life as an adult: a man is expected to accomplish certain stages in this period, such as leaving the family home, starting work and supporting himself, marrying, and becoming a father.

The young adult male

Young men are in a period of learning, adjustment, and decision-making that leads them toward defining and committing to a choice of lifestyle. Biologically speaking they are adult, but this does not mean that they have made firm decisions in terms of careers, family, and work; psychologically, the assumption is that they will have gotten through the changes brought about by adolescence, such as social freedom, emotional and sexual stability, an integrated identity, and the ability to make commitments.

This is a time when physical capacity reaches its peak efficiency, along with manual dexterity and greater visual accuracy. At this stage, men are in the prime of life; they achieve the peak of their coordination, balance, agility, strength, and endurance.

As long as they develop it, men reach their maximum muscular strength between the ages of 25 and 30.

The body functions perfectly, and such complaints as arise sort themselves out; in other words, young men do not usually suffer illnesses or serious medical conditions, which is why they generally worry little or at all about their health.

Despite the fact that men's physiques are at their peak at this stage, it must be borne in mind that some aspects of male capacity begin to decline from around the age of 30.

After overcoming the egocentricity of adolescence, they become able to empathize with others, share experiences, and behave altruisti-

cally, and they can then establish a responsible relationship with a partner and even take on fatherhood. As a result of discovering his identity and his increasing self-assurance, a man will share with others, whether at work or in his love life, that he has already acquired the capacity to adapt and become involved. At around the age of 30, he tends to reconsider

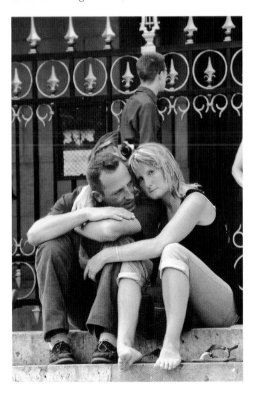

Young men are in a period of learning, adjustment, and decision-making that leads them toward defining, and commitment to, a choice of lifestyle.

his past life and the decisions that he has taken: his choice of partner, his career, etc. New avenues are taken, and commitments are either reinforced or changed. An adult male feels the need for his life to have a solid and committed basis to it in order to achieve stability, which is why he reconstructs and reorganizes it.

The level of productivity increases at around age 20, which has a direct effect on young men's work, the aim of which is to generate income, recognition, and fulfillment. However, the working role brings with it certain problems, particularly in the family setting: there may be a conflict between fatherhood and professional success.

Within the context of mental well-being, stress is a frequent problem resulting from tension, internal and external pressures caused by the demands of work, family, and social relationships, and the dynamics of a lifestyle characterized by constant, accelerating changes. In turn, this can lead to the body's defenses lowering, increasing susceptibility to infectious diseases.

Sex

In this period of a man's life he may either have an active sex life in a stable relationship or enjoy sexual relationships with different partners. Relationships of the latter type come with a higher risk of catching sexually transmitted diseases (STDs), such as syphilis, gonorrhea, or HIV, as well as impersonal and unsatisfactory sexual experiences due to an absence of love and today's unrealistic media stereotyping, which fails to provide fulfillment in reality.

Another consequence of irresponsible sex is unwanted pregnancy, which can result in abortion, forced marriages, or even a complete change in direction to cope with new responsibilities.

Diet

For young adults, diet is affected by various factors, such as food fads, having little time to eat, lack of culinary experience, fast food, alcohol consumption, etc. All these things can result in a man not following a balanced diet, and this can have an effect on his nutritional state of health. There are a number of health risk factors associated with diet: a high consumption of saturated fats, sodium, and alcohol, together with a low intake of fruit and vegetables, can cause premature heart disease. An imbalance can exist between the intake of protein and the energy burnt up through physical activity. This imbalance can lead to a person becoming overweight or even obese, a problem which is currently on the increase. Obesity is linked to heart disease and becomes more acute in combination with other factors, such as smoking, raising the risk of mortality.

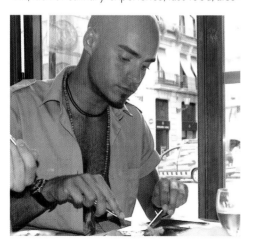

The world of work

A man's productivity increases around the age of 20–25, and this has an effect on work.

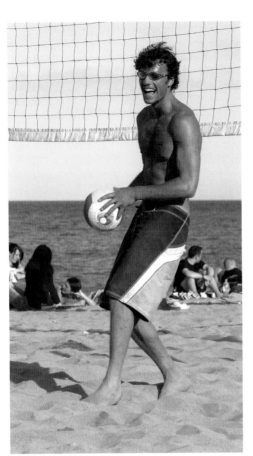

opportunities to establish emotional relationships with members of the opposite sex. At times, however, the burden of work or the quest for professional success results in him putting recreational activities second, which can make his life monotonous and also complicate couple relationships.

Drugs

These days, the most commonly consumed drugs are tobacco and alcohol, as well as the illegal ones. Both drinking and smoking are habits that generally start in adolescence and are continued for years. A young man can be significantly attracted to such habits, in part because they may fit in with socially accepted behavior, seem appealing, and be endorsed by the media and his group of friends. Young smokers and drinkers are often unaware of the genuine risks that these habits pose to health and to others.

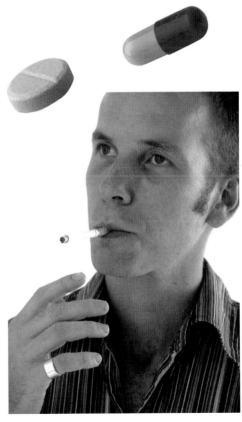

Work is good for earning money, recognition, and feeling fulfilled. However, the world of work comes with certain problems attached, such as stress, lack of time for leisure and development of personal life, conflicts with parenting, etc.

Exercise

Young men frequently take part in some type of exercise; team sports, gym training, swimming, etc., are some of the typical forms of exercise at this stage of life. These activities bring with them as many psychological benefits as they do physical ones. Generally, the motivation underlying this exercise has more to do with aesthetics than it has to do with health. Men take up sports to try to achieve athletic physiques and better muscular development.

Leisure time

A young man's leisure time is determined by his need to widen his circle of friends and for

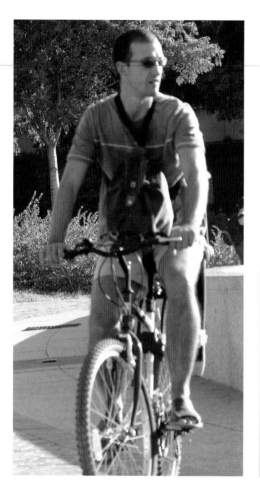

The middle-aged adult male

In middle age, which covers the period from 40–45 up to 60–65, a man's attention is again focused on himself: the search for balance in his emotional and intellectual development, consistency, personality, self-esteem, personal autonomy, etc. A time of crisis sometimes arises during this stage, resulting from a growing awareness that the first half of adulthood is over, that his children are growing up, and that old age beckons closer every day.

▟ N.B.

- An increase in mental skills occurs (thought, comprehension, and knowledge), while at the same time motor functions may start to diminish.

- This is a time when a change in roles occurs: instead of parents looking after their children, the children begin to look after their own parents.

- Intimacy in a couple's relationship can be lost in early adulthood; in middle age, however, a couple can rediscover each other once the children have reached adolescence.

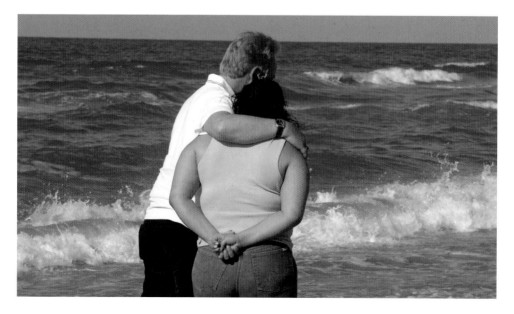

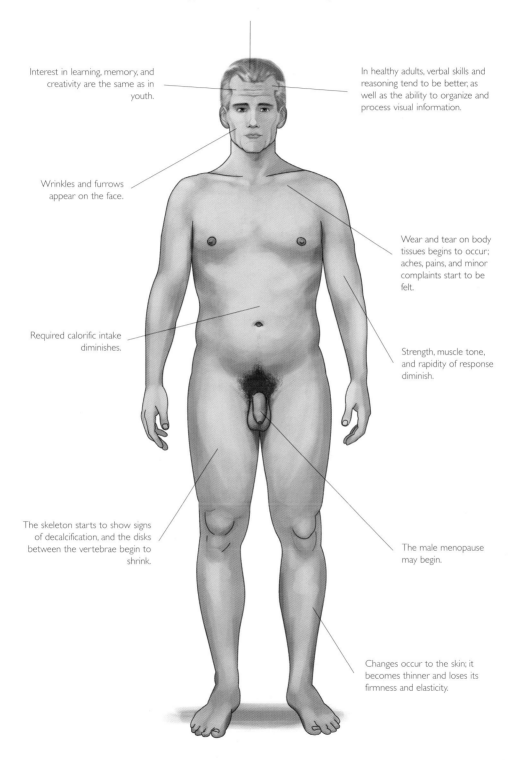

Hair growth slows down; it may start thinning, gray hairs begin to appear, and it loses its luster and body.

Interest in learning, memory, and creativity are the same as in youth.

In healthy adults, verbal skills and reasoning tend to be better, as well as the ability to organize and process visual information.

Wrinkles and furrows appear on the face.

Wear and tear on body tissues begins to occur; aches, pains, and minor complaints start to be felt.

Required calorific intake diminishes.

Strength, muscle tone, and rapidity of response diminish.

The skeleton starts to show signs of decalcification, and the disks between the vertebrae begin to shrink.

The male menopause may begin.

Changes occur to the skin; it becomes thinner and loses its firmness and elasticity.

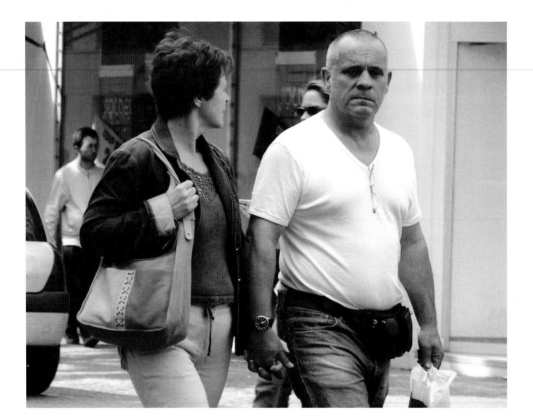

The mature adult male

It is important for a man at this stage of life to achieve a balance between satisfying his own needs and satisfying the needs of those whom he is supporting, whether it be parents or chil- dren. For that reason it is useful for him to understand the changes that he is undergoing, accepting them as part of a human being's development and growth, and to try to maintain a healthy life both emotionally and physically.

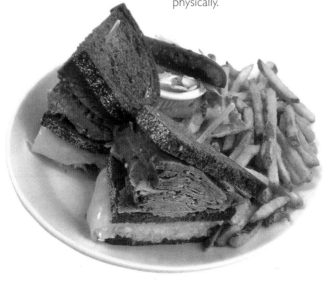

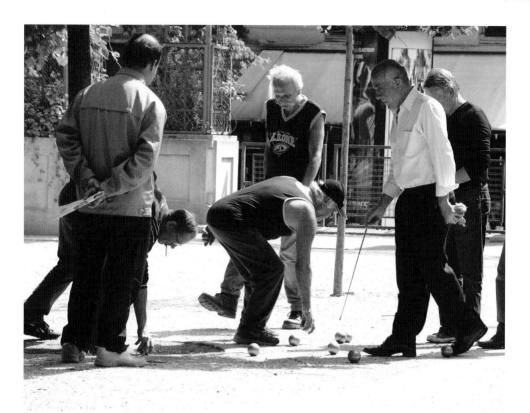

Diet

The imbalances or harm that food can cause often result in gastrointestinal problems, which can turn into more serious conditions, especially when complaints arise with the gallbladder, liver, or pancreas. The most common issues for mature males are being overweight, high blood pressure (hypertension), and arthritis. Obesity causes problems that are generally aggravated by habits such as smoking or drinking. At this stage of life, the body slows down and a man's energy requirements diminish. As time goes by, he can become increasingly sedentary.

Physical activity

Very often, men of this age devote a great amount of energy to all kinds of activities, frequently involving the community and civic responsibilities. In his fifties, a man often has to confront doubts about his abilities, whether physical, social, or work-related, and tends to fight to maintain everything that he has achieved over the years. Often this can result in men committing themselves to excessive activity or, conversely, retreating and assuming a more passive role that centers on domestic or work-related activities. Closely related to this is the importance that a man of this age attaches to appearing and feeling youthful. Self-esteem can be affected when faced with the first signs of old age. Sometimes, in order to maintain his self-esteem, he will use a wide range of resources and methods to prolong a more youthful appearance: gym training, surgery, cosmetic surgery, weight-loss centers, facial products, hair dye products, wearing toupees, or undergoing treatments to conquer baldness, etc.

Sex

The menopause can affect the sex life of men as well as women. At this stage in life, neither ability nor sexual desire is lost and pleasure can be experienced with greater freedom, given that the risk of pregnancy no longer exists. As far as family life is concerned, this is when children are reaching adulthood, and

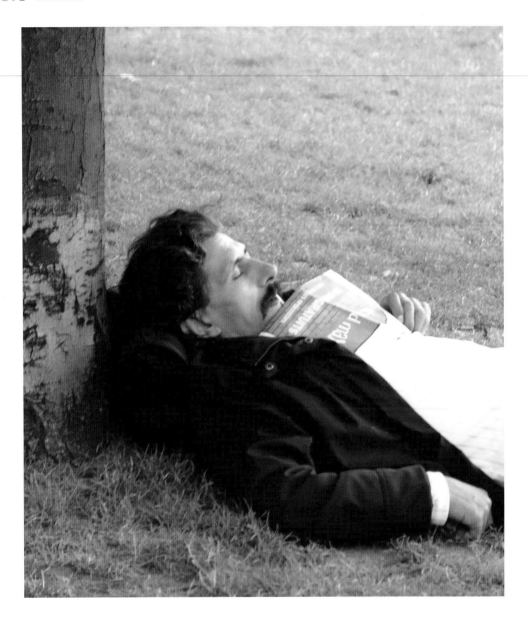

parents have to adjust to living on their own again as the children leave home. At this time, male physical health can be more susceptible to the effects of psychological factors than to the effects of physiological ones. The incidence of problems with erections increases significantly after the age of 50, usually due to factors such as work and money worries, physical or mental fatigue, overindulging in food and drink, or exaggerated concerns about sexual failure.

Insomnia

Among the most common problems encountered by adult males is insomnia, or the difficulty of getting to sleep and staying that way through the night. Sleep apnea, in which breathing is interrupted for a few seconds, is just as important. It causes an individual to wake up throughout the night and, consequently, results in a lack of proper rest.

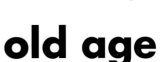

old age

Old age is the final stage in life and is the phase during which the body's organs start losing their capacity to adapt to the external factors that affect the body. In general, old age begins from the age of 65 to 70. The diagram below includes some of the main changes that occur at this time of life.

Men in old age

respiratory system
Through the course of a person's life, the respiratory system is vulnerable to lesions caused by infections, atmospheric pollution, and allergic reactions. These factors are even more damaging than the physical decline expected as a normal part of the ageing process. With the passing of time, the bronchial passages lose their elasticity, causing difficulty in breathing. Breathing requires greater effort for the old, because they rely increasingly on using the diaphragm to force air in.

cardiovascular system
In old age, cardiac energy diminishes due to a stiffening of the arteries and a slow-down in the network of blood vessels. This stagnation in blood flow raises blood pressure and causes an increase in the quantity of fluid traveling toward the interstitial tissue, which gives rise to the formation of edemas. Arterial blood pressure increases, blood flow to the brain reduces, peripheral resistance increases, the walls of the heart become enlarged. The old are more susceptible to suffering from low blood pressure and abnormal heart rhythms (arrhythmia).

muscular and skeletal system
The loss of skeletal and muscle mass is a common phenomenon with age and results in many disruptive conditions, such as osteoporosis (brittle bones), degenerative osteoarthritis, and a loss of strength and resistance.

skin
With the passing of the years, the skin suffers progressive and irreversible degeneration, both in terms of its morphology as well as function. These changes become more obvious when a person is in his thirties, with visible evidence of wrinkles, dryness, and blotchiness, etc., which are the hallmarks of skin in old age. The ageing process that affects the skin does not occur evenly or homogeneously; it depends on racial background and atmospheric conditions and can also differ in different parts of the same person's body.

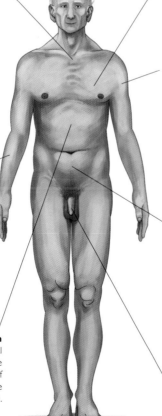

digestive system
The most important changes to the digestive system that happen with age are: chewing becomes less effective; less saliva is produced; the sense of taste declines; digestion becomes slower; gastric juices and enzymes diminish; the intestinal wall loses its elasticity; and there is less mobility in and reduction of blood flow to the intestines.

immune system
Infectious diseases are one of the principal causes of illness and mortality in the old. There is an increase in susceptibility to instances of tumors and a progressive reduction in the body's immune response.

urogenital organs
The kidneys degenerate and, consequently, their ability to filter urine diminishes. Furthermore, the pelvic muscles swell up and the bladder's ability to function properly diminishes, which can result in incontinence. The prostate increases in size, and urination often becomes difficult as a result.

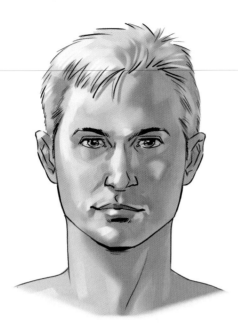

size, and color of such blemishes are affected by a person's exposure to the sun.

The skin can shrink, become dry, and form wrinkles. Although these wrinkles are inevitable by a certain age, it is likely that smoking and exposure to the sun encourage their appearance.

Some men's ears may enlarge slightly, probably due to the growth of cartilage. As they grow older, some men may well notice an increasing amount of hair growing from their ears.

The number of sebaceous glands diminishes, as does their activity. Earwax dries up, causing plugs to form obstructions in the ear canal, which in turn contributes toward deafness.

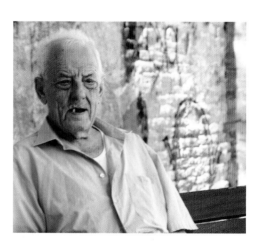

Facial changes

As with the rest of the body, the typical features of the face and neck change with age: muscle tone is lost, taking on a flaccid appearance; the cheeks and cheekbones lose their tautness; the nose lengthens slightly and becomes more prominent. A greater number of liver spots appear on the skin. The quantity,

The eyebrows and eyelashes turn gray. The skin around the eyelids becomes looser, and wrinkles appear, which produces the effect known as "crows'-feet."

Bags can develop under the lower eyelids, and sunken eyelids can even develop, restricting vision.

The iris, the colored part of the eye, loses its pigmentation; it is because of this that the majority of old people have gray or clear blue eyes.

The wearing down and loss of teeth causes the lips to appear wrinkled as well. The jawbone deteriorates, causing it to shrink in size, which, in turn, makes the forehead, nose, and mouth seem more pronounced.

The gums also retract, which contributes to the appearance of dental problems and alterations to the mouth.

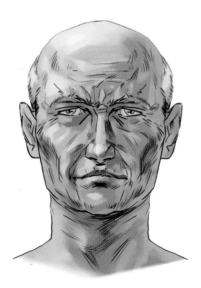

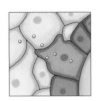

colorless air bubbles replace the melanin

Hair and nails

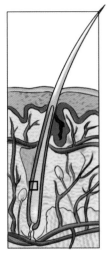

Changing hair color is probably one of the most obvious signs of ageing. The hair owes its color to the presence of melanin, a pigment produced by the hair follicles and these occur in fewer numbers because of the ageing process.

Hair usually begins to turn gray after age 30, although this varies widely from person to person. Gray hairs generally start to show at the temples and extend toward the upper part of the scalp. The hair becomes increasingly pale and, ultimately, it loses all color entirely, turning white. By the age of 40, the majority of men will have some gray hairs. Body and facial hair turns gray as well, albeit later, in general, than hair growing from the scalp. Armpit hair, chest hair, and pubic hair may turn less gray or even not at all.

The appearance of gray hair is determined by your genes. Gray hairs tend to appear earlier in Caucasians and later in those of Asian origin. The amount of hair that a man has on his head and body is also genetically determined. However, almost all men experience hair loss in old age, as well as a reduction in its speed of growth. The hair fibers become smaller and contain less pigment; thus the thick, coarse hair of a young adult male changes with age into hair that is fine, thin, and lighter in color. Furthermore, the ability of hair to regenerate is also reduced; in other words, many hair follicles simply stop producing new hair.

The nails also change as the ageing process advances: they grow more slowly and turn pale and brittle; their color may change from translucent to yellowed and opaque. Toenails, in particular, can become hard and coarse, and they frequently become ingrown, while the tips of the fingernails become easily split and broken.

The eye

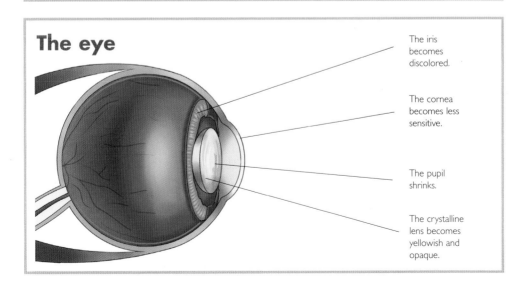

The iris becomes discolored.

The cornea becomes less sensitive.

The pupil shrinks.

The crystalline lens becomes yellowish and opaque.

Sensory changes

When people become old, their senses— their sight, hearing, smell, taste, and touch—become increasingly less acute, making it difficult for them to distinguish details.

Sensory changes can have a major impact on the quality of life, because problems with communication frequently arise as a result, interest in ordinary pleasures is lost, and social relationships diminish, leaving the old feeling isolated.

All of the senses receive information from external sources. This information is converted into a nervous impulse and is transported to the brain, which interprets it as a sensation. Everyone requires a minimum level of prior stimulation in order to perceive any type of sensation. This minimum intensity of stimulation is referred to as the "threshold." This threshold increases with age, which means that the old require greater levels of sensory stimulation in order to notice things.

While changes to sight and hearing are the most significant, all of the body's senses can be affected by ageing.

The older people get, the more their auditory structures deteriorate: the eardrum thickens and the miniature bones inside the ear, as well as other structures, are affected and, typically, it

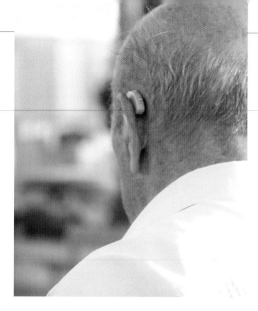

becomes less and less easy to keep your balance.

Hearing capacity reduces gradually, especially with regard to high-frequency sounds and in particular for people who were exposed to a lot of noise in their youth. This age-related hearing loss is referred to as "presbycusis."

The occurance of some degree of hearing loss in old age is virtually inevitable, and it is estimated that 30 percent of all people over the age of 65 show signs of significant deterioration to their hearing.

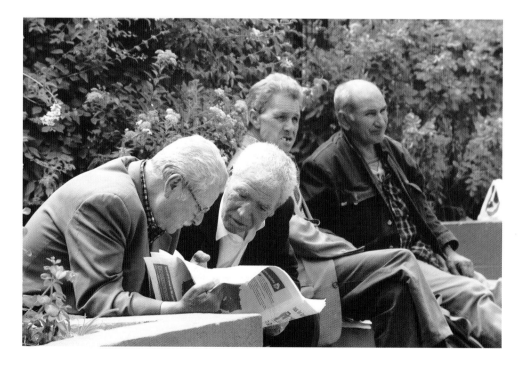

All structural elements of the eye change over time: the cornea's sensitivity diminishes, such that lesions can occur unnoticed. At around the age of 60, the pupil will have shrunk in size by a third compared to how it was at the age of 20.

The pupil loses its capacity to change in size in response to the level of darkness or brightness. The crystalline lens becomes yellowish, less flexible, and slightly opaque; the structure of the eyeball also alters, and the eye becomes sunken in its orbit. The ocular muscles atrophy, preventing the eye from making a full rotation.

Visual acuteness and the field of vision are also affected with the passage of time.

The number of taste buds on the tongue reduces as one ages, making it harder to distinguish flavors.

The sense of smell also diminishes to a greater or lesser extent, especially after the age of 70, and can be related to the loss of nerve endings in the nose.

The waning senses of smell and taste can be accompanied by a loss of interest and pleasure in food. Some old people may stop looking after their personal hygiene once the sense of smell deteriorates.

In old age, a person may display changes or a reduction in the ability to detect sensations of

N.B.

- The joints become stiffer and less flexible.
- The muscles also alter with the passage of time: they lose their tone and their capacity to contract.
- Strength and resistance change due to the loss of muscle mass; however, resistance can increase thanks to changes undergone by the muscle fibers.
- Involuntary movements, tics, and tremors appear.

pain, vibration, cold, heat, pressure, and contact. It is difficult to know whether these changes are related to ageing itself, or whether they are related to medical conditions associated with old age.

As one gets older, skeletal mass or density is lost, because bones become depleted of calcium. They become more fragile and are susceptible to a greater risk of fracture.

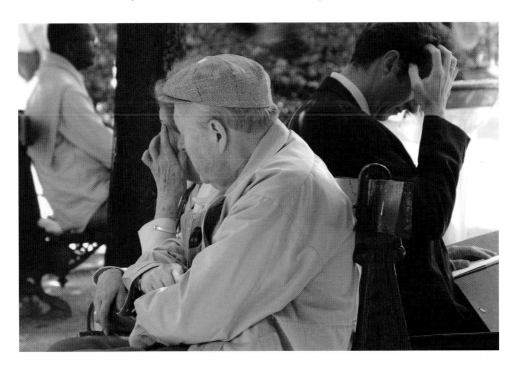

The spinal column is formed by vertebrae, which are separated by gelatinous vertebral disks acting as cushions. Ageing gradually causes these disks to lose fluid, which makes them shrink. As a result, the torso diminishes in size and thus height is reduced. Moreover, the vertebrae also lose calcium and other minerals, which can give rise to curvature and compression of the spinal column.

Some bones, such as the shoulder blade, become porous.

The larger arm and leg bones, despite being more fragile as a result of decalcification, do not change in length, which is why they can seem out of proportion to the reduced size of an old person's torso.

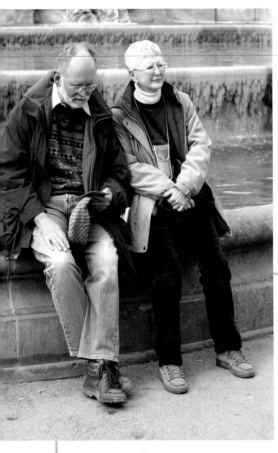

The male menopause

The male menopause is the progressive decline in a man's sexual capacity as he grows older, in tandem with his other bodily functions. In the same way as women experience their menopause, men also start to lose their sexual potency; however, in the case of men, this is not defined by such an abrupt change or by the completion of a cycle. Neither does the male menopause present a decisive limit on a man's capacity to procreate, which is still possible even at a very advanced age.

The conjunction of changes that characterizes the male menopause involves the progressive decrease in the amount of male hormones produced in the body. The reduction in androgens has an impact on a number of processes in the male body, but its consequences are most particularly evident in terms of a man's sexual capacity. Androgens also affect a man's state of mind

and can provoke irritability, anxiety, and even depression.

Men entering the male menopause may show signs of:

- Hypogonadism: a natural and progressive reduction in the function of the testicles with a progressive decline in the amount of testosterone produced.

- Decline in the quality of semen and the capacity of sperm to fertilize an egg. Ejaculations reduce in volume and energy.

- Reduction in erection owing to a more rapid loss of penile vasodilation (supply of blood to the penis). There is a greater need for physical stimulation and arousal requires more time.

- Orgasm undergoes changes, becoming less intense and not lasting as long.

- Reduced production of other hormones, such as growth hormone (somatotropin produced in the hypothalamus) and secretions from the adrenal glands (noradrenalin, adrenalin, and corticosteroids—a combination that plays a central role in the body's response to stress).

- Gynecomastia, meaning the growth or enlargement of breast tissue.

- A reduction in muscle mass and an increase in the accumulation of body fat can be produced as a result of some of these changes. This can give rise to increased levels of cholesterol and a tendency to obesity, as well as a higher risk of suffering from heart diseases.

Looking after your health: regular general checkups

A man's health is his most precious asset and is often what he considers least. Having regular checkups is invaluable for maintaining a good state of health, allaying concerns and, in the worst-case scenario, discovering whether you are suffering from an illness in good time.

Routine checkups

There are various reasons for a man to have regular health checks:
- To check on his state of health.
- To see whether he is carrying a contagious illness.
- To see if he has a hereditary disease.

Checkups are also very important for the early detection of various serious conditions in their incipient phase, which increases the likelihood of curing them.

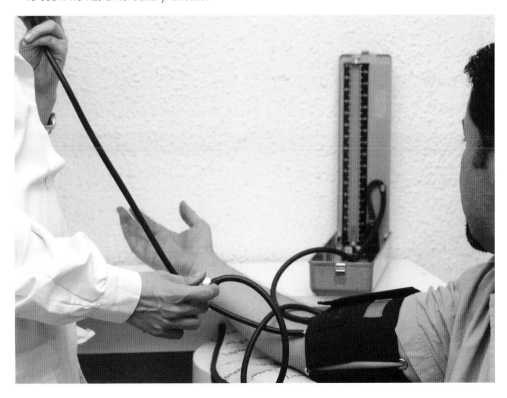

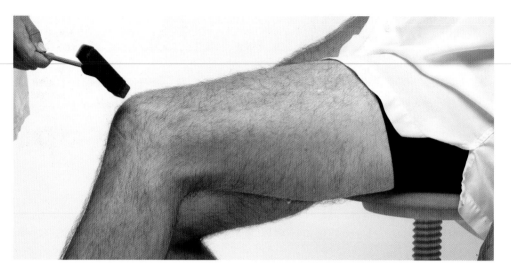

Physical appearance

Physical condition refers to a person's basic state of health. Through a simple assessment of a patient's physical appearance, a practitioner can see whether any disease or abnormality might exist. For example, a thin bluish line around the lips might suggest a heart or respiratory condition; if the face is blotchy, it may be a sign of alcoholism or dermatological problems.

Medical history

Before a medical examination, a practitioner will usually ask a series of questions about any clinics where you have registered previously, whether you have suffered from any illness, whether there is any history of illness in your family, and what your lifestyle entails—such as whether you smoke, suffer from insomnia, etc.

"Auscultation" is an exploratory technique that uses a stethoscope or phonendoscope to amplify sounds in the body. By using this simple technique, heart and lung functions can be analyzed and any circulatory problems can be detected.

Testing reflexes

This is a simple technique to check whether the nervous system has suffered any damage. One of the best known of these tests is the knee-jerk reflex in which a rubber hammer is used to tap the tendon below the kneecap, thus causing the leg to jerk in an involuntary reflex. This reflex action is either quite violent or not produced at all if nerves in the spine have been damaged.

 N.B.

You should not restrict visits to your doctor to those times when your symptoms clearly leave you no other choice. Everybody should undergo regular medical checkups—once a year—irrespective of age or state of health, if only to discount the possibility of some illness or to prevent one from taking hold.

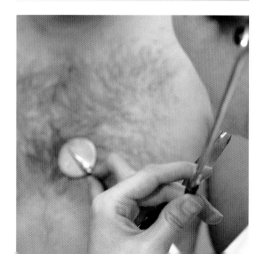

TESTS DURING NORMAL CHECKUPS

Test	Frequency	Reason	Greater frequency
weight	In any medical examination, especially those involving children and adolescents.	Many illnesses involve either weight loss or weight gain.	When weight changes dramatically and unintentionally, i.e. if you have not gone on a specific diet.
height	In any medical examination, especially those involving children and adolescents.	Many illnesses cause development in children and adolescents to decelerate or accelerate.	If you are suffering from any growth-related condition.
blood pressure	For adults, once a year.	This checks the health of the heart and circulation.	If you suffer from high or low blood pressure, or if you are taking any medication that can affect blood pressure.
blood sugar	This is checked in every blood test.	This shows the level of glucose in the blood. A high level may indicate diabetes.	If you suffer from some complaint, such as diabetes, or if you are taking medication.
cholesterol and triglicerides	For adults, once every five years. However, this should be checked once a year if you are a smoker, overweight, or in old age.	This indicates the condition of the blood vessels and the likelihood of suffering a heart attack.	If there is a history of high cholesterol in your family, if you have a high level of cholesterol, or if you are taking certain medications.
urine	In any medical checkup.	This indicates the health of your kidneys and whether you are suffering from any type of infection or diabetes.	If you suspect some type of urological complaint or a urinary infection.
prostate	For adults aged 50 or over, once a year. (Either through a rectal examination or a urine sample.)	This shows whether you are suffering from any prostate-related condition.	If you are suffering from a prostate-related condition or inconveniences, or if you are having difficulty passing urine.
other specifically male-related tests	From adolescence onward, you should self-examine your testicles each month, and visit a urologist once a year.	Detection of any male urogenital conditions.	If you feel discomfort, suffer from some medical condition, have a family history of cancer, suspect you may be infertile, have problems with ejaculation, or suffer from erectile dysfunction.

Eye tests

Eye tests are very important, especially during childhood when many problems can still be corrected before they become irreversible.

Adults, especially those over 40, should have their eyes examined every two years to check for any deterioration in vision due to ageing, to prevent and treat this if necessary, and thus maintain a person's vision at its optimum capacity.

People suffering from complaints such as high blood pressure or diabetes should visit

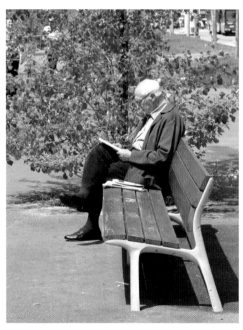

A test to determine color vision. The Ishihara color test seen here is used to test a person's ability to distinguish red from green. If he is unable to do this, he is diagnosed with red-green color blindness, also referred to as Daltonism. This is a genetic disorder that is much more common in men than in women.

their optometrist once a year, as these types of condition also affect sight.

An urgent visit to an ophthalmologist is required if you feel sharp eye pain, if you start seeing double, or if sight becomes patchy, as well as if you are seeing black spots, circles of colors, or bright flashes of light.

Visual acuteness is usually verified using the Snellen chart placed at a distance of 20 feet from the person under examination. A person with normal vision must be able to read up to the penultimate line.

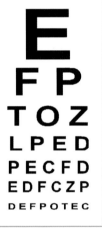

Presbyopia, or tired vision, affects almost all people above the ages of 40 to 45. At that age, the crystalline lens hardens, thus losing its elasticity, and it becomes impossible to focus on near objects. At present, the only solution to this problem is to use glasses or corrective lenses.

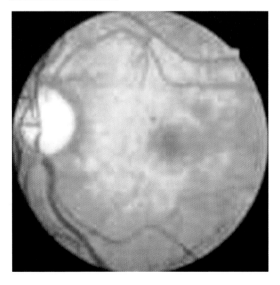

An ophthalmoscope allows the interior of the eye to be examined. It consists of an instrument that, with the aid of strong light and lenses, enables details of the inner eye to be observed, allows diagnosis of conditions such as detachment of the retina, macular degeneration, inflammation of the optic nerve, or any problems with the eye's blood vessels.

TESTS PERFORMED IN AN EYE CHECKUP		
Test	**What this is**	**What it causes**
Myopia	Short-sightedness. The image focuses in front of the retina.	It prevents clear vision of distant objects.
Hypermetropia	Long-sightedness. The image focuses behind the retina.	It makes it difficult to focus on near objects. The effort made in focusing causes visual fatigue.
Astigmatism	The cornea is ovoid in shape. The lack of convergence creates more than one point of focus and thus diffuses vision.	Poor vision both nearby and at a distance.
Presbyopia	This defect occurs when the muscles that hold the crystalline lens become more rigid and the eye loses its ability to focus, especially on near objects.	This is a natural defect and generally occurs as one grows older. Difficulty with reading or seeing near objects typically starts after the age of 40.

Hearing tests

Hearing problems have become commonplace in modern society.

Without being aware of it, more and more people are suffering from hearing loss every day because of the noise pollution that surrounds us.

The noise produced in our streets, at work, and even at home often exceeds 100 decibels, which is damaging to the inner ear.

If you notice problems when speaking on the phone, if you need to turn up the volume on the radio or television, if you do not understand conversations, or if you confuse some of the words spoken to you, it is a good idea to go for a hearing checkup.

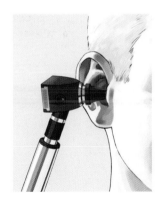

The Weber test

The Weber test uses a tuning fork, which is tapped gently and then held aloft on either side of the head to determine the capacity to hear sound transmitted through the air.

Afterward, the tuning fork is tapped again and placed on the temporal bone, located just behind each ear, to determine the capacity to hear sound transmitted through bone.

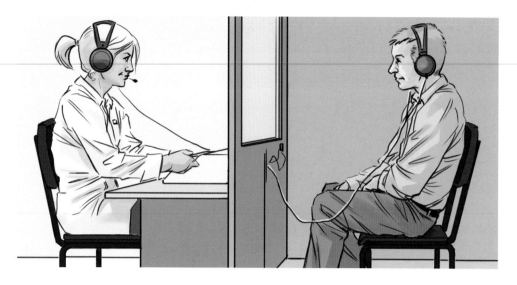

Hearing

Hearing is produced when sound waves are transmitted to the ears' internal nervous system and from there to the brain. The sound waves can travel to the inner ear through the air (via the ear canal, the ear drum, and the bones of the inner ear) or through bone (via the bones that surround and lie behind the ears).

Audiometer testing

An audiometer is a piece of equipment that transmits sounds at different frequencies and levels of intensity. The person being examined is placed in an isolation booth. The volume of the sound is progressively reduced until the person can no longer detect it. The data obtained indicates whether there is any hearing deficiency in the various ranges of frequency audible to the human ear.

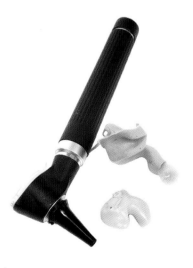

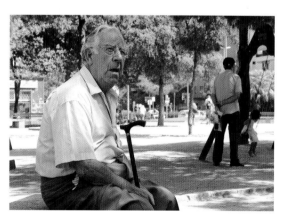

In old age, many people lose their sensitivity to higher-frequency sounds, which can result in their inability to follow conversations and can even plunge them into a state of confusion. Nevertheless, a solution exists for this reduction in hearing sensitivity. Hearing aids that amplify sound help older people to hear better. Men usually suffer greater hearing loss in old age than women.

▗▘ Who needs to have a hearing test?

- Children
- Any child or adolescent suffering from language difficulties.
- Anyone who has difficulty following a conversation or who hears noises in the inner ear.
- All older people showing signs of confusion.
- All people in situations with high noise levels, such as construction workers or employees in factories and workshops.

Blood tests

Blood tests are more commonplace nowadays. Few people have not undergone one, and few are unaware of them. They are used in routine health checks or to rule out the presence of diseases, as well as to determine a person's blood type should they ever need a blood transfusion. Blood tests are used routinely to help in the diagnosis of illnesses or to check on a person's health.

Many common, frequently occurring illnesses, such as anemia, diabetes, or any type of infection, can be detected through blood tests. They can also be used to detect less common and more serious types of illness, such as leukemia or other types of cancer.

PARAMETERS	NORMAL VALUES
Red blood cells	
Erythrocytes	4–5.5 million per milliliter
Hemoglobin	12–16 grams per deciliter
Hematocrit	37–52%
Mean corpuscular volume (MCV)	80–99 femtoliters
Mean corpuscular hemoglobin (MCH)	27–32 picograms
Mean corpuscular hemoglobin concentration (MCHC)	32–36 grams per deciliter
Platelets	
Platelets	135,000450,000 per milliliter
Mean platelet volume (MPV)	9.6 femtoliters
White blood cells	
Leukocytes	4,500–11,000 per milliliter
Neutrophils	42–75%
Lymphocytes	20.5–51.1%
Monocytes	1.7–9.3%
Eosinophils	0–1%
Basophils	0–0.2%
Erythrocyte sedimentation rate	
ESR	less than 5 to 20 in the first hour (depending on age and sex)

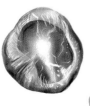

BASIC BLOOD TEST			
	What is it analyzing?		**What is it for?**
complete (full) blood count	Red blood cells White blood cells Platelets	Transportation of oxygen Immune system Blood clotting	Determines the state of the three principal cell types circulating in the blood
biochemical test	Glucose	Sugar	Biochemical analysis can provide a picture of liver and kidney function, because it analyzes the substances that they produce.
	Urea and creatinine	Kidney function	
	Transaminases: • AST (SGOT) • ALT (SGPT) • GGT	Liver function	
	Sodium (Na) Potassium (K) Chlorine (Cl)	Cell metabolism	
clotting tests	Prothrombin clotting time (Quick's test) Activated partial thromboplastin time (APTT) INR (International normalized (clotting) ratio): measures the effectiveness of anticoagulant medication Erythrocyte sedimentation rate (ESR)		Fundamental tests to establish whether the blood is clotting properly. It is essential to know this if someone needs to undergo surgery.

white blood cells

platelets

red blood cells

Basic blood test

A basic blood test is used to determine the levels of different substances that circulate in the bloodstream.

It consists of two parts: a complete blood count, or breakdown of the blood's composition (white blood cells, red blood cells, and platelets), and a biochemical analysis that identifies substances dissolved in the blood, such as the amount of glucose, urea, sodium, and potassium.

Although it is possible to determine a large number of substances in blood, a basic blood test is used to show the most important ones affecting general health or the body's most important organs.

Standard values exist for each substance or parameter. If the concentration of a substance rises above the standard level, it is referred to as a surplus; if it falls below that level, it is referred to as a deficiency.

In-depth analysis of blood

When it is necessary to analyze a patient's general state of health in more detail, a doctor will ask for information on a greater number of substances in the blood.

More specific or fuller blood testing requires larger amounts of blood to be taken and a more complex laboratory process.

Each specialist needs information on a set series of substances related to his area of expertise. As a result, each specialist requires a different type of analysis to be performed.

Blood is just another of a human being's bodily tissues, but, unlike the others, it is composed for the most part of water, which allows it to be fluid and circulate through the entire body.

NORMAL LEVELS FOR THE MOST COMMON BIOCHEMICAL PARAMETERS

Biochemical parameters	Normal levels
Glucose in blood	70–105 milligrams per deciliter (for children: 40–100 mg/dl)
Uric acid	adult males: 4–8.5 milligrams per deciliter adult females: 2.5–7.5 mg/dl (children: 2.5–5 mg/dl)
Urea	7–20 milligrams per deciliter (children: 5–18 mg/dl)
Creatinine	adult males: 0.7–1.3 milligrams per deciliter adult females: 0.5–1.2 mg/dl (children: 0.2–1.0 mg/dl)
Direct bilirubin	0.10.3 milligrams per 100 millliters
Total bilirubin	0.3–1.0 milligrams per 100 milliliters
Indirect bilirubin	less than 1.0 milligrams per milliliter
Alkaline phosphatase	30–120 units per liter
Gamma GT	Men: 8–38 units per liter Women: 5–27 units per liter
GOT	5–32 milliunits per milliliter
GPT	7–33 milliunits per milliliter
Cholesterol	100–200 milligrams per 100 milliliters
High-density lipoproteins (HDL)	Men: more than 45 milligrams per 100 milliliters Women: more than 55 mg/100 ml
Low-density lipoproteins (LDL)	60–180 milligrams per 100 milliliters
Total proteins	6.4–8.3 grams per deciliter
Albumin	3.5–5.0 grams per deciliter
Calcium	8.5–10.5 milligrams per 100 milliliter
Potassium	3.5–5 millimoles per liter
Sodium	135-145 milliequivalents per liter
Phosphorous	2.9–5.0 milligrams per 100 milliliters

Urinalysis – examination of the urine

Urine contains water and a multitude of other substances, each of which provides a key to understanding an individual's health. Urinalysis can be complicated, because it may require the use of a wide variety of techniques and protocols according to the type of information being sought on a particular condition.

Urine can be analyzed just like any other fluid or liquid in the human body. Since urine is a product of the body's metabolism, it holds a great deal of information on many illnesses. Another reason for using urine as part of a basic diagnostic test is the ease with which a sample can be obtained.

A sample of urine passed first thing in the morning is usually requested, because this sample will be the most concentrated.

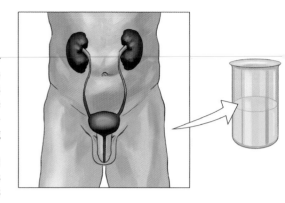

Before giving a urine sample, men should wash their hands and the head of the penis to prevent any lack of hygiene from contaminating the sample and thus to safeguard the sample's reliability.

DIFFERENT TYPES OF URINALYSIS	
Urinoscopy	The most elementary way of studying urine is direct observation. This is referred to as "urinoscopy" or "uroscopy." A reliable specialist will be able to discern the symptoms of certain illnesses simply by looking.
Urine sedimentation	Urine sedimentation is the most basic analytical test. It is used to assess the presence of solid matter. The traditional method is to observe a sample of centrifuge-separated urine under the microscope. Taking the premise that urine should contain virtually no cells or solid matter, any sign of sediment usually indicates a medical condition and points to an illness of some sort.
Urine dipsticks	Reactive dipsticks are moistened with urine, producing a series of reactions that changes the color of the treated blotting paper that coats the sticks. Each dipstick contains reagents that relate to a particular type of change in the urine. These dipsticks are 99 percent reliable in detecting erythrocytes (red blood cells) or leukocyte-nitrites (infections), which makes them an extremely valuable means of investigation.
Urine biochemistry	Urine biochemistry consists of studying the substances contained in it, just as for blood. There should not be any glucose or bilirubin. A biochemical urine study can be done using one sample or using urine collected over a 24-hour period.
Special urine testing	In general, this is an attempt to detect toxins (drugs and poisons), stimulants, or doping agents and substances eliminated in certain types of (metabolic or hormonal) illness. The urine sample is treated in a specific manner for each type of toxin or substance that requires analysis.
Urine culture	Urine culture is a specialized type of analysis. It is used in an attempt to establish whether an infection is present and, if so, to identify the microorganism responsible and thus propose the most effective antibiotic to counteract it.
Urine cytology	This consists of analyzing the cells expelled in the urine. To assess this, it is necessary to collect urine samples over a three-day period.

Coronary health – the heart and blood pressure

Prevention is better than cure. Cardiac problems are among the greatest risks that men encounter in adult life. It is very important to have routine checkups performed to assess your coronary health and the condition of your circulation.

Blood pressure

Measuring blood pressure consists of checking the pressure generated by the heart as it pumps blood through the arteries (systolic pressure) and the pressure present in the arteries when the heart is in repose between beats (diastolic pressure).

Blood pressure varies from person to person depending on age, weight, and an individual's physical and emotional state. Nobody's arterial blood pressure remains at a constant level; it varies according to the time of day, the body's level of exertion, or the type of emotion being experienced.

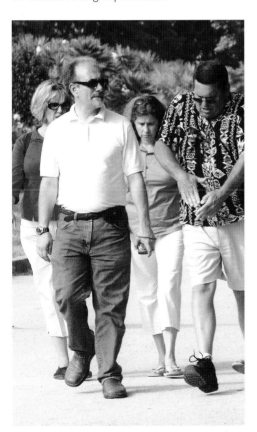

◾ How is blood pressure taken?

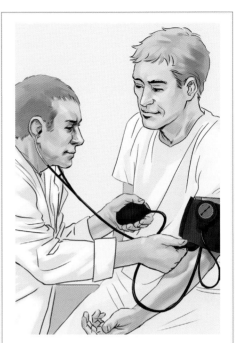

A device known as a sphygmomanometer is used to take blood pressure. There are many different types of these, but in general they all include a squeezable rubber bulb linked to an inflatable cuff for the upper arm with a pressure measuring device connected to it that employs either a column of mercury or some type of gauge. Sphygmomanometers include a normal stethoscope, which may either be integrated as part of the equipment or may come as a separate component. It is advisable to feel relaxed when having your blood pressure taken. You should not smoke or drink anything containing caffeine immediately beforehand, otherwise the pressure reading could appear artificially high.

High blood pressure (hypertension) is a condition without symptoms. As a result, the more time that passes before it is diagnosed and treated, the greater the risk is that a person will suffer a heart attack or stroke, heart failure, or even a kidney-related condition.

Electrocardiograms

- An electrocardiogram is a graphic representation of the electrical energy that works the heart. During the cardiac cycle of pumping blood from the heart and refilling it, a recognized pattern of alternating electrical impulses reflects how the heart is functioning.

- An electrocardiogram is a tool that allows us to record the heart's electrical activity. It is used to measure the rhythm and regularity of heartbeats and to detect any possible medical conditions.

- The electrocardiogram is indispensable for the diagnosis of cardiac arrhythmia and allows information to be gathered on the presence of former or recent coronary disease and other heart-related problems.

- The process is completely painless and takes only a few minutes to perform.

- Normally, a patient is reclining and relaxed when an electrocardiogram is done; however, it can also be performed with a patient undergoing physical activity (an exertion or effort test).

- A portable version also exists: the Holter monitor. This is used to record a patient's electrocardiograms 24 hours a day.

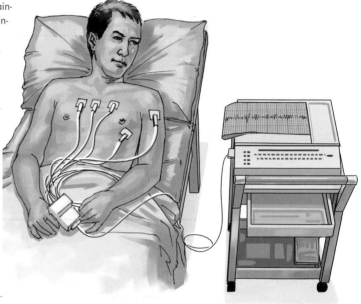

NORMAL AND ELEVATED LEVELS OF BLOOD PRESSURE IN MEN				
	Systolic	Systolic	Diastolic	Diastolic
Age	Normal	High	Normal	High
16–18	105–135	145	60–86	90
19–24	105–140	150	62–88	95
25–29	108–140	150	65–90	96
30–39	110–145	160	68–92	100
40–49	110–155	170	70–96	104
50–59	115–165	175	70–98	106
60+	115–170	190	70–100	110

Checks on the urinary tract and bowel and conditions specific to men

Urological (urinary tract) examinations permit the early detection of a range of diseases, such as renal and prostate cancer. Identifying such conditions at an early stage can be vital to a patient's health. In other words, these are checkups that you should never forget.

Urological checkups

Urology is the area of medicine that studies the urinary tract and the male reproductive system: in other words, the kidneys, bladder, urethra, prostate, testicles, and penis.

Urological checkups in childhood concentrate on diagnosing possible medical conditions, such as phimosis (constriction of the foreskin), hydroceles (swellings in the scrotum), cryptorchidism (undescended testicle), and penile abnormalities, such as an epispadias, as well as urinary tract conditions.

In adolescence, these checkups are performed to diagnose any changes or medical conditions, such as phimosis, hydroceles, varicoceles and other testicular conditions, such as tumors, sexually transmitted diseases, and all of the urological complaints that can occur.

Middle-aged men are checked in order to diagnose and treat conditions such as prostatitis, sexually transmitted diseases, erection or ejaculation-related dysfunctions or changes, hydroceles and other testicular complaints, the presence of blood in urine (hematuria) or in semen (hemospermia), fertility problems, and other urological conditions, such as problems with urination or the urinary tract.

For men aged 50 or more, these checkups are used for the early diagnosis and treatment of prostate enlargement (benign prostatic hyperplasia), prostate cancer and other tumors associated with the urinary system, erection problems: impo-

tence and other dysfunctions, the presence of hard lumps on the penis that cause pain or curvature (Peyronie's disease), hydroceles, as well as any other medical conditions that may occur in the urinary tract or in relation to the kidneys.

In men over the age of 70, apart from the bladder-related problems, impotence, and sexual dysfunctions that can occur, the principal objective is to provide early diagnosis and treatment for benign or malignant tumors that mainly affect the prostate, the bladder, and the penis, thus permitting a better quality of life through treatments that are less aggressive and more easily tolerated, which enable any diagnosed illness to be cured quickly and easily.

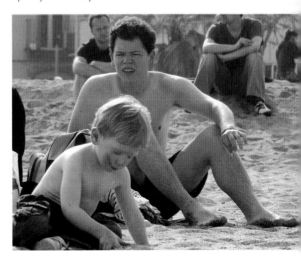

N.B.

A urine checkup needs to be performed in the following cases:
- If there is blood in your urine.
- If you suffer from recurrent urinary infections.
- If you have difficulty when starting, maintaining, or stopping urination.
- If you suspect a bladder-related tumor or cancer.

It is advisable to have a prostate checkup if:
- You notice blood in semen or urine.
- You suffer from recurrent urinary infections.
- You have difficulty when starting, maintaining, or stopping urination.
- You suspect a bladder-related tumor or cancer.
- You are given an early diagnosis of prostate cancer.
- You are over 45 years of age.
- You are over 40 with a history of cancer in your family.

It is a good idea to have your genitals examined if:
- Your erections change or become dysfunctional.
- There is blood in your semen.
- There are changes in your ejaculation (premature, delayed, etc.)
- You feel pain in or notice inflammation of the testicles.
- You suffer from frequent fungal infections.
- You suffer from phimosis (constriction of the foreskin).

It is appropriate to have your kidney function examined if:
- You are suffering from kidney pain.
- You have urinary infections.
- You have gallstones or kidney stones.
- You have cardiovascular or arterial conditions.

Urograms

Intravenous urograms or pyelograms are performed by injecting a contrast agent (dye) into a vein in the arm. Afterward, a series of x-rays is taken at regular intervals while the dye passes through the kidneys, ureters, and bladder.

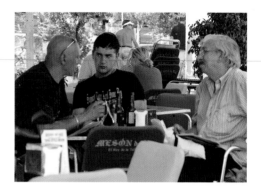

Rectal examinations

A digital (with the fingers) rectal examination assesses the condition of the prostate by touch. It is not only used to detect prostatic anomalies but is also used to detect hemorrhoids, anal fissures, and anomalies in feces, such as visible or occult (hidden) blood.

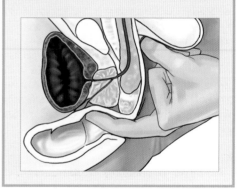

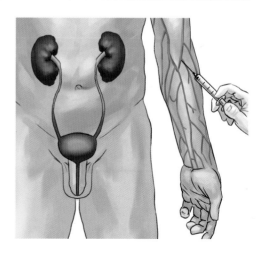

Prostate checkups

This is recommended for men aged between 50 and 70. If there is any family history of prostate cancer, you are advised to start having these checkups from the age of 40. Moreover, a prostate examination should be included in the checkup of any man with symptoms that involve urination problems.

What does a prostate checkup involve?

Medical history

As with any checkup, the urologist will ask a series of questions in order to establish your medical history and circumstances. Questions include how often you need to urinate, whether you have difficulties or suffer inconvenience when urinating, whether there has been any blood in your urine, etc.

Physical examination

A digital (finger) rectal examination is required in order to assess the condition of the prostate. This presents two issues: the aversion felt by many men to such an examination and the test's lack of sensitivity and specificity.

This technique, in isolation, is not 100 percent effective in the early detection of prostate cancer, but its value is indisputable when combined with other tests, such as identifying PSA (prostate specific antigen) in the blood.

Analysis

Analysis of urinary sedimentation. This can distinguish urinary infections from prostate conditions that may produce similar symptoms. In addition, it is also used to identify any presence of blood in the urine.

Measurement of creatinine in blood. This involves an analysis that gives an overview of a patient's kidney function. Both this and the previous test form part of a routine urological checkup.

PSA. The prostate specific antigen (PSA) is a protein produced by the prostate's epithelial cells and, among other things, increases its concentration in blood if a prostatic tumor is present. The problem here is that although high levels of PSA occur in patients with cancer, patients who simply have an enlarged prostate (benign prostatic hyperplasia) also have high levels of the antigen. In other words, it is not unusual for patients with high levels of PSA merely to be suffering merely from an increase in prostate size, rather than cancer. Although this test does not provide definitive proof of cancer, it is of great value if performed in combination with other tests.

Uroflowmetry

This is a simple test that causes no discomfort and allows objective and quantifiable data to be collated on the pattern of a patient's urination.

It consists of urinating into a container via a funnel (a uroflowmeter), which measures the amount of urine expelled over time.

Urograms (pyelograms)

Urograms use a series of x-rays to study the urinary system.

▪▪ Cystoscopy

Cystoscopy is a procedure in which a flexible endoscope with optical fibers (cystoscope) is inserted into the urinary bladder via the urethra. The bladder is filled with water and its interior is inspected. The image seen through the cystoscope can also be seen on a monitor. This technique is used to diagnose and assess urinary tract conditions, cancer of the bladder or urethra, prostate enlargement, possible causes of pain when urinating, or recurrent bladder infections.

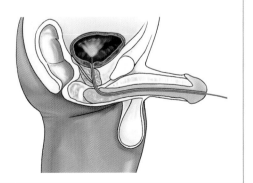

This technique employs a particularly dense contrast agent (dye) that shows up on x-rays in order to highlight differences between the kidneys, or any other anomaly.

This test also analyzes the size and shape of the bladder.

An intravenous urogram (IVU) is the radiological procedure most typically employed to assess the kidneys and is used to study a multitude of problems, including:

- Kidney pain
- Suspected kidney stones.
- Blood in the urine.
- Suspected obstructions.
- Suspected congenital abnormalities.

A mild laxative is usually given before the test in order to empty the intestine, as a full intestine may otherwise obscure the x-ray images required for diagnosis. Patients have to lie down on an x-ray table. An x-ray is taken of the kidneys and the bladder area before administering the contrast agent. Next, the dye is injected into the arm or via the back of the hand. It circulates through the blood until it reaches the kidneys, where it fills the kidney's filtration system and passes through its principal ducts toward the bladder.

A series of x-rays is taken in order to follow the course taken by the dye (normally one x-ray every five minutes, later every 20 minutes, and a final x-ray after the bladder has been emptied).

It may be necessary to obtain additional x-rays in order to be sure of the precise location of an obstruction.

Sigmoidoscopy and colonoscopy

Sigmoidoscopy: rectal and sigmoid colon examination

A sigmoidoscopy is performed to view the lower part of the bowel (large intestine) using a special optical device.

It is a technique that most patients find uncomfortable. Although it is not generally painful, it does cause some discomfort similar to that felt with intestinal gas. This discomfort arises from the interior of the bowel being inflated with air in order to dilate it, thus enabling better observation.

The examination takes no longer than 10–15 minutes, does not require anesthesia, and can be done as an outpatient.

Sigmoidoscopy involves inserting a sigmoidoscope into the lower bowel. This is a tube that contains a specially adapted micro-camera, and it simultaneously inflates the lower bowel with air in order to open it up for examination. The sigmoidoscope is gently guided upward an inch or so at a time and is afterward retracted while the physician carefully inspects the mucous lining in the search of any abnormalities, such as inflammation, polyps, or tumors.

If any suspicious lesions are found, biopsy samples are taken for study under the microscope.

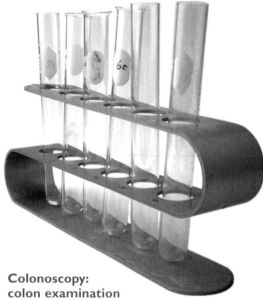

Colonoscopy: colon examination

The large intestine is divided into the colon and the rectum. Although the rectum and the lower part of the colon can be viewed directly using small plastic or metal tubes, the remainder of the intestine has to be examined using other methods: radiological tests, such as basic x-rays or barium enemas, and endoscopic examinations, such as colonoscopy.

Colonoscopy allows examination of the mucous membranes that line the colon and, therefore, it is used to investigate blood loss, changes in bowel movements, abdominal pain, and anomalies detected in other examinations, such as x-rays, which require confirmation by direct visual means or a tissue sample to be

INTERNATIONAL QUESTIONNAIRE AND GRADING FOR PROSTATIC SYMPTOMS AND QUALITY OF LIFE

	Never	1 out of every 5 times	1 out of every 3 times	1 out of every 2 times	2 out of every 3 times	Almost always
When finishing urination during the past month, how many times have you had the feeling that your bladder was not emptying completely?	0	1	2	3	4	5
During the past month, how many times have you had to urinate more than once in under two hours?	0	1	2	3	4	5
When urinating during the past month, how many times has your flow been interrupted or intermittent?	0	1	2	3	4	5
During the past month, how many times have you had difficulty suppressing the desire to urinate?	0	1	2	3	4	5
When urinating during the past month, how many times has your flow been weak?	0	1	2	3	4	5
During the past month, how many times have you had to squeeze or strain in order to urinate?	0	1	2	3	4	5
	None	Once	Twice	3 times	4 times	5 times or more
During the past month, how many times have you had to urinate each night between the time of going to bed and the time of getting up in the morning?	0	1	2	3	4	5

QUALITY OF LIFE BASED ON URINARY SYMPTOMS

	Excellent	Satisfactory	Fairly satisfactory	Indifferent	Fairly unsatisfactory	Poor	Very poor
If your pattern of urination was the same as it is now for the rest of your life, how would you rate it?	0	1	2	3	4	5	6

used for laboratory testing and obtained through a biopsy.

A whole range of changes can be detected by this means, such as inflammation or ulceration of the intestine's mucous membranes, polyps (benign tumors), hernias, and tumors of all kinds.

If necessary, the physician may take tissue samples (biopsies) for later analysis.

Patients must take a laxative on the day before the examination in order to guarantee a clean and emptied intestinal tract. Failure to do so could render the examination incomplete, and thus its results could be incorrect or

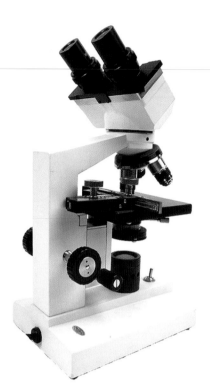

inconclusive. You are not allowed to eat or drink anything for six hours prior to the examination.

Colonoscopy does not require hospitalization and lasts between 20 and 40 minutes.

It is usually necessary to administer a sedative in order to produce a drowsy and relaxed feeling while the examination is performed.

A person must lie still on one side during the procedure. The colonoscope is then lubricated with a gel and gently inserted via the anus into the rectum and then the rest of the large intestine. The colonoscope is able to inflate the intestine gently with a little air to obtain a better view of its lining.

This may give an uncomfortable feeling of abdominal pressure to the person under examination, including an irrepressible desire to break wind, but it is important to resist until the physician has collected all of the required images and samples!

The collection of tissue samples (biopsies) should not cause any pain.

Patients can return home after a colonoscopy, although if a large piece of tissue has been removed, such as a polyp, it may be necessary to stay in hospital for observation for a few hours in case of any consequent loss of blood.

▪▪ **The colonoscope**

cialist clear vision. The colonoscope is also able to inflate the colon with air or deflate it if necessary, and it is also fitted with tools that enable a certain degree of long-range maneuverability so that the specialist can also perform localized therapeutic interventions, such as biopsies.

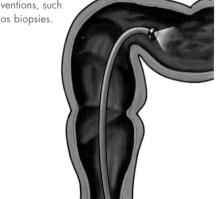

The colonoscope is a flexible, fine tube with a fiber-optic camera measuring approximately 3 feet in length. It is designed to take images of the interior cavities into which it is inserted, and these images can be in video format. It is equipped with a powerful light to give the spe-

diet and nutrition

Eating is, and has always been, one of humanity's great pleasures. A healthy, balanced diet does not mean eliminating that pleasure. Food should be based on sensible consumption: i.e. eating everything in a balanced fashion. There is no such thing as "bad" or "inappropriate" food. Proper nutrition requires that we consume all kinds of food, in the right proportions. Greater knowledge about nutrition and an understanding of what a balanced diet means and how it is composed allows us to identify easily those foods that are most suitable for our health.

Why do we eat?

The body's nutritional needs

When we ingest food, that is to say when we eat, we not only satisfy our appetites, but we also provide the body with the nutrients it needs for functioning properly and thus for life.

Nutrients are substances that the body requires to carry out its functions, and it can obtain these nutrients only through food.

Therefore, food is used in order to:
• Fuel our energy requirements.

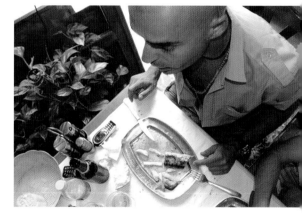

It is important for proteins to account for between 12 and 15 percent of the total calories in your dietary intake

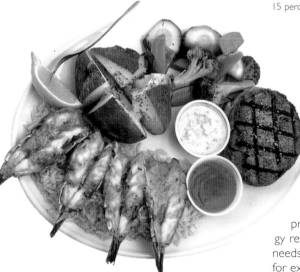

• Maintain and enable the growth of the body and its component parts.
• Regulate the vital processes that allow the body to function properly.

The body's energy needs

An exchange of energy is needed for the body to carry out all of its biochemical processes. This energy comes from the carbohydrates, fats, and proteins in ingested food. A person's energy requirement is the quantity of energy that needs to be ingested in order to compensate for expended energy, or calories.

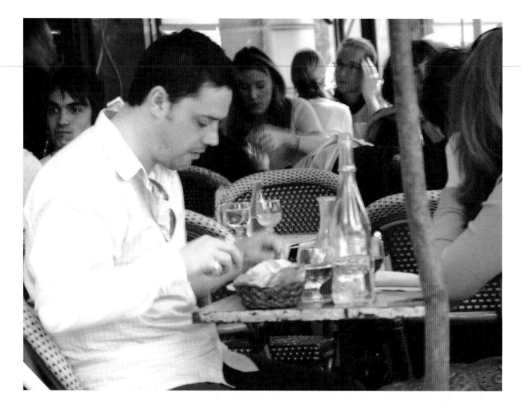

A healthy, balanced diet accompanied with moderate physical exercise can prevent cardiovascular diseases, obesity, or diabetes, among other conditions. Although awareness of these recommendations is high among a large percentage of the population, they are often not followed in day-to-day life.

What are calories?

- Living organisms need an input of energy in order to perform all their functions. In humans, this energy derives from cell oxidation of the carbon and hydrogen contained in nutrition.

- You could say that carbon and hydrogen are like "coals" that produce heat on burning. Oxidation is equivalent to the burning process, and the energy obtained from it is equivalent to the heat that it generates. This energy is measured in units called calories.

- A calorie is the unit of heat required to increase a gram of water by one degree Celsius. Nutrition is measured in terms of kilocalories; a kilocalorie is 1,000 calories. Confusingly, when discussing nutrition, a kilocalorie is usually described simply as a calorie, often with a capital "C." If food packaging shows calorie values, kilocalories are what is meant.

- Each group of nutrients supplies a distinct level of energy. Therefore, while a gram of glycides (proteins) provides, on burning, approximately four calories, a gram of lipids (fats) produces nine.

- Not all ingested substances end up producing energy. For example, the function of some is to participate in chemical reactions or to rebuild bodily structures. This is the case for vitamins, minerals, fiber, and water.

Energy in food

Proteins

Proteins are the principal structural component in cells and, thus, the body's tissues. In other words, they form the foundation for developing the skeleton and muscle.

Proteins are essential for growth and the body's development:

• They maintain and repair tissue.
• They are involved in the production of metabolic and digestive enzymes.
• They are the essential components of certain hormones.
• They take part in the body's defense mechanisms, as they form a structural part of the immune system's antibodies.
• They are involved in blood clotting processes.

Carbohydrates

Carbohydrates, or sugars, are very important to diet because of their energy potential, their ability to sweeten, and their high fiber content.

The most important source of carbohydrates is found in vegetables. For example, glucose is found in fruits and vegetables; fructose in fruits

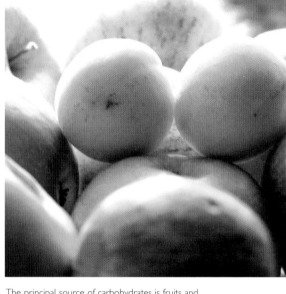

The principal source of carbohydrates is fruits and vegetables.

and honey; sucrose in beets, sugarcane, or in fruits and vegetables; starch in grains, tubers, peas and beans, fruits, and other vegetables.

The recommended daily intake is five or more portions (one portion = half a cup) of vegetables and citrus fruits, and six portions that include bread, grains, and peas and beans. This reduces fats, and thus calories, and increases the consumption of fiber in the daily diet.

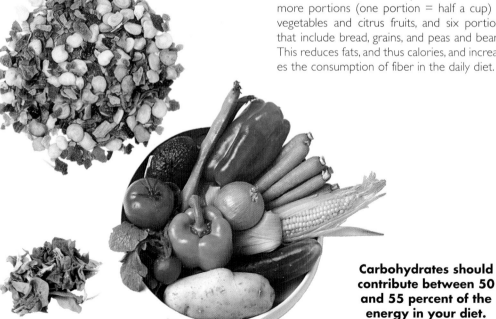

Carbohydrates should contribute between 50 and 55 percent of the energy in your diet.

59

Fiber

Fiber is a combination of substances derived from plants, for the most part sugars, which do not dissolve during the digestion process. Fiber creates mobility in the intestine by increasing bulk and softening residues. Because it delays the absorption of nutrients, it prevents sudden rises of glucose levels in the blood. It also supplies a low amount of energy by absorbing the fatty acids that are produced during the fermentation process through the action of the intestinal flora, and it stabilizes and cleans the large and small intestines.

The recommended daily intake of fiber is about 1 ounce, because it has a proven role in protecting against high blood cholesterol (hypercholesterolemia), diabetes, obesity, colon conditions, and even some types of cancer. Children are recommended to eat about a third of an ounce for every 50 pounds of body weight.

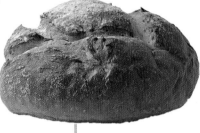

Proteins are composed of amino acids and are found mainly in milk and dairy products, eggs, meat, and fish. Legumes (peas and beans), grains, nuts, and dried fruit also contain proteins; these are called vegetable proteins and are of less biological value.

Fats

Fats, or lipids, provide the body with energy and are essential for it to function properly:
- They form part of the structure of cellular membranes.
- They transport liposoluble vitamins to the cells (A, D, E, and K).
- They store energy.

They are involved in the blood-clotting processes.

However, whether lipids are beneficial or deleterious to health depends on their type and how much is ingested.

Saturated fatty acids

These derive mainly from animal fats, such as butter, cheese, fat in meat, eggs, and some vegetable oils used in industrial bakeries. Excessive consumption of these types of fats raises cholesterol and triglyceride levels and poses a risk factor for heart disease.

Unsaturated fatty acids

These are divided into:
- Monounsaturated fats: found principally in olive oil, dried fruit, nuts, and seeds.
- Polyunsaturated fats: these are essential fatty acids, because they cannot be synthesized by the body and thus have to be supplied through a person's diet; they are found principally in oily fish, some root vegetables, and high-energy foods.

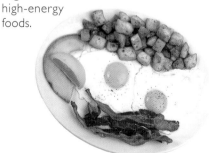

Unsaturated fatty acids are part of our recommended dietary intake and are very important for pregnant women, children, and older people.

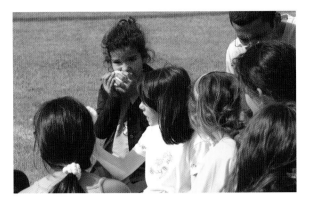

Unsaturated fats help to reduce LDL cholesterol levels (referred to as "bad cholesterol") and increase HDL (or "good cholesterol"). These types of fats have a preventive and therapeutic effect on diseases such as cancer, inflammatory illnesses, and skin conditions.

RECOMMENDED DIETARY INTAKE OF FATS	
Total fats (% of energy)	30–35%
Saturated fatty acids	7–8%
Monounsaturated fatty acids	15–20%
Polyunsaturated fatty acids	5%
Cholesterol	<300 milligrams per day

◢ The importance of water

Water is the principal component of living organisms. At birth, 75 percent of the human body is water; by adulthood, it is approximately 60 percent. Roughly 60 percent of that water is found within the body's cells, while the rest circulates in the blood.

Water also has the job of eliminating waste substances produced by the body's chemical and physical processes, its cellular metabolism, and it plays a vital role in regulating body temperature.

Water is also produced from the body's processing of nutrients. For example, the oxidation of one gram of fat results in one gram of water.

It is very important to consume a sufficient amount of water each day for the body's assimilation processes to function properly and, above all, for the elimination of the cellular metabolism's waste products.

The human body needs some 6 pints of water a day, approximately half of which is obtained from food and the other half from drinking.

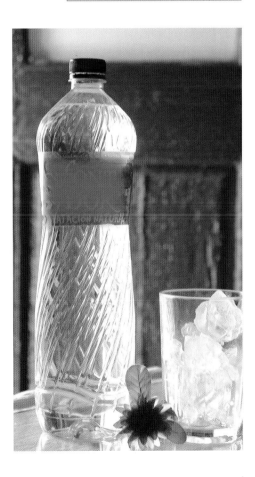

Vitamins and minerals:
their functions and where they are found

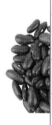

LIPOSOLUBLE VITAMINS	PHYSIOLOGICAL FUNCTION	FOODS THAT CONTAIN THEM
Vitamin A	Involved in visual mechanisms, the metabolism of steroids and cholesterol, and maintaining the immune system. Moreover, it is very important during development of an embryo.	Dairy products, liver, eggs, and oily fish, such as tuna or sardines.
Vitamin D	Involved in mineralizing bones, as it helps the absorption of calcium.	Oily fish, such as salmon or tuna, cod-liver oil, eggs, and dairy products (although in small amounts).
Vitamin E	A powerful antioxidant.	Vegetable oils, nuts and dried fruit, kitchen vegetables, green vegetables, and grains.
Vitamin K	Important in regulating the mineralization process and involved in blood-clotting mechanisms.	Green vegetables, such as spinach, broccoli, and cabbage, and in soy and olive oil.

HYDROSOLUBLE VITAMINS	PHYSIOLOGICAL FUNCTION	FOODS THAT CONTAIN THEM
Vitamin C	Essential in order to form and maintain collagen. A powerful antioxidant and involved in processes that tackle infections and toxins.	Fruits, such as strawberries, kiwi fruit, and citrus fruits; kitchen or green vegetables, such as peppers, Brussels sprouts, radishes, or broccoli; liver and kidneys, milk, and meat.
Thiamine	Involved in metabolizing carbohydrates and plays an important role in the nervous system.	Grains, legumes (peas and beans), green vegetables, fruits, and dairy products.
Riboflavin	Facilitates the energy supply required for biological processes.	Liver, milk and cheese, eggs, green vegetables, and grains.
Vitamin B6	Involved in metabolizing amino acids.	Red meat, dairy products, grains and bread, nuts, legumes, and fruit.
Folic acid	Plays an important role in embryonic development, in metabolizing amino acids, and prevents anemia.	Liver, green vegetables, fruit, grains and bread, nuts, such as peanuts and hazelnuts, and beer.
Vitamin B12	Essential for numerous enzyme-related reactions.	Meat, fish, eggs, and dairy products (in lesser quantities).

MINERALS	PHYSIOLOGICAL FUNCTION	FOODS THAT CONTAIN THEM
Iron	Allows oxygen to be transported and the storage of oxygen in muscle tissue.	Meat, fish, dairy products and, to a lesser extent, kitchen and green vegetables.
Zinc	A mineral essential to the function of a great number of enzymes and also involved in regulating gene expression.	Red meat and seafood.
Calcium	Fundamental to the skeleton and for enzyme activation. Involved in blood clotting processes and in the transport of membranes.	Milk and milk-products, grains, fruit, and green-leaf vegetables.
Phosphorus	Important in replenishing metabolic energy and regulating enzymes.	Fish, grains, and nuts.
Magnesium	Essential in biosynthesis processes and neuromuscular activity.	Nuts, whole grains, green-leaf vegetables, legumes, chocolate.

A healthy, balanced diet

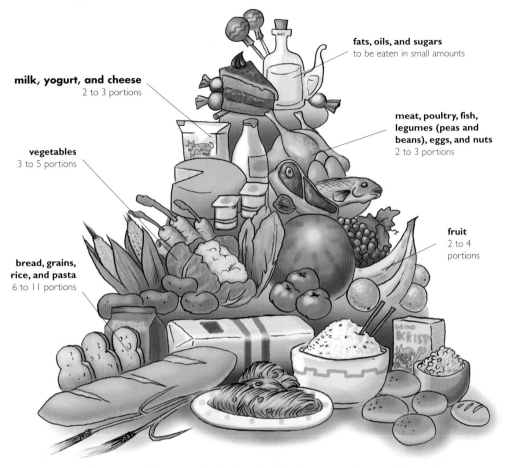

fats, oils, and sugars
to be eaten in small amounts

milk, yogurt, and cheese
2 to 3 portions

meat, poultry, fish, legumes (peas and beans), eggs, and nuts
2 to 3 portions

vegetables
3 to 5 portions

fruit
2 to 4 portions

bread, grains, rice, and pasta
6 to 11 portions

The food pyramid shows the foods that should underpin our diets and the products that should be eaten in moderation.

N.B.

- The World Health Organization (WHO) has laid down the following proportions:Carbohydrates should form at least 55–60 percent of total calorific intake.
- Fats should not exceed 30 percent of total calorie intake.
- Proteins should make up the remaining 15 percent of a person's diet.
- Daily alcohol consumption, even if not high, supplies the body with additional calories. If this calorific excess is not successfully eliminated, it is deposited in the body as fat.

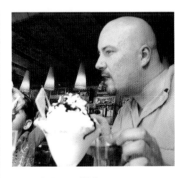

Although these guidelines seem easy enough to follow, the world's most developed societies do not eat a properly balanced diet, and their intake of fats and proteins is much greater than the recommended allowance.

All nutrients are essential for the body to function properly, but they all provide a different type of diet depending on the category of foods to which they belong and the proportion in which they are eaten, and it is this that determines a healthy or less healthy diet.

To eat a balanced diet, it is important to understand the correct proportions for each type of food.

It is better to speak of a healthy, balanced diet rather than an ideal diet, because an ideal diet does not exist per se. Eating has to be adapted to individual requirements, depending on physiological characteristics, age, and health.

A balanced diet must contain all the categories of food and the amounts of nutrients necessary to enable the body to perform all its functions normally.

Food consumption should not be excessive, because excess creates imbalance, such as increased cholesterol or higher blood pressure.

■ Mediterranean diet

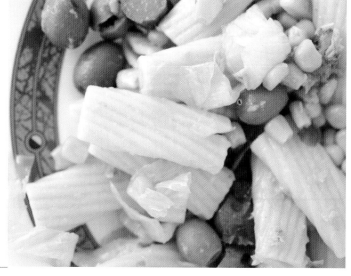

- The Mediterranean diet fulfills the requirements and recommendations for a balanced, healthy diet.

- This is a diet based on the eating habits in the countries bordering the Mediterranean Sea. Although the countries may be very different from one another, their foods share many common characteristics.

- The Mediterranean diet makes good use of fats. Virgin olive oil contains 80 percent oleic acid (a monounsaturated fatty acid) and 14 percent saturated fatty acids. Monounsaturated fatty acids increase the level of HDL cholesterol in relation to LDL cholesterol; HDL protects against the build-up of plaques (patches of fatty material) on the arterial wall, which cause atherosclerosis, commonly referred to as hardening of the arteries. The Mediterranean diet is rich in pasta, vegetables, and fruit and, as a result of consuming a large amount of legumes (lentils, chickpeas, and beans), it contains an adequate percentage of carbohydrates.

- Fish is eaten to the same degree as meat, thus increasing the intake of polyunsaturated fats in relation to saturated fats.

- Furthermore, Mediterranean cuisine uses herbs and spices that aid the digestion of food.

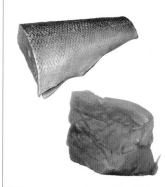

Vegetarian diet

- Not all vegetarians are the same. They can be divided into three principal groups:
  - Lacto-ovo vegetarians, who consume milk, eggs, and vegetables.
  - Lacto vegetarians, who consume milk and vegetables.
  - Strict vegetarians, or vegans, who consume only vegetables.

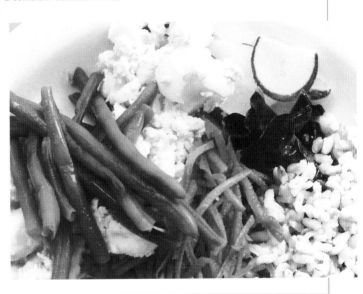

- Experts maintain that vegetarians enjoy a good state of health. Problems only arise vegans, as they can suffer from deficiencies of certain nutrients caused by a lack of essential amino acids, iron, and vitamins B2, B12, and D.

- Vitamin B12 does not exist in vegetables; human beings obtain it from meat, milk, or eggs. Furthermore, milk and eggs are our principal source of calcium, thus people who do not eat these products can also miss out on a sufficient calcium intake.

- Another deficiency in the diet of strict vegetarians comes from their difficulty in obtaining enough iron—present in meat and eggs —because the iron in vegetables is less easily absorbed.

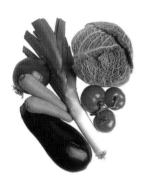

Diet throughout the various stages of life

A man needs to adapt his diet to the changing requirements of his body and to the different phases of his development.

A different amount of calories is needed in childhood compared with the amount needed in adulthood or old age. Each phase of development involves particular nutritional priorities, which are important and need to be understood in order to avoid problems, such as malnutrition or osteoporosis (brittle bones).

Correct nutrition is essential in unusual circumstances such as illness, a period of stress, or increased physical activity.

Childhood

In the first few years of life, the pattern of growth is very high and, therefore, energy and nutritional requirements are also high. Any imbalance or deficiency can cause weakness or illness.

It is very important for school-age children to follow a balanced diet and to avoid, or at least control, their fat intake—especially those fats that come from pastries—in order to avoid cholesterol and childhood obesity.

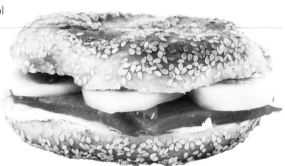

The recommended daily allowance is:
- Two to four glasses of milk and milk products.
- One portion of meat and another of fish.
- One or two daily portions of rice or pasta.
- Two to four pieces of fruit each day.
- Three to five portions of vegetables.
- Three eggs a week.

Eating out

Today's working environment obliges many of us to eat out. But eating out does not have to be synonymous with putting on weight or not following a balanced diet.

- Here is some advice for avoiding dietary imbalance.
- Try to keep your daily menu varied, consisting of two courses plus a dessert.
- It is important for some of the main dishes to be composed of vegetables, either as the main ingredient of the first course or as an addition to the main course.
- Always try to eat at a restaurant at the same time of day; this helps your body to develop a better digestive rhythm. Eating food slowly and thorough chewing is also an aid to better digestion.
- Avoid fast food. It provides few nutrients and will put on more pounds.
- Avoid dishes that contain extremely fatty sauces.
- Choose main courses that have been prepared on a griddle or roasted, as this type of cooking results in dishes with less fat.
- Avoid dishes accompanied by fattening sauces or side orders, such as tomato ketchup, Russian salad, or French fries. Instead, replace these with green salads.

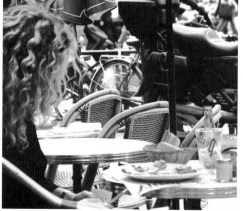

- Avoid alcoholic spirits. Apart from being bad for your health, they are also fattening. Instead, substitute wine, beer, or cider, which have lower alcohol content, are less fattening and, in moderation, can even be beneficial to health.
- Replace heavy desserts with seasonal fruits.

Adolescence

A multitude of changes occur in adolescence: rapid growth, a redistribution of body fat and muscle mass, and sexual maturity. These changes affect girls as much as boys, although for girls they are usually less pronounced and of shorter duration. During this phase, nutritional requirements should be specific depending on a person's sex.

Boys' musculature usually develops far more; their skeletons are larger and their growth phase is longer. Consequently, their protein consumption should be higher to compensate for their significantly greater physical growth. Therefore, it is important for protein to supply between 12 and 14 percent of an adolescent's energy. As far as fats and carbohydrates are concerned, the proportions should be the same as for adults.

Minerals are also very important during this stage, particularly calcium, iron, and zinc.

Half a pint of milk provides more than 250 mg of calcium; cheese and yogurt are also good sources. You should remember that substances such as sugar, caffeine, and fiber make it more difficult for the body to absorb calcium, while vitamin D, magnesium, lactose, and protein make it easier.

Iron is necessary for the development of muscle tissue and blood vessels. Meat provides

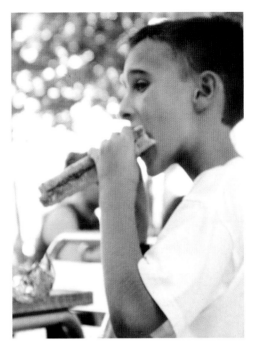

Eating habits are established in childhood. If children are introduced to a balanced diet from the very beginning, they are highly likely to maintain the same eating patterns in adulthood. Certain changes have recently been observed in the eating habits of school-age children in the developed world. They seem to be eating more fat, fewer carbohydrates, and less fiber, because their diets lack grains, green vegetables, and fruit.

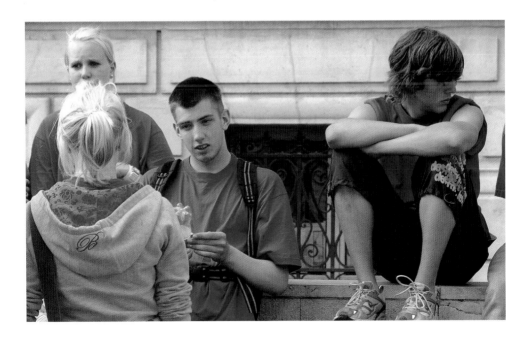

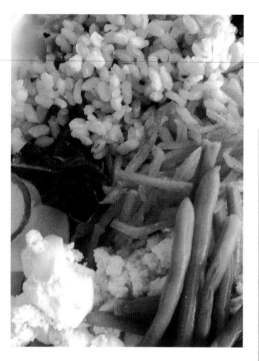

A balanced diet is essential from earliest childhood, as is avoiding, or at least controlling, the intake of fat, particularly fats in bakery products (Danish pastries, cookies, etc.), in order to avoid excess cholesterol and childhood obesity.

20 percent of iron ingested, and 5 percent comes from fruit and vegetables. Iron-rich foods include offal, sesame seeds, egg yolks, legumes, and some dry foods, such as almonds.

When a diet is poor in zinc, skin lesions can appear, hair can fall out, and wounds heal more slowly. Foods rich in zinc include shellfish, veal, nuts, vegetables, and bananas.

Vitamins are very important at this stage of life, especially those relating to growth, such as vitamin A, vitamin D, and the vitamin B complex.

Senior citizens

It is as important for senior citizens to follow a balanced diet as it is for any adult.

The recommended daily intake is between 3 and 5 portions of vegetables, each with an average uncooked weight of between 5 and 7 ounces.

The body's metabolic and activity levels decrease and, consequently, so do the body's calorific requirements, which is why it is important to avoid eating too much sugar or fat and thus prevent obesity and the buildup of cholesterol.

However, the opposite is true with regard to protein, more of which is required in old age. Dairy products, fish, and eggs must be eaten more often.

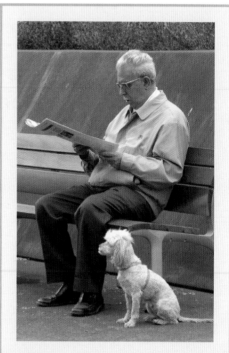

Some advice for senior citizens

- Older people who are overweight or with high levels of cholesterol are advised to drink skim or low-fat milk.

- Older people suffering from high blood pressure should keep their salt intake to a minimum, as well as alcoholic drinks and caffeine.

- Older people are at a greater risk of dehydration; therefore, it is a very good idea to get into the habit of drinking at least 4 pints of water every day.

Nutritional abnormalities: anorexia, bulimia, orthorexia

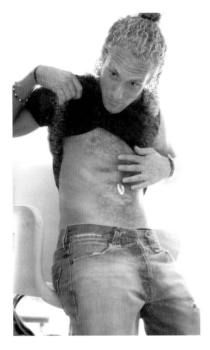

Anorexia and bulimia affect men as well. In recent years, there has been an increase in the number of men affected, now estimated to be around one man for every ten women.

Children and adults suffer from these conditions, but the time of greatest risk continues to be during adolescence, which is the period in which five out of every hundred teenagers develop some type of nutritional disorder. These conditions are very serious and complex.

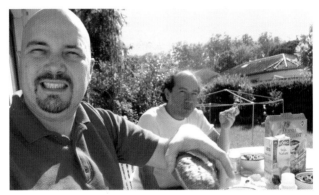

The cult of the body beautiful

The male obsession with the body beautiful started in the 1980s, when men began to be targeted by the fashion and cosmetics industry, which until then had not fully exploited men as a consumer group. Furthermore, women, who had by then become fully integrated within the workplace, started to change their priorities about the ideal man: a man's social status began to be less important to them than his physical appearance. Faced with this type of pressure, men were compelled to join this trend for the aesthetic ideal.

Nowadays, it seems that social success requires a man to be up to date on the latest fashion and style trends, while he also concentrates on achieving the ideal physique.

This concern about appearance has been a double-edged sword for men: the desire to have a "perfect 10" body—supposedly equipping you with a guarantee of victory and success (in life, with women, etc.)—can turn itself into an obsession. In recent years, cases of anorexia and bulimia in men have increased by 20 percent,

and new, exclusively male-related, psychological conditions have appeared: "fitness fanatic syndrome," or those obsessed with body building, and "compulsive jogger syndrome"—a condition that compels those who suffer from it to spend hours running when they believe they have overeaten.

Statistics show that cases of men suffering from bulimia (episodes of uncontrolled binge eating followed by vomiting or overuse of laxatives or diuretics) are double those of men with anorexia.

Both of these nutrition-related conditions have very similar symptoms in both sexes; however, men show a greater obsession for physical exercise and losing all-over body weight, while women are more obsessed with slimming particular areas of their bodies. Although this shows that men may have a more realistic perception of their bodies than women, they also suffer greater fear and shame about admitting they have a problem, given that these problems are typically (albeit erroneously) identified as female conditions.

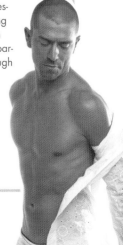

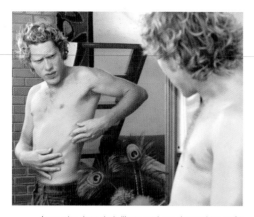

Anorexia can be seen as an axtreme alteration to eating habits and/or behavior.

Anorexics deny their illness and see themselves as fat despite often having a skeletal appearance.

Anorexia and bulimia

Anorexia (nervosa) involves a serious change in self-perception brought about by a terror of putting on weight and becoming obese, and aggravated by the insecurity felt about confronting this as a problem.

Anorexics are usually obsessed with food and everything related to it. Typically, they will snack on things, especially candy, drink large amounts of coffee and/or smoke.

Bulimia is a psychological condition characterized by episodes of voracious hunger or, which amounts to the same thing, short periods of time when bulimics eat large amounts of food—binge eating—which is always followed by behavior aimed at preventing weight gain: vomiting, use of diuretics, and laxatives.

Both anorexia and bulimia are serious chronic conditions that require continuous treatment monitored by specialists (pediatricians, psychiatrists, psychologists, child psychiatrists, endocrinologists, dieticians, etc.) in order to prevent relapses and complications.

These complex conditions are usually also accompanied by manifestations of depression and anxiety.

One of the major differences found between men and women with bulimia is that

Adult men with the highest risk of suffering bulimia are those who have been obese and lost weight since, yet who are still scared about putting it back on again.

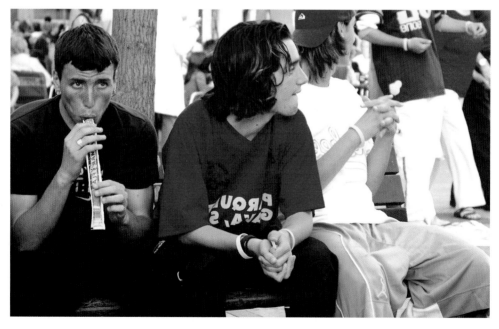

65 percent of men with bulimia nervosa have had a history of obesity, while only 20 percent of bulimic women have a history of obesity.

There are other non-specific eating disorders, which also cause problems and have parallels to anorexia and bulimia but do not correspond exactly to all the features of these conditions.

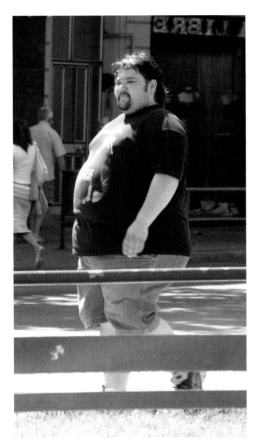

Those who are most susceptible to suffering an eating disorder fall into two groups: boys with an obesity problem and adolescents struggling with the acknowledgement of their homosexuality.

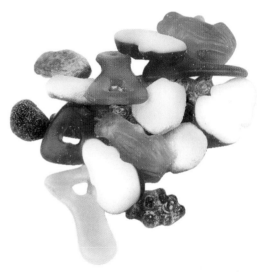

ANOREXIA SYMPTOMS	BULIMIA SYMPTOMS
Terror of putting on weight.	Repeated episodes of binge eating in which a great amount of food is consumed in a short space of time accompanied by a sense of loss of control.
Distorted image of one's own body, or seeing oneself as fat despite being very thin.	Behavior to compensate for binge eating in order to avoid gaining weight (vomiting, use of medication, exercise, fasting).
Weight falling below normal until reaching the point of malnutrition.	Self-image and self-esteem are conditioned by weight, size, and body shape.

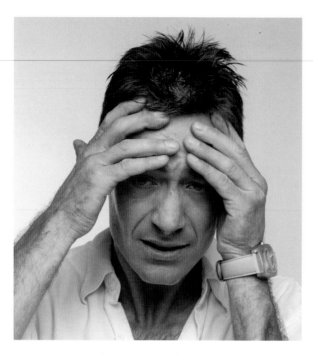

What are the causes of anorexia and bulimia?

The causes of anorexia and bulimia are still not known for certain.

A range of psychological, physical, educational, and social factors can cause a collapse of self-esteem and loss of control.

A restrictive, slimming diet can trigger the problem if these factors are there in the background.

Genetic factors may also exist, given that the closest relatives of a patient with anorexia (his parents, children, siblings) are 6–10 times more likely to develop an eating disorder.

Furthermore, any family history of depression increases a person's risk of suffering anorexia or bulimia.

▪ What other problems may accompany anorexia and bulimia?

- A range of medical complications and physical risks due to severe malnutrition can arise, such as digestive tract conditions (due to binge eating, vomiting, use of laxatives), heart problems due to malnutrition, biochemical changes (low levels of potassium or sodium in the blood), endocrine or hormonal changes, and calcium-deficient bones.

- Other psychiatric problems frequently arise connected with eating disorders. Anorexia is linked to depression, dysthymia (chronic depression), and obsessive-compulsive disorder. Patients with bulimia frequently suffer from depression, anxiety, and addiction problems or difficulty in controlling their impulses (compulsive shopping, kleptomania, self-harming, and sexual promiscuity).

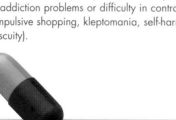

It is thought that part of the problem may lie in the body's regulation of the hormone serotonin; antidepressants known as selective serotonin re-uptake inhibitors (SSRIs) improve the levels of this neurotransmitter and have been shown to be useful in the treatment of bulimia.

Treatment and prognosis

The first step is to see a specialist in order to undergo a weight-gain regime and be re-educated about diet and food. This process should be adhered to rigidly with frequent checkups so that weight gain is achieved gradually.

Other problems that may result in eating disorders need to be analyzed and dealt with, such as anxiety about school or issues with parents or friends. Psychiatric treatment combines patient education, group and one-on-one psychotherapy, and family therapy.

In some cases, the patient can be helped using medication. For example, some antidepressants can have a positive effect on binge eating, vomiting, and, of course, feelings of depression, as well as treating other problems associated with anorexia and bulimia.

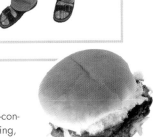

Anorexia is a serious illness with up to a 6-percent risk of death over a 10-year period (due to suicides and complications involving malnutrition), particularly if left untreated. However, up to 60 percent of anorexics and 50 percent of bulimics who receive treatment recover within 10 years.

It is often a chronic condition, with some people continuing to present problems 5 to 10 years after their initial diagnosis. It is crucial to receive proper treatment at an early stage in order to avoid complications, but this will not always prevent the problem from turning into a chronic condition.

Compulsive eating

• This is an illness that involves eating large amounts of food without any self-control. Sufferers subject themselves to frequent and desperate bouts of binge eating, unable to rein themselves in even though they feel full. Unlike bulimics, compulsive eaters do not induce vomiting afterward, nor do they take laxatives or diuretics.

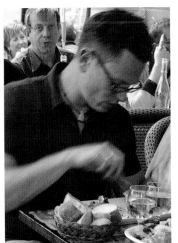

• It is common for compulsive eaters to be obsessed with starting diets; typically, however, they break these diets soon after beginning. The majority of sufferers are obese, although people of normal weight can be afflicted with this condition as well. More than half of these patients are obsessed with their weight, feel guilty about their lack of self-control, and exhibit the symptoms of depression. Moreover, they come to develop complications, such as gastrointestinal complaints, bladder problems, cardiovascular conditions, high blood pressure, high levels of cholesterol, or diabetes.

Orthorexia

This eating disorder is characterized by an obsession regarding specific types of food or entire food groups which sufferers believe are bad for their health and, therefore, must be eliminated systematically from their diet. Anorexics and bulimics are fixated on food quantity, while orthorexics are fixated on its presumed quality. Orthorexics have disproportional concern about what is healthy, natural, or organic. The problem surfaces when a person adopts an extreme choice of diet. This obsession ends up producing physical and psychological distress, as well as feelings of guilt in the event of committing some dietary "transgression." Orthorexics usually suffer complications such as depression, anxiety, aggression, anemia, fatigue, or a weakened immune response.

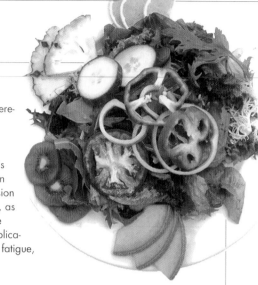

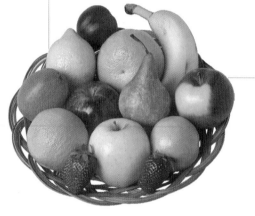

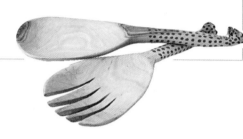

Obesity

What is obesity?

This is a chronic illness characterized by an excess of fat that in turn translates into weight gain. Obesity is the developed world's most common metabolic disorder.

Obesity is a chronic illness that occurs when there is an excess of adipose tissue in the body: in other words, excess body fat. Moreover, apart from the more obvious problems that obesity presents, experts affirm that its most negative effects result in a rapid worsening and aggravation of medical conditions such as diabetes, high blood pressure, coronary diseases, and even some types of cancer, such as those affecting the digestive system.

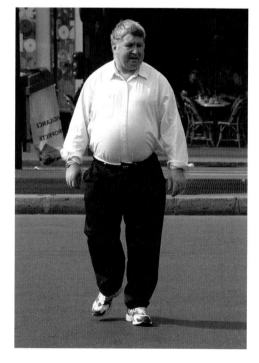

According to international criteria, people are categorized as overweight or obese when their body mass index (BMI) exceeds normal levels.

The BMI is obtained by dividing weight in kilograms (kg) by height in meters squared (m²).

For example, a man who is 5 feet 7 inches (1.7 m) tall and who weighs 165 lbs (75 kg) has a BMI of $75 \div (1.7 \times 1.7) = 75 \div 2.89 = 25.95$.

A BMI between 18.5 and 24.9 is considered normal. A person is overweight if this figure is

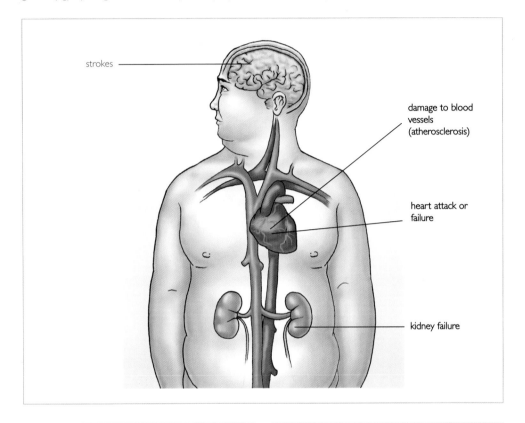

strokes

damage to blood vessels (atherosclerosis)

heart attack or failure

kidney failure

BMI	GRADE OF OBESITY
<18.5	Underweight
18.5–24.9	Normal weight
25–26.9	Overweight grade I
27–29.9	Overweight grade II (pre-obese)
30–34.9	Obesity type I
35–39.9	Obesity type II
40–49.9	Obesity type III (severe or morbid obesity)
>50	Obesity type IV (extreme obesity)

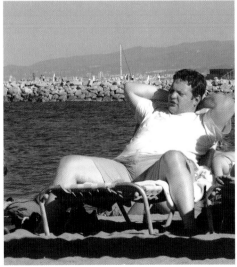

between 25 and 29.9, and he is classified as obese if the figure reaches 30 or above. However, you need to take into account the fact that different individuals with the same BMI may have a greater or lesser quantity of adipose (fatty) or lean (muscle) tissue depending on their build or sex.

Abdominal obesity, which consists of a build up of adipose tissue around the waist, is another concept to bear in mind. In order to detect this kind of obesity, measurements are taken of the circumference of the waist and hips. The ratio determines the presence of abdominal obesity. Men are considered obese if this ratio exceeds a value of 0.9. For example, a man with a waist measurement of 35½ inches and a hip measurement of 27½ inches has a waist to hip ratio of 1.28. Therefore, he has abdominal obesity, even though his total weight is normal.

There are two distinct types of obesity, depending on the distribution of body fat:
- Android obesity: this is localized in the face, neck, torso, and upper part of the abdomen. It is most common in men.
- Gynoid obesity: predominates in the lower abdomen, hips, and buttocks. It is most common in women.
- In general, people with abdominal obesity present a greater long-term risk of high blood pressure problems, diabetes, and heart disease.

HEIGHT feet/inches	OVERWEIGHT lbs	OBESITY lbs	SEVERE OBESITY lbs
4 ft. 9 in.	> 116 lbs	> 139 lbs	185 lbs
4 ft. 11 in.	> 124 lbs	> 149 lbs	198 lbs
5 ft. 1 in.	> 132 lbs	> 159 lbs	212 lbs
5 ft. 3 in.	> 141 lbs	> 169 lbs	226 lbs
5 ft. 5 in.	> 150 lbs	> 180 lbs	240 lbs
5 ft. 7 in.	> 159 lbs	> 191 lbs	255 lbs
5 ft. 9 in.	> 169 lbs	> 202 lbs	270 lbs
5 ft. 11 in.	> 179 lbs	> 214 lbs	286 lbs
6 ft. 1 in.	> 189 lbs	> 226 lbs	302 lbs
6 ft 3 in.	> 199 lbs	> 239 lbs	318 lbs
6 ft. 5 in.	> 209 lbs	> 251 lbs	335 lbs

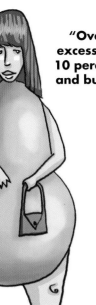

"Overweight" and "obesity" are the terms used to describe excessive body weight. "Overweight" refers to people who are 10 percent above the body weight that is normal for their height and build. "Obesity," on the other hand, refers to people whose weight is 20 percent above recommended levels.

Causes of obesity

The appearance of obesity has many causes. Apart from environmental factors, such as poor diet and lack of exercise, there are also genetic and biological factors (some diseases) which can cause it to arise. The environmental factors that cause obesity concern the amount of calories that an individual consumes. If someone consumes more calories than he needs, taking into account his basic energy consumption and his level of physical activity, the excess is deposited in the form of fat, which is the process that develops into obesity.

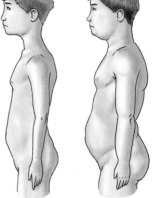

FACTORS THAT AFFECT BODY SIZE

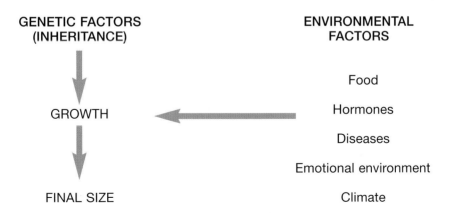

GENETIC FACTORS (INHERITANCE)	ENVIRONMENTAL FACTORS
GROWTH	Food
	Hormones
	Diseases
	Emotional environment
FINAL SIZE	Climate

Overweight boys and teenagers are more likely to be overweight as adults.

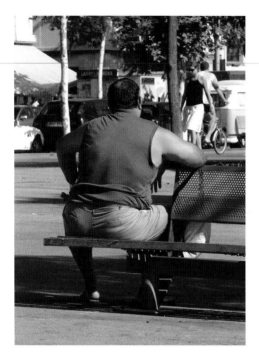

When treating someone for obesity, it is necessary to ensure that weight loss is achieved over the long term and thus reduce the risk of diseases affecting the heart, metabolism, and blood vessels, and possibly premature death as a result.

Is obesity an illness?

Whether or not obesity is an illness is still the subject of debate. What is certain is that obesity gives rise to a range of medical conditions:

- Conditions relating to the joints (arthritis, degenerative osteoarthritis), knees, spinal column, pelvis, etc.
- High arterial blood pressure (risk of stroke/brain hemorrhage)
- Enlargement of the heart and heart failure
- Diabetes
- Peripheral arterial/vascular conditions (deficient blood circulation, varicose veins)
- Long-term breathing problems
- Deterioration of kidney and liver function
- General biological deterioration and premature aging
- Sexual dysfunction
- Emotional conditions (anxiety, feelings of inferiority, depression)
- Hormonal imbalances

Advice for losing weight:

- Eat five or more types of fruit and vegetables each day. Vegetables can be eaten raw or cooked in a steamer.
- Eat dairy products, salad dressings, and cheese rarely or only if low in fat.
- Don't eat vegetables with gravy, sauces, butter, or margarine.
- Remove fat and skin before cooking meat.
- Instead of frying, it is better to broil, boil, or oven-roast your food.
- Do not eat more than four eggs each week.
- Do not follow rigid or fashionable diets that force you to eat less than 1,200 calories a day.

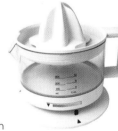

- Avoid eating rich, sugary foods, such as cakes, cookies, and pastries.
- Avoid bottled or canned fruit juice, as it is often high in calories.
- Weigh yourself once a week. Do not worry about minor variations in weight over the course of a day.
- Drink around 2 quarts of water a day.
- You must not lose more than 1–2 lbs a week. Some weeks, you may lose no weight at all. This

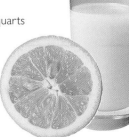

is normal. The important thing is not to lose motivation and to carry on with the diet.
- Do not skip any meals.
- Limit your alcohol intake. Alcoholic drinks are high in calories.
- Eat slowly, sitting down, and without distractions. Watching television or reading during meals means that you are not paying attention to what you are eating.

- Avoid snacking on nuts, potato chips, French fries, and pastries.
- Vegetables make healthy snacks instead of rich, fatty comfort foods that are high in calories.

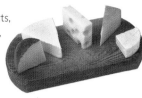

- Do some kind of aerobic exercise two or three times a week.

■ Treatment

- The best way to treat obesity is to prevent it from occurring in the first place. It is important to identify at an early stage when people are beginning to put on weight.
- Physicians feel that obesity should be treated as a chronic illness that requires long-term treatment with nutritional standards, modification of eating habits, physical exercise, and, if necessary, drug therapy.
- The latest therapeutic approach is based on encouraging weight loss as well as a control program for illnesses and diseases that

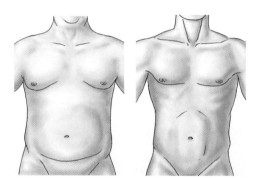

result in heart and circulation problems and conditions affecting the body's ability to metabolize food.

- The expression "ideal weight" has been replaced by "recommended weight"; the number of pounds that an obese person sheds is not as important as the amount of body fat lost. Small, long-lasting losses that ensure metabolic improvement are better.
- Surgical treatment. There are two types of surgery for obese patients: those that reduce the amount of food ingested, or the amount that can be digested, and surgery that essentially treats an obese person's physical appearance. The first type includes surgery or special procedures to reduce the size of the stomach or to reduce the amount of small intestine in which the absorption of food occurs. These types of procedure are not without risk and major discomfort for the patient, which is why they are only recommended either in cases of severe obesity or for patients who have tried other forms of therapy and they have failed.

Hyperlipidemia

Hyperlipidemia refers to a group of changes to the metabolism of lipids (fats), which typically cause increased levels of fats to be circulating in the bloodstream.

Of these fats, the two most important types are triglycerides and cholesterol.

These fats can build up when produced in excess or when metabolism is deficient. With accumulations of such fats there is a significant risk of furring of the arteries (atherosclerosis).

Fats flow through the blood-stream attached to certain protein molecules known as lipoproteins. The most important of these are chylomicrons, very low-density lipoproteins (VLDLs), low-density lipoproteins (LDLs), and high-density lipoproteins (HDLs).

LDLs carry cholesterol to body tissue, and these are referred to as "bad cholesterol" when at a high level. Conversely, HDLs carry cholesterol to the liver and are referred to as "good cholesterol."

Although there are different ways of classifying hyperlipidemia, for the sake of simplicity it can be broken down into hypertriglycerides (an increased concentration of triglycerides), hypercholesterolemia (increased levels of cholesterol), and mixed hyperlipidemia (in which there is an increase in the levels of both cholesterol and triglycerides).

These conditions can occur at any age. Hereditary hyperlipidemia can appear very early in life.

Hyperlipidemia can be classified as either primary or secondary: primary when it is the result of a particular change in the lipid metabolism, and secondary when it is produced as the result of another disease or taking certain types of medication.

Many diseases cause lipids to increase—such as diabetes mellitus, hypothyroidism, nephrotic syndrome, post-hepatic (obstructive) jaundice, lupus erythematosus, and alcoholism, as do treatments using beta-blockers, etc.

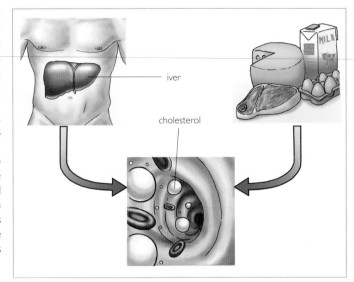

liver

cholesterol

The majority of LDL cholesterol is found in the bloodstream. It is dangerous for too much to be circulating in the blood, because it then accumulates on the arterial walls. In combination with other substances, it can start to form atheromatous (lumpy) plaques. This is what is described as atherosclerosis.

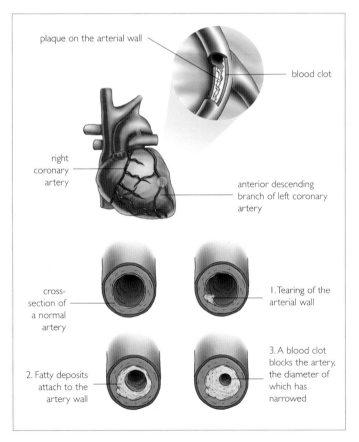

plaque on the arterial wall

blood clot

right coronary artery

anterior descending branch of left coronary artery

cross-section of a normal artery

1. Tearing of the arterial wall

2. Fatty deposits attach to the artery wall

3. A blood clot blocks the artery, the diameter of which has narrowed

N.B.

Triglycerides and cholesterol derive from food and from its synthesis by the liver. Both types fulfill different physiological functions in the body.

Episodes of abdominal pain can ensue when triglycerides are at high levels. This is due to inflammation of the pancreas and/or an increase in the size of the liver and spleen. Fatty deposits under the skin (known as "eruptive xanthomas") may also be present.

If the increase in the levels of cholesterol and/or triglycerides is chronic, this constitutes a significant risk factor for the development of furring of the arteries (atherosclerosis). For that reason, high blood cholesterol (hypercholesterolemia) can result in the development of coronary artery disease (angina, heart attacks), strokes, and peripheral artery disease.

People showing evidence of hyperlipidemia should follow an appropriate dietary regime that is based on restricting the intake of saturated or animal fats.

Moreover, it is important to maintain a normal body weight; in other words, it is just as important to avoid being underweight, as it is to avoid being overweight or obese.

It is sensible to take regular physical exercise, because this helps to improve the lipids' metabolism.

If the hyperlipidemia persists after a period of three months, treatment with drugs becomes necessary. The drugs usually administered to treat high blood cholesterol (hypercholesterolemia) are called "statins," and those used to treat high blood levels of triglycerides (hypertriglyceridemia) are called "fibrates" or "fibric acid derivatives."

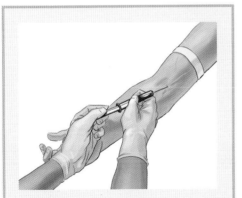

Having a blood test

In the majority of cases, an increase in the level of lipids in the blood does not produce any acute symptoms, which is why it can be detected only by means of a blood test. Under normal circumstances, the concentration of total cholesterol and of triglycerides in the bloodstream should be less than 200 mg/dl, while HDL cholesterol should be over 35 mg/dl.

Diabetes

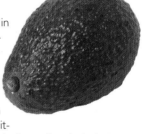

Diabetes is a disease in which the body is incapable of using and storing glucose properly. This results in above-normal levels of glucose remaining in the blood. In turn, this situation alters the metabolism of carbohydrates, lipids (fats), and proteins.

It can arise as a result of the body producing a very low amount of insulin (the hormone produced by the pancreas that has the job of regulating the amount of sugar in the blood), or because of a resistance to insulin, or for both reasons.

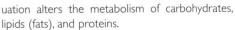

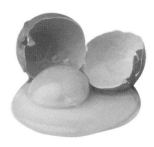

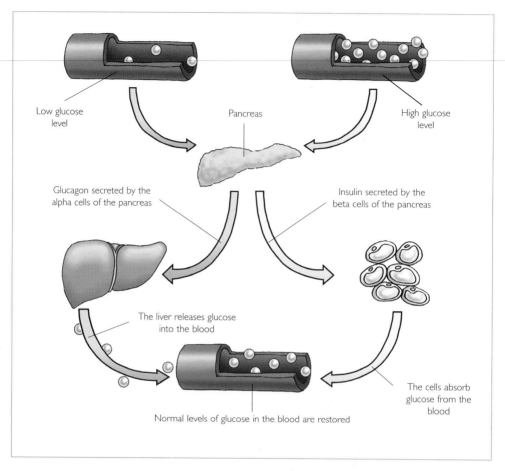

Low glucose level

Pancreas

High glucose level

Glucagon secreted by the alpha cells of the pancreas

Insulin secreted by the beta cells of the pancreas

The liver releases glucose into the blood

The cells absorb glucose from the blood

Normal levels of glucose in the blood are restored

◼ Diet for a healthy heart

This diet involves reducing your intake of animal fats and replacing meat with fish, eating a greater amount of fruit and vegetables, and using olive oil instead of other cooking oils.

Good food:

The principles underlying beneficial food are that it should contain low levels of saturated fatty acids, low levels of salt, and be low in calories. Fruit, vegetables, lean meat, poultry, oily fish, vegetable oils, and grains are all good foods.

Bad food:

Food with a high content of saturated animal fats raise cholesterol levels and have an adverse effect on the heart. These include egg yolks, butter, pork, sausages, lard, whole milk, or high-fat cheeses. Similarly, very salty food, canned food, or shellfish can raise blood pressure. High-calorie foods eaten to excess encourage obesity, which, over time, will cause serious damage to the heart.

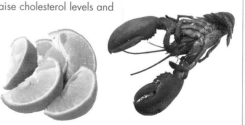

In order to understand diabetes, it is important to comprehend the normal process for metabolizing food:

Glucose—a sugar used by the body as a source of energy—enters into the bloodstream.

The pancreas produces insulin, the function of which is to transport the glucose from the bloodstream to the muscles, the body's fatty tissue, and the liver cells, where it is used as a source of energy.

People with diabetes have high glucose levels, either because the pancreas is not producing enough insulin, or because the muscles, fat, and liver cells are not responding normally to the insulin—or for both of these reasons simultaneously.

How our bodies use insulin and glucose

When functioning normally
- Insulin is essential in enabling glucose to enter cells and be converted into energy for the body.

Type 1 diabetes
- In type 1 diabetes, the beta cells in the pancreas do not produce insulin, and thus glucose is unable to enter the body's cells.

Type 2 diabletes
- In type 2 diabetes, the beta cells in the pancreas do not produce enough insulin for all of the available glucose to enter the body's cells.

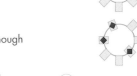

glucose   insulin   cell

Risk factors that can give rise to diabetes

- Family history of diabetes (parents or siblings)
- Obesity
- Being aged 45 or above
- Belonging to certain ethnic groups (particularly African Americans or Hispanics)
- High blood pressure
- High triglyceride levels in the blood
- High cholesterol levels in the blood

Types of diabetes

There are three major types of diabetes:
- Type 1 diabetes: this is generally diagnosed in childhood. The body produces little or no insulin. In such cases, daily injections of insulin are necessary in order to survive.
- Type 2 diabetes: this type is much more common than type 1 and relates to approximately 90 percent of all cases of diabetes, generally appearing in adulthood. The pancreas produces insufficient insulin to maintain normal levels of blood glucose; this is often due to the fact that the body has a poor response to insulin. Many people with this type of diabetes do not even realize that they have it, despite it being a serious condition. This type of diabetes is becoming increasingly common due to more of us living longer, a rise in obesity levels, and lack of exercise.
- Gestational diabetes: this involves an increase during pregnancy in the level of blood glucose of non-diabetics. This occurs only very rarely, in a small percentage of cases.

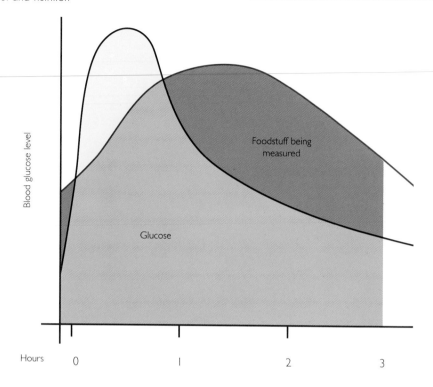

Blood glucose level

Foodstuff being measured

Glucose

Hours   0   1   2   3

When a high level of glucose is present in the blood it produces a need to urinate frequently, excessive thirst, hunger, fatigue, weight loss, and blurred vision. However, because type 2 diabetes develops slowly, some people with high sugar levels do not show any symptoms at all.

At present, there is no cure for diabetes. The immediate objective in treating it is to stabilize sugar levels in the blood and to eliminate the symptoms and conditions associated with hyperglycemia (high blood sugar). In the long term, an attempt is made to prolong and improve the patient's quality of life, to alleviate symptoms, and to prevent any complications that might arise over time, such as heart-related conditions and kidney failure.

The treatment of diabetes includes: insulin injections, a rigorously controlled diet, and administering certain drugs to help control blood sugar levels.

What is the glycemic index?

When we eat any kind of food that is rich in glucose, the blood's glucose level progressively increases as the sugars contained in that food are digested and assimilated. The speed at which food is digested and assimilated depends on the type of nutrients from which it is composed, the amount of fiber present, and the composition of the rest of the food present in the stomach and intestines during digestion. For any given food, these factors are gauged using the glycemic index. This index relates to the relationship between the area below the curve obtained over time for the absorption of a given quantity of pure glucose and the curve obtained over time for the absorption of glucose from the same quantity of a given foodstuff. Difficult though the index may be to establish, it is easy to interpret: peaks show rapid absorption, while troughs indicate slow absorption. Diabetics have to avoid sudden increases of glucose in their blood.

Ten pieces of advice about diabetes

- Control the amount of glucose in your blood. Choose food with a low glycemic index. Avoid pure sugar, and eat whole grains and high-fiber foods.
- Maintain a satisfactory body weight. Excess body fat makes it more difficult for people with type 2 diabetes to use their own insulin.
- Eat a balanced amount of carbohydrates (65 percent), proteins (15 percent), and fats (30 percent). A person in generally good health does not need to go on high-protein, ketogenic, or any other type of diet that alters the recommended balance of nutrients.
- Avoid rich food and cholesterol.
- Food should be fresh and as unprocessed as possible. Avoid ready-made meals from supermarkets, mass-produced pastries and frozen foods, canned food, etc.
- Foods that are high in fat should be eliminated from your diet or reduced in quantity: e.g. hamburgers, pizzas, frankfurters, delicatessen sausages and cold cuts, lard, margarine, nuts, high-fat salad dressings, donuts, cheesecakes, and animal fats in general.
- Food should provide a sufficient quantity of essential nutrients (vitamins, minerals, essential fatty acids, etc.).
- Eat off a smaller plate so that your portions do not become excessive.
- Control the amount of sodium in your diet. The kidneys are the organs most commonly affected by diabetes due to the additional work they have to perform when insulin levels are insufficient.
- Take regular physical exercise.

Dietary aims for diabetics

A diabetic's diet is extremely important: it helps control the metabolism and thus reduces possible problems that might arise over the long term. In cases of diabetes mellitus type 1, involving children and adolescents, it is essential for them to receive the nutrition necessary to guarantee proper development and to integrate the administration of insulin within a daily regime of meals and exercise.

When diabetes is being treated using oral antidiabetic drugs or insulin, it is very important to spread the intake of sugar evenly throughout the day in order to avoid either a sudden increase or a dip in sugar levels.

Furthermore, the diet must also be tailored to keep diabetics at the recommended weight for their age, sex, and height.

Gout or hyperuricemia (excess uric acid)

This is a metabolic condition that results from defects in the metabolism of proteins—especially the "purines"—producing an increase in the amount of uric acid in the bloodstream. This increase causes uric acid to be deposited on the joints in the form of crystals, which produce painful swellings, particularly in the feet and legs.

Sometimes, these crystals form tangible clusters—known as "tophi"—or leave deposits in the kidneys, causing renal colic (a pain commonly caused by kidney stones) or functional disorders.

This disease is four times more common in men than in women. It can appear at any time from adolescence into old age, although it tends to affect men between the ages of 35 and 50 and women over 50.

The principal risk factor, apart from being male and in middle age, is having high levels of uric acid in the blood: the higher the level, the greater the risk. Other factors that give rise to gout are obesity, high blood pressure, alcohol, certain medications, and a diet comprising the rich foods that lead to (high levels of) uric acid.

The symptoms of gout usually appear in the form of attacks of intense pain and swollen joints—gout being one of the causes of acute arthritis.

FOOD TO AVOID IN YOUR DIET IF YOU SUFFER FROM GOUT	FOOD THAT YOU CAN EAT
Animal offal: brains, kidneys, liver, tongue	Eggs and refined cereals and tubers
Red meat and game	Poultry, such as turkey or chicken
Among the various types of fish, avoid anchovies, sardines and herrings, trout and salmon.	White fish
Shellfish	Dairy products: milk, yogurt, cheese, and other dairy products
Pork-based products and pâtés	Fruit and vegetables
Among the various types of vegetable, avoid celery, watercress, asparagus, cauliflower, spinach, mushrooms, dried peas and beans, lettuce, lentils, parsley, and radishes	Peas and green beans in moderation

Without treatment, an acute episode can last several days. These episodes tend to recur and can affect any joint in subsequent attacks. If gout is left untreated, these attacks can develop into a chronic condition and restrict a person's quality of life.

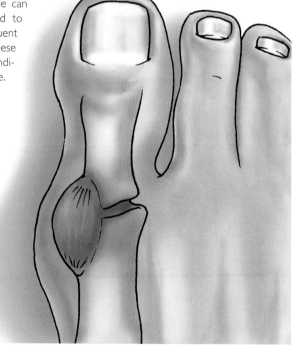

The joint most commonly affected by gout is the big toe, but it can also appear in other toe and foot joints, the ankles, and, less commonly, the knees or wrists.

Emotional well-being

Everyone has felt anxiety or stress at some time. The reasons for it can vary: being in love, examinations, work, the birth of a child, a sporting competition, public speaking, bereavement, or a marital separation, etc. The heart and breathing accelerate, blood pressure rises, a feeling of nausea ensues, the muscles tense up, and the pupils dilate. Although this state of alertness can be of use in confronting certain daily situations and responding to danger, when it occurs in a continuous and uncontrolled manner, stress and anxiety have a deleterious effect on health and, as a result, quality of life.

What is anxiety?

Anxiety is an emotional state in which people feel worried, apprehensive, and fearful.

People affected feel anxious when facing situations that are beyond their control, anything new or unanticipated, or situations that seem threatening or dangerous.

When anxiety cannot be brought under control or persists over a period of six months or more, it is treated as a disorder and requires specialist help.

Anxiety can produce different symptoms, such as:
- Shortness of breath or a feeling of asphyxiation
- Palpitations
- Pain or tightness in the chest
- Giddiness or dizziness
- Nausea or stomach upsets
- Hot flashes or goose flesh
- Fear and panic
- Pins and needles or numbness
- Shivering or trembling
- Feeling of unreality
- Feeling out of control
- Excessive sweating

An anxiety or panic attack is a sudden and inexplicable situation that is not based on any specific cause but which arises spontaneously.

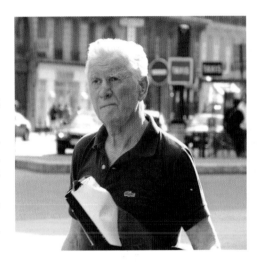

It is usually the result of more general problems that have been building up over a period of time until they unleash an attack.

People suffering such attacks suddenly experience feelings of terror faced with an exaggerated sense of danger and the proximity of death.

Although a panic attack is very difficult to control when it arises, a person must first and foremost attempt not to overdramatize the situation.

Often it is the very feeling of panic that causes the attack in the first place, and a vicious circle can develop.

A panic or anxiety attack is a situation that involves the appearance of a relatively sudden sensation of intense fear, often without any apparent rational cause, accompanied by significant physical distress and a range of symptoms that can vary from one person to another.

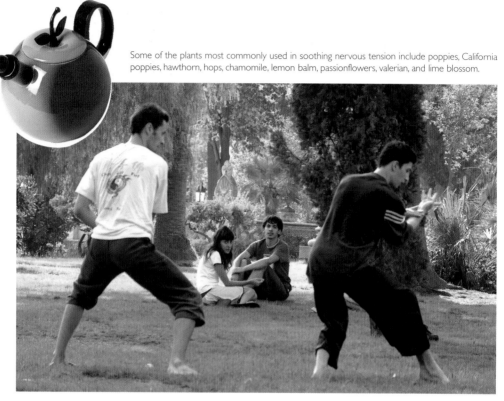

Some of the plants most commonly used in soothing nervous tension include poppies, California poppies, hawthorn, hops, chamomile, lemon balm, passionflowers, valerian, and lime blossom.

When someone is undergoing an anxiety attack, it is essential for people surrounding that person not to become agitated and to remain calm. It is very important for anyone suffering an attack to feel that a person he trusts is remaining calm and keeping a cool head, so as not to intensify his sense of panic.

What is stress?

Stress is a state of major nervous tension that can be due to overwork, uncompleted tasks or goals, anxiety, divorce, the death of a friend or relative, etc.

It usually manifests itself through a range of responses that include everything from prolonged fatigue and exhaustion to headaches, gastritis, and ulcers; and it can even produce psychological disorders.

There is a normal level of stress that cannot be eliminated from a person's life, because it constitutes the basic essence of who that person is. It can even be a positive influence, if you know how to deal with it effectively.

When stress turns into a prolonged and intense response to something, it can begin to produce serious physical and psychological problems.

When the body becomes unable to free itself of the changes that this produces, a person can enter into a state of chronic stress.

Types of work-related stress

Excessive workload. This is one of the major types of stress. It requires the worker to operate at a much faster rhythm than his body and mind will allow. The most immediate consequences of this situation are tiredness, anxiety, irritability, tension, loss of concentration, and signs of confusion.

Inadequate terms of employment. Essentially, this boils down to low pay conditions, job insecurity, and poor diet. These conditions, far from being a motivational force or providing a worker with incentives, generate a constant feeling of unhappiness in him. By degrees, this is transformed into a crisis, ultimately causing major work-related stress.

Inappropriate physical or environmental conditions in the workplace. Poor lighting, ventilation, and temperature, as well as excessive noise, can provoke a decline in physical and psychological well-being, preventing a person from functioning normally at work.

High level of responsibility at work. Sufferers of stress are usually people who are frequently involved in high-level decision-making. This produces fatigue, anxiety, and the impossibility of enjoying a social or family life. Individuals also find that it causes them sleep disorders, creates the theoretical conditions for succumbing to addictions (e.g. smoking, alcoholism), generates a loss of sexual desire, and produces serious irritability.

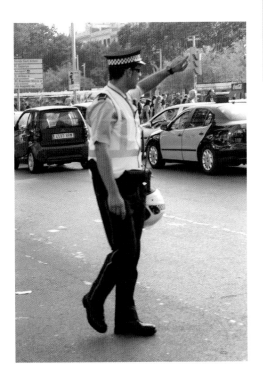

Symptoms of stress

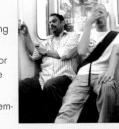

- Difficulty in getting to sleep
- Frequent feelings of wanting to cry
- Feeling tired or drowsy all the time
- Feeling bad-tempered
- Difficulty in concentrating and making decisions
- Appearance of nervous ticks
- Frequent headaches and muscular pains
- Inability to talk with other people
- Sudden mood swings
- Feeling deadlocked and incapable of action
- Drinking or smoking to excess
- Suffering from attacks of rage
- Losing interest in sex
- Constantly having gloomy and pessimistic thoughts
- Loss of appetite
- Lack of enthusiasm

Changes to the natural rhythm of life. People suffering from this type of stress are essentially workers without regular working hours whose schedule changes frequently. This results in the body failing to adapt to the rhythm of work and, consequently, an increased level of stress. Signs pointing to the appearance of this type of stress include anxiety, irritability, fatigue, loss of concentration, decreased sexual desire, and difficulties in relationships with friends and family.

What is "mobbing"?

Mobbing is a modern term to describe harassment, ganging up on someone, bullying, or psychological attack. It is an extreme form of psychological harassment that one or usually more people may exercise systematically on another person over a lengthy period of time. This pressure is usually found in the workplace, but is as easily identified in other environments, such as within the family, at school, or between members of a neighborhood. Mobbing is caused by major disagreements, differences, or conflicts of any type between work colleagues, irrespective of rank. When trying to put a stop to a mobbing situation, you should speak first with your supervisor or the department responsible for health and safety, if such exists.

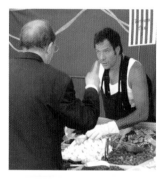 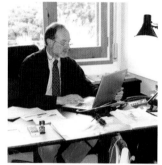 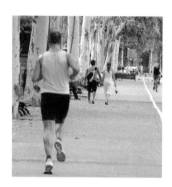

Stress in the home

Times of tension and stress occur in the majority of homes, and these situations can throw the emotional well-being of family members off balance. Stress can arise because of being constantly required to satisfy the demands of children or other family members. Or it may arise as the result of some specific upheaval, such as the death of someone in the family.

A rebellious child, or one who is leaving the family nest or suffering from an addiction, can cause a high level of stress in the family.

Emotional or sexual problems, a serious illness, moving house, an excessive workload, having children, or money problems are just some of the situations that generate stress and problems between couples and can even lead to their break-up. When a couple is faced with such a difficult period in their lives, it may be necessary to ask for help from a professional. The intention of marriage therapy is to provide support and put forward solutions in an attempt to improve the relationship.

Children also feel anxiety, and incidences of anxiety attacks among them are on the increase.

Stress cannot be thought of as an illness per se but rather a physical and mental response by someone when he finds it difficult to adjust or adapt to changes in his circumstances. Stress is one of the body's natural defense mechanisms. It can be a positive and healthy factor if it is low in intensity, because it not only stimulates and encourages us to do things, but also to do those things well.

What is "burn-out"?

Burn-out is a type of chronic emotional stress that occurs in the context of the workplace and is thought to affect thousands of employees, although they do not always report it. In the main, it affects people who work face-to-face with the public or others, such as health workers, teachers, social workers, the police, firefighters, and all those whose work involves serious commitment. It is usually induced by unrecognized effort beyond the call of duty, lack of motivation, failure to meet with expectations, dull routine, and work-related stress.

A change of address or school, the death of a relative, or a parental separation can create situations of fear in children, which, if not dealt with in time, can turn into traumas that resurface in adulthood. Although stress may be a normal experience—involving fear, sadness, or loneliness—if it recurs systematically and its effects are acute and exaggerated, it can begin to turn into a more serious condition. It is essential to help children who are affected by this, thus enabling them to conquer their problems successfully.

What is "technophobia"?

This is a new type of disorder based on a resistance to accept technological advances. It is estimated that this will affect one in three employees involved with new technology at some point in their working lives. Technophobia is commonly seen in librarians, office workers, and executives. Its cause is a lack of skill at dealing with new information technology and corporate demands, resulting in the belief that you are going to be fired as a consequence.

Practical advice for dealing with work-related stress

- Maintain a positive outlook.
- Agree to a position at work that suits your personality.
- Find out precisely what work is involved in the position you are accepting so that you realize what the demands on you will be.
- Organization is a factor fundamental to avoiding stress: plan your time, meet your deadlines, determine which tasks have priority, avoid interference, keep a diary, etc.
- It is important to know what your priorities are and to avoid the frustration of being unable to meet your objectives.
- Working in a team is a good means by which to avoid stressful situations, as it provides you with support and shares out the workload. Furthermore, striking up bonds of friendship with the work team generates a better working atmosphere.
- Creating a decent environment in which to work is essential; think about lighting, temperature, and ventilation.
- It is a good idea not to bring work home with you, as you need to find time to disconnect from work and give some priority to your private and family life.
- Vacations are important in allowing your body and mind to relax and recuperate.

Effects of stress on the body

Anxiolytics

Anxiolytics, often referred to as sleeping pills or tranquilizers, include all types of medication prescribed to treat anxiety attacks; however, they can also be dangerous. It is not recommended to take such tranquilizer treatments for any longer than four weeks; otherwise, a dependency on the medication can soon develop.

How to control stress and anxiety

- Think positively
- Get your problems out into the open
- Laugh
- Follow a balanced diet
- Take up physical exercise or a sport
- Practice relaxation techniques
- Learn breathing exercises
- Plan and organize your time effectively
- Get proper sleep
- Avoid addictive substances

Excessive stress weakens the system and can affect a range of our organs and bodily processes. It can give rise to a variety of disorders and illnesses.

mouth
People feeling weakened by prolonged stress can develop disorders relating to the gums, teeth, and the appearance of mouth ulcers.

hair
Hair loss and some types of baldness are directly related to stress.

brain
Stress can induce many mental and emotional disorders. Prolonged stress can cause depression, obsessive-compulsive disorders, nervous breakdowns, anxiety attacks, insomnia, eating disorders, etc.

immune system
Prolonged stress can weaken the immune system, causing greater vulnerability to colds and infections.

heart
Stress increases the risk of someone experiencing heart-related problems, high blood pressure, and heart attacks.

muscles
A person undergoing major stress suffers more from pulled muscles, muscular overload, and any nervous tics may be accentuated.

lungs
Emotional difficulties aggravate the symptoms of asthma and respiratory problems.

skin
Skin also suffers under stress. Someone who is stressed can develop skin conditions, sudden eczema, or psoriasis.

digestive system
Stress causes or aggravates illnesses, such as gastritis, ulcers, or irritable bowel syndrome.

reproductive organs
Stress is the most frequent cause of problems relating to erections and ejaculation, as well as being responsible for changes to a man's desire for sex.

bladder
Many men in different stress-related situations suffer from irritable bladder (urge incontinence).

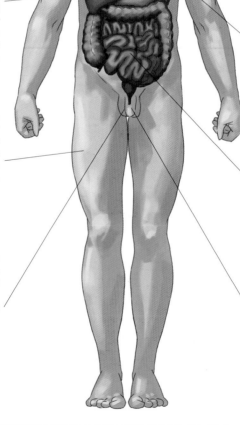

Breathing exercises

Knowing how to breathe properly can also help with relaxation. Getting into the habit of regular, deep breathing can be an effective remedy for tension. Here is one way of doing this:

- Remove your shoes and socks, and sit on a stool or chair in a quiet room. Keep your feet resting flat on the floor.
- Allow the chair to take your full weight, and notice how your body and shoulders relax.
- Breathe slowly and deeply, ensuring that you take twice as long to exhale as you do to inhale.
- Repeat the exercise over a period of at least five minutes. It is normal to feel a little dizzy, because your body will be hyperventilating, but interrupt the exercise if you feel uncomfortable.
- Try to keep your mind blank while you concentrate on maintaining the rhythm of your breathing.
- Practice this exercise twice a day or whenever you feel anxious.

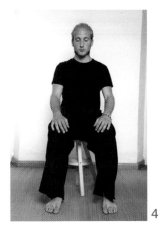
1

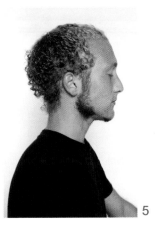
2

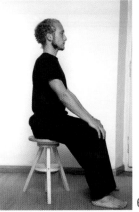
3

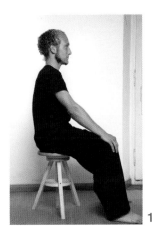
4

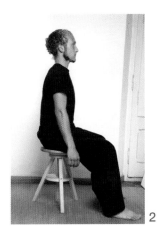
5

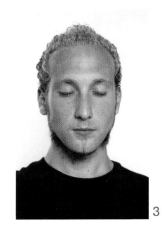
6

Depression

Depression is one of the greatest afflictions in present-day society. All over the world, regardless of race or culture, millions of people suffer from this illness, which arises when discouragement, resignation, and frustration overwhelm the individual.

Alcohol and drugs disguise depression in men more commonly than they do in women. Similarly, the socially acceptable tendency of being a workaholic can also act as a cover for depression. It is not unusual for men to manifest depression through displays of irritability, anger, and discouragement instead of, as may seem more likely, through feelings of hopelessness or vulnerability.

The World Health Organization (WHO) predicts that by 2020 depression will have become the second greatest cause of disability in the world after heart/arterial diseases (heart attacks, heart failure, and strokes). It held fourth place in 2000.

In recent years, depressive illness has increased more in for men than for women.

Some 80 percent of cases of depression begin gradually. Sometimes it happens with such stealth and with such an absence of any concrete signs that it can go unnoticed, even by the person affected. Delayed sleep phase syndrome, in which a person's body clock regularly causes them to wake up extremely late in the day, and

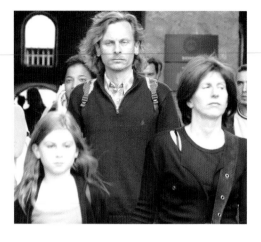

Men are less likely to suffer from depression than women; however, men tend to be less forthcoming about admitting to it.

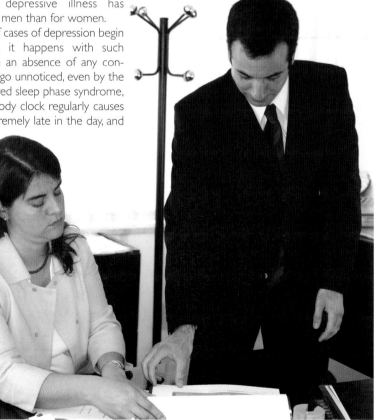

behavioral conditions, such as sexual promiscuity or violent behavior, often mask manifestations of depression.

Symptoms of depression go beyond changes in mood: many depressed men feel neither sad nor depressed; nor do they nurture thoughts of suicide. However, they may show signs of apathy, loss of energy, sexual dysfunction, social withdrawal, bad temper, disinterest in personal appearance, and changes to sleep patterns, together with major fluctuations of these symptoms throughout the day.

It is important for a man suffering from depression to understand and accept the idea that depression is a real illness and that, as such, it requires treatment.

What is depression?

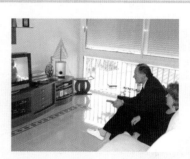

- A depressive disorder is an illness that affects the body, mood, and way of thinking. It affects the way that a person eats and sleeps, and how he sees and values himself, as well as the way in which he sees the world around him and handles his life.

- A depressive disorder is not the same as a temporary state of sadness.

- Depression does not indicate personal weakness.

- Emotional disorders are extremely variable: they range from the lows that your mind sinks into every so often throughout life to serious, prolonged clinical syndromes.

■ Symptoms of depression

- Changes to the sleep pattern: a major increase in the number of hours spent asleep or awake (insomnia).
- Changes in eating habits and weight: overeating or loss of appetite.
- Loss of interest in sex.
- Loss of physical energy, greater fatigue, and irritability.
- Inexplicable aches and pains.
- Reduced interest and pleasure in everyday activities and in life in general.
- Difficulty with concentration and making decisions.
- Feelings of vulnerability and hopelessness.
- Changes in attitude: especially loss of interest in friends, family, work, and pastimes.
- More time spent thinking about the past and past mistakes; feelings of blame and thoughts of death.

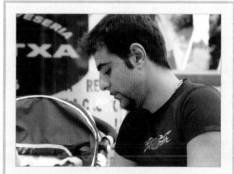

Types of depression

Although many types of depression exist, they fall into two basic categories:

- Exogenous depression, which is caused by an external factor that affects an individual, e.g. a divorce or the death of a friend or relative;
- Endogenous depression, in which feelings of unhappiness and isolation are not caused by any external factor or a specific, established fact.

▪▪ Causes of depression

There is no one single cause of depression. Depression can be caused by one or more factors, and some people are more likely to suffer from it than others. Here are some of the most common factors:

- **Family history:** The risk of suffering from depression is increased if there is a history of the illness in your family—you may therefore have inherited a biological predisposition to it. However, not everyone who has a family history of depression will go on to suffer from the illness, which suggests that additional factors causing depression are also at work.

- **Biochemical factors:** It has been shown that the brain's biochemistry plays a significant role in depressive disorders. For example, people with serious depression have an imbalance in certain chemical substances in the brain (neurotransmitters).

- **Stressful situations:** The death of a relative or friend, a chronic illness, relationship difficulties, financial problems, a separation, or a divorce can all give rise to the symptoms of depression, which, if they persist, can lead to clinical depression.

- **Seasonal affective disorder (SAD):** It has been observed that some people develop episodic depression during the winter months when the days are shorter. It is possible that a reduction in the hours of daylight may affect the balance of certain chemical compounds in the brain.

- **Personality:** People with a negative outlook on life, low self-esteem, lack of self-control, and a tendency to worry excessively are liable to suffer from a depressive disorder of some kind. The personal characteristics of each individual can heighten the effect of stress or interfere with the person's natural capacity to cope with or recover from adversity.

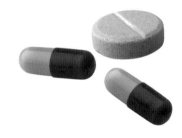

Treatment

The majority of people with a depressive disorder can be cured if they receive proper treatment and help for their condition. There are a number of very important factors with regard to treating depression correctly:

The support of family and friends: It is extremely important to receive solid support from the family and from friends.

Antidepressants: These are drugs that affect the brain's neurotransmitters, such as seratonin, noradrenalin, and dopamine. The level of these substances decreases in patients suffering from depression. The purpose of these drugs is to return these substances back to normal levels. However, it takes over two weeks before a patient starts to feel any effect, and there can be side effects, such as nausea and drowsiness.

Psychotherapy: This treatment can be extremely beneficial for people whose depression is a result of their personality or a bad experience that they have had.

Cognitive-behavioral therapy: This involves a form of therapy that helps you to think positively and raise your level of self-esteem.

▪ A little self-help

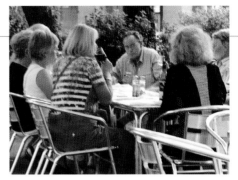

- Set yourself realistic goals, taking your depression into account, and do not attempt to take on an excessive amount of responsibility.
- Split up your tasks into manageable pieces, work out your priorities, and do only what you can, when you can.
- Try to be in company: confiding in someone is always better than being alone and not talking to anyone.
- Exercise, go out with friends, see a movie, and participate in an activity of some sort (recreational, religious, social, or anything else). Physical activity and mental stimulation help to conquer depression.

Group therapy is a way of bringing feelings out into the open. This type of psychotherapy can provide major support for people suffering from depression.

- You should not expect an immediate cure for your depression. Your state of mind and energy will recuperate gradually.
- It is advisable to postpone important decisions until your depression improves. Before making important changes to your life, such as changing jobs, marriage, or divorce, it is sensible to talk with people close to you who can be objective about the situation.
- Be aware that your negative thoughts are going to be replaced by positive ones as soon as your depression starts to respond to treatment.

Alcoholism

Without doubt, the problem of alcoholism has become one of the most widespread social phenomena of recent times. Alcohol is the most commonly used psychoactive drug in the world. At present, its abuse has reached huge proportions both in the developed and developing world, and it can be linked to dozens of secondary effects, the most serious and immediate of which, from a clinical point of view, is the illness of alcoholism itself.

In general, people suffering from severe alcoholism undergo periods of alcohol tolerance and alcohol withdrawal. Tolerance is necessary to imbibe increasingly large quantities of alcohol in order to achieve the desired effect: in other words, to become inebri- ated. Withdrawal occurs when consumption is reduced or halted completely.

What is "delirium tremens"?

Delirium tremens refers to an acute physical response as the result of a sudden withdrawal from the use of alcohol. During such attacks, an alcoholic suffers serious hallucinations. This state of delirium is associated directly to withdrawal. Delirium tremens begins with episodes of anxiety, bewilderment, insomnia, nightmares, heavy perspiration, and deep depression. It generally starts to disappear 12–24 hours after initial abstinence, but if it persists can lead to serious disorders and even death.

■ Alcoholism

- Alcoholism refers to the prolonged, excessive consumption of alcohol resulting in total dependence.
- Alcoholism is a chronic illness, which interferes with both mental and physical health. It also has a detrimental effect on personal relationships, including family and work-related responsibilities.
- Alcohol dependency happens gradually and in stages. At first, an individual goes through an initial phase of tolerance to alcohol, which causes him to consume ever-increasing amounts of it.
- The next phase is signaled by a deterioration of memory (a drinker suffers blackouts) related to alcohol consumption, and subsequently a loss of self-control occurs at which point he is no longer able to stop drinking even though he may want to do so.
- Withdrawal symptoms develop because the brain has adapted itself physically to the presence of alcohol and cannot function properly without its consumption. The symptoms of alcoholic withdrawal range from a higher body temperature, higher blood pressure, and a faster pulse, to feelings of unease, anxiety, psychosis, convulsions, and even death.
- There are many reasons why a person may be driven to drink alcohol to excess. Some people drink to relieve stress, to reduce tension, to reach a feeling of well-being, to raise their sense of self-esteem, or to overcome obstacles in their day-to-day lives. Because of its capacity to reduce stress and because of its pleasant effects, alcohol represents an easy option, but one that is difficult to give up once it becomes a habit. Studies have shown that many people with alcohol-related problems have a strong genetic predisposition to the illness, although so far the genes responsible for this have not been discovered. Moreover, it is known that certain areas of the nervous system are a determining factor in alcohol addiction.

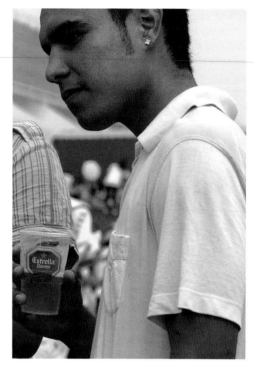

Alcoholism is a type of drug dependency. As with all such addictions, dependency is both physical and psychological. Physical dependency is apparent when alcohol tolerance becomes ever greater and illnesses develop associated with its consumption.

Alcoholism is the prevalent drug addiction in many countries. It affects a large number of people, generally adults, but at the same time, and increasingly so, it is also affecting teenagers. Not only are they becoming alcoholics, but also issues related to the consumption of alcohol, such as road accidents, family and school problems, alcohol poisoning, etc., are increasingly affecting adolescents.

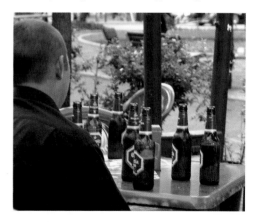

For some people, serious symptoms of anxiety, stress, or depression that are untreated can lead to inappropriate behavior, such as drinking too much, overeating, smoking, or taking non-prescription drugs. All of this is to alleviate emotional tension. In the long term, however, this sort of behavior serves only to reinforce and worsen the problem.

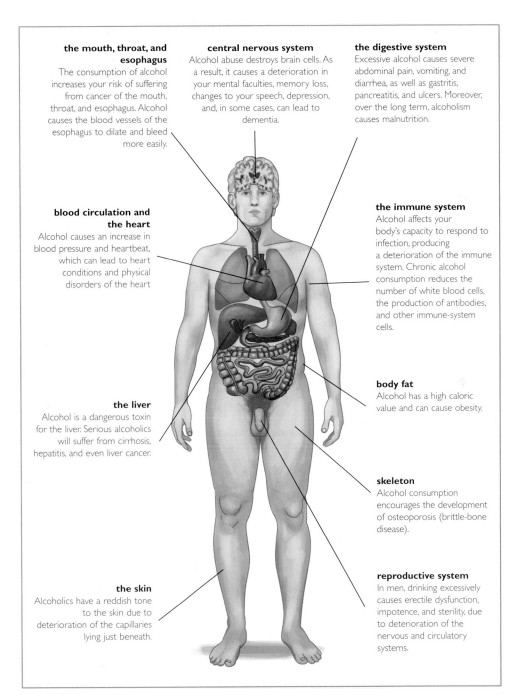

the mouth, throat, and esophagus
The consumption of alcohol increases your risk of suffering from cancer of the mouth, throat, and esophagus. Alcohol causes the blood vessels of the esophagus to dilate and bleed more easily.

central nervous system
Alcohol abuse destroys brain cells. As a result, it causes a deterioration in your mental faculties, memory loss, changes to your speech, depression, and, in some cases, can lead to dementia.

the digestive system
Excessive alcohol causes severe abdominal pain, vomiting, and diarrhea, as well as gastritis, pancreatitis, and ulcers. Moreover, over the long term, alcoholism causes malnutrition.

blood circulation and the heart
Alcohol causes an increase in blood pressure and heartbeat, which can lead to heart conditions and physical disorders of the heart

the immune system
Alcohol affects your body's capacity to respond to infection, producing a deterioration of the immune system. Chronic alcohol consumption reduces the number of white blood cells, the production of antibodies, and other immune-system cells.

the liver
Alcohol is a dangerous toxin for the liver. Serious alcoholics will suffer from cirrhosis, hepatitis, and even liver cancer.

body fat
Alcohol has a high caloric value and can cause obesity.

skeleton
Alcohol consumption encourages the development of osteoporosis (brittle-bone disease).

the skin
Alcoholics have a reddish tone to the skin due to deterioration of the capillaries lying just beneath.

reproductive system
In men, drinking excessively causes erectile dysfunction, impotence, and sterility, due to deterioration of the nervous and circulatory systems.

How to overcome alcoholism

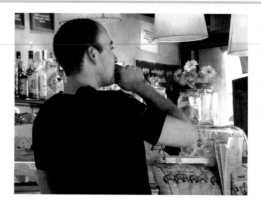

Alcoholism can be treated. With help and willpower, it can be overcome without relapses.

- Treatment of people who are addicted to alcohol begins with getting them to recognize that they have a problem. Alcoholism is associated with denial: people with the illness frequently deny that they need help, and often need to be persuaded by friends and family to seek treatment. Purely voluntary acceptance of the need for treatment is very unusual.

- The second phase of treatment is detoxification. The availability of alcohol is removed from the patient, who is kept under supervision. If necessary, tranquilizers and sedatives are administered to alleviate and control the effects of withdrawal.

- Rehabilitation programs are designed to help sufferers, once they have detoxed, to continue to abstain from alcohol. These programs include advice, psychological support, help while at hospital or treatment center, and health care. Part of the therapy concentrates on teaching people about alcoholism and its effects.

- Alcohol-aversion therapies also exist, which use drugs that interfere with the metabolism of alcohol, and these produce very unpleasant effects for up to two weeks after treatment, even if you drink only a very small amount.

Symptoms of alcoholism

- Increasing tolerance to the effects of alcohol.
- Daily or frequent need for alcohol in order to perform day-to-day functions.
- Loss of ability to control, reduce, or avoid drinking alcohol.
- Drinking alone.
- Making excuses for drinking.
- Episodes of memory loss linked to alcohol consumption.
- Deterioration of social and family relationships and of responsibility at work.
- Missing days at work.
- Mood swings.
- Behavior that attempts to conceal alcoholism
- Hostility when talking about your drinking.
- Lack of appetite.
- Not paying attention to physical appearance.

- Nausea and vomiting.
- Abdominal pain.
- Cramps.
- Sluggishness and trembling.
- Reddening of the face and appearance of dilated blood capillaries on the face, especially on the nose.
- Confusion and fainting.
- Convulsions, tremors, and nervous ticks.
- Fatigue.
- Insomnia.
- Bewilderment.
- Hallucinations.
- Abnormally rapid heartbeat.
- Sweating.
- Weeping fits.

Drug addiction

Illegal drugs include a highly divergent range of substances from a pharmacological and chemical point of view. The factor common to all of them is that they give the people who use them a pleasing sensation—so much so that they are encouraged to take them again and again.

What is a drug?

Drugs are used for many things, but some are "mind-altering," insofar as they have the capacity to modify the way a man's body functions so that his behavior, judgment, conduct, perception, or state of mind are affected. Drugs are not in themselves either good or bad.

What is an addiction?

An addiction describes a person's pressing and uncontrollable need to take any particular substance. This dependency can be physical and/or psychological in nature. Psychological dependence refers to a need created through contact with a drug, which causes an individual to feel a compulsion to experience the effects that the drug produces. Physical dependence, on the other hand, is produced by changes that the body undergoes in adjusting to the presence of a drug.

Cannabis

Cannabis comes from the hemp plant (*Cannabis sativa*), and its psychoactive effects derive from one of its principal agents: tetrahydrocannabinol (THC). It is most typically taken as hashish (resin) or marijuana (the dried flowers). Its effects are: relaxation, loss of inhibition, hilarity, a sensation of the passage of time slowing down, drowsiness, changes in sensory perception, difficulty in expressing yourself, memory loss, and a reduction in the ability to concentrate and the capacity to comprehend. Furthermore, it causes an increase in appetite, dryness of the mouth, shining, bloodshot eyes, increased heartbeat, increased perspiration, and uncoordinated movement. Prolonged use results in depression, anxiety attacks, apathy, respiratory problems, hormonal disorders, and infertility.

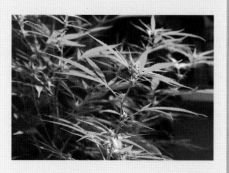

How do you know whether someone is taking drugs?

Certain signs can be taken as reasons for suspicion. They do not always mean that someone is abusing drugs, but they can help to identify someone who is:

- Sudden changes in personality and habits.
- Unusually bad temper. Irritability. Sensitivity.
- Sudden downturn in quality of schoolwork or productivity at work.
- Lack of care about personal appearance and hygiene.
- Disappearance of objects of value or money from the home.
- Trembling, insomnia, drowsiness or doziness, incoherent speech.
- Depression, apathy, lack of motivation.
- Inability to carry out own tasks and responsibilities.
- Withdrawal from usual group of friends.
- Antisocial behavior (lying, stealing, arguing, etc.)
- Attacks of nerves.
- Loss of appetite.

Heroin and opium

Heroin is a substance extracted from the opium poppy (*Papaver somniferum*) and is similar to other opiate derivatives, such as methadone, morphine, or codeine, etc. Heroin is a substance that creates serious dependency—both physical and psychological. It can be smoked, inhaled, or injected. The initial effect that heroin produces is one of euphoria, well-being, and pleasure. It eliminates pain and suppresses hunger. Prolonged use causes personality changes, memory loss, constipation, tooth decay, anemia, insomnia, loss of sexual desire, infections linked to the use of syringe needles, a growing tolerance to the drug that requires the consumption of increasing amounts to achieve an effect, increased dependency, and an unpleasant withdrawal syndrome.

Cocaine

Cocaine is a drug extracted from the leaves of the coca bush (*Eritroxilon coca*). It is a stimulant, since it works by activating the central nervous system. Cocaine that is sold as a drug is in fact cocaine hydrochloride and is in the form of a white powder that is either snorted or injected. Crack cocaine is cocaine hydrochloride that has been altered through a simple chemical process to obtain crystals that, when heated, crack and produce fumes that can be breathed in. Initially, cocaine produces a euphoric feeling, talkativeness, greater sociability, mental acceleration, hyperactivity, increased sexual desire, a sense of greater energy, less need to sleep, and suppression of appetite. Chronic usage causes fatigue, apathy, psychological disorders, such as depression and paranoia, major psychological dependency, irritability, insomnia, perforation of the cartilage separating the nostrils, chronic sinusitis, heart attacks, cerebral hemorrhages (strokes), and heart conditions.

Amphetamines

An amphetamine is a drug that stimulates the central nervous system. It comes in the form of pills or capsules in a variety of shapes and colors. It produces feelings of alertness and confidence, and it increases energy levels and feelings of self-esteem. It also removes feelings of hunger and the need for sleep. One of the most commonly used amphetamines is amphetamine sulfate, also known as speed. Amphetamines can be swallowed, snorted, or injected. They are often mixed ("cut") with other drugs to enhance them or bulk them out. Speed is usually in the form of a powder and, like cocaine, is inhaled. The effects caused by taking amphetamines are: agitation, euphoria, an increased feeling of self-esteem, verbosity, being persistently vigilant and on the alert, aggression—as well as loss of appetite, increased heart rate, insomnia, dryness of the mouth, increased perspiration, and twitching of the jaw. Chronic use leads to malnutrition due to loss of appetite and a greater susceptibility to illnesses and infections as a result. It also leads to chronic fatigue, psychotic episodes similar to schizophrenia, delusions, major psychological dependency, high blood pressure, irregular heartbeat, circulation problems, and gastrointestinal disorders.

LSD and magic mushrooms

LSD is lysergic acid diethylamide: a hallucinogenic or psychedelic drug that is extracted chemically from the ergot fungus found on rye.

It is odorless and colorless and has a slightly bitter taste. It is commonly sold in the form of tiny squares of blotting paper impregnated with LSD. These squares are either swallowed or chewed. The effects of LSD are unpredictable. They depend on the quantity taken, personality, state of mind, the user's expectations, and the environment in which the drug is taken. LSD produces serious mental changes, such as paranoia, hallucinations, anxiety, depression, and panic attacks. A person can become reckless or act out of character due to the fact that it alters one's perception of reality. On the physical level, it causes the pupils to dilate, raises body temperature and blood pressure, and causes insomnia, tremors, and loss of appetite. Many users experience repeat hallucinogenic sensations without even taking the drug. These "flashbacks" occur suddenly and can happen days or months after having last taken LSD.

Designer drugs

The chemical name for the drug ecstasy is MDMA or methylenedioxymethamphetamine, although pills available on the street can be adulterated with other substances, sometimes making them very dangerous. Ecstasy belongs to the family of drugs known as stimulants. It causes a mixed experience somewhere between stimulation and altered perception. Its initial effects are ones of sociability, empathy, euphoria, less inhibition, increased sexual desire, verbosity, restlessness and anxiety, higher heart rate, dry mouth, increased perspiration, trembling, dehydration. Long term, it causes anxiety attacks, depression, psychosis, excessive increase in body temperature, convulsions, heart disorders, blood clotting problems, thrombosis, strokes, and heart failure.

Tranquilizers

The benzodiazepines are drugs prescribed for anxiety disorders or insomnia, although these pills are sometimes abused because of the relaxing effect that they produce. For example, diazepam is a pharmaceutical drug that can cause dependency if used for longer than two weeks. Normally, these drugs are prescribed only for very brief periods and at low dosages. After prolonged use, their intake has to be reduced gradually in order to avoid severe withdrawal symptoms.

Barbiturates

Barbiturates are sedatives available on prescription for cases of epilepsy and anxiety. They are used for their sedative and calming effect. They can make it difficult to speak, coordinate movement or balance properly, and cause drowsiness. Regular use results in dependency, and very unpleasant symptoms ensue if they are suddenly withdrawn.

Solvents or glue

Solvents are volatile substances, such as glue, liquid detergents, lacquer, paints, and nail polish remover. Their inhalation produces hallucinations and feelings of well-being. Physically, they cause the pupils to dilate, headaches, skin flushes, and confusion. Chronic use causes inflammation and ulceration around the nose and mouth, brain damage, kidney and liver-function problems, fluid on the lungs (pulmonary edema), chronic conjunctivitis, circulation and heart problems, and even asphyxiation during inhalation.

Bodybuilding drugs

Some athletes abuse anabolic steroids in order to develop their physical strength and increase their muscular physique. Because they increase an athlete's capacity to recuperate from any physical exercise, they take them in order to train harder and for longer. Their use is very dangerous, because they cause greater aggression, acne and other skin conditions, testicular atrophy and impotence, changes in growth of body hair, baldness, kidney malfunction, and aberrant sexual behavior.

Compulsive behavior

The concept of drug addiction is widely understood, but the term "addiction" is increasingly becoming accepted as having application where no physical substance exists. This refers to (obsessive-) compulsive behavior, such as in the cases of pathological gambling or compulsive shopping.

■ How to distinguish an enjoyable activity from compulsive behavior

An interest, hobby, or pastime becomes an addictive-type compulsion when it turns into something harmful and irrational, despite knowing the negative consequences that are associated with it, or when feelings of deprivation ensue if the activity is not carried out (withdrawal syndrome). This compulsion can be defined as a loss of self-control and interest in any other type of activity. These compulsions occur when a certain type of normal behavior is carried out beyond reason, intensely, and repeatedly, and it usually implies a significant financial cost. Furthermore, this behavior has a direct effect on a person's family, social life, and work.

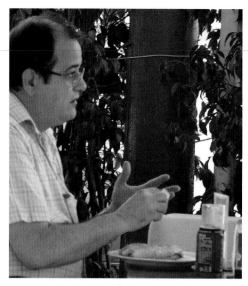

Many people channel their anxieties through compulsive eating. This disorder can result in severe depression. Almost 30 percent of patients suffering from obesity have undergone changes in eating behavior that take the form of compulsive eating disorder.

Sex addiction

Addiction to sex is one of the compulsions least admitted to and least visible in society.

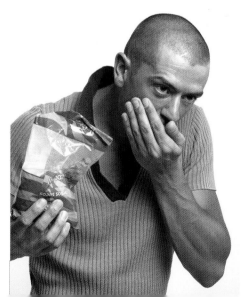

Over the past few decades, however, there has been a steady increase in the number of people asking for help due to consequences resulting from this addiction: from financial and work-related problems to broken relationships, anxiety attacks, and depression.

Unlike other addictions, a dependency on sex can take a variety of forms, from compulsive masturbation to rape, pedophilia, and other forms of sexual violence, and in between it can include promiscuity, with heterosexual and homosexual partners or both, frequent encounters with strangers, a constant reliance on pornography, prostitution, and telephone sex lines, exhibitionism, voyeurism, etc.

In the majority of cases, compulsive sexual behavior is produced in the mind, where sexual fantasies and erotic thoughts are trans-

Some people are addicted to candy (chocolate), dairy products (unable to sleep without drinking a glass of milk), bar snacks (e.g. compulsively eating potato chips without being able to stop), and even eating non-food substances, such as earth (geophagia), feces (coprophagia), or ice.

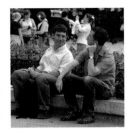

formed into avenues of escape from problems. As with other forms of addiction, dissatisfaction ensues after initial pleasure, together with deep feelings of guilt and shame

Compulsive behavior related to food

Many men suffer from stress and anxiety caused by a range of factors, such as problems at work, in their relationships, or with the family. This anxiety can channel itself into an irrepressible urge to eat. Compulsive eaters may suffer from serious problems, such as depression, obesity, and heart disease. These conditions may develop into extremely serious ones and are illnesses that require not only psychological support but also treatment with drugs in order to reduce anxiety.

Gambling addicts

Compulsive or pathological gambling involves an increasing inability to resist the urge to gamble, leading to behavior that caus-

Treatment for sex addiction is based on redirecting a person's sexual behavior and thus reducing the feelings of anxiety and guilt that are so common among sex addicts. The intention is for the patient to control his urges and to become aware of his problem.

Kleptomania

This refers to a compulsion or irresistible urge to possess objects and items that do not belong to you. Usually, these items are of little value or use to the person concerned. Five percent of the shoplifters identified in stores and shopping malls are kleptomaniacs. This condition is far more common among women than it is among men.

When a kleptomaniac enters a store, he experiences a buildup of tension that can be dispelled only if he steals an object of some kind. Afterward, this gives rise to successive feelings of well-being, release, and then remorse.

Kleptomania can be associated with conditions such as depression and anxiety, and eating or personality disorders.

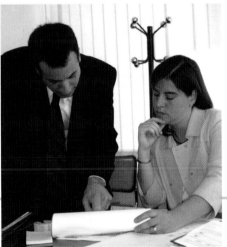

Workaholics

The distinction between hard workers and workaholics is not so much the amount of time that they devote to their work but the attitude they have toward undertaking work-related activities.

The term "workaholic" can be applied to people who show signs of obsessive behavior toward their work, returning hurriedly to work, and constantly putting their work first before all other responsibilities and activities, such as the family, friendships, leisure, and relaxation. These people tend to work until they reach the point of exhaustion, which over the long term can give rise to a host of problems affecting physical health as much as mental health and personal life.

Workaholics display a personality problem that usually involves feelings of low self-esteem, insecurity, anxiety, the need to escape from personal issues or family responsibilities, etc.

es serious harm to the individual, his family, and working life. Gambling addiction can occur at any time in a person's life. A variety of biological, psychological, and social factors can affect the development of this compulsion and predispose an individual to this type of behavior. Clearly, having access to gambling opportunities and to money is also important. A gambling addict loses control over his behavior and willpower. When the gambler notices the effects on family, friends, and work, it only makes him take even greater refuge in gambling.

Addiction to electronic games

A new type of compulsion has surfaced in recent years: the addiction to video and computer games. This type of dependency is characterized by a loss of self-control that results in playing these games in a obsessive-compulsive manner. The disorder is most common among people with low levels of self-control—typically adolescents—who are impulsive in nature, have short attention or concentration spans and low self-esteem and often, suffer from depression.

Emotional obsessive-compulsive behavior

Some people suffer from a form of behavior that makes them over-anxious about forming relationships, because they feel worthless and are terrified of abandonment. This prevents them from maintaining a healthy degree of intimacy and makes them unable to establish and sustain constructive relationships with others, including members of their own family and those closest to them. These disorders, very

■ Compulsive shopping

Being addicted to shopping could be defined as a form of unplanned and spontaneous behavior in which a person feels the irrepressible desire to acquire objects that are mainly unnecessary or even repeat purchases. A compulsive shopper feels a sense of anxiety or irritation that can be assuaged only if a purchase is made; and feelings of guilt follow on swiftly from the initial feeling of pleasure.

This represents an increasingly worrying problem in today's consumer-culture society in which value is attached to the ownership and showing off of things.

Typically, the items that men purchase are usually leisure-related, such as computer technology, videos and DVDs, stereo equipment, and automobile accessories. It is typical for interest in a purchase to wane immediately after an item is bought, to the extent that items are frequently hidden, hoarded without even being unwrapped, given away as gifts, returned, destroyed, or even sold on.

It is notable that many compulsive shoppers are in fact clinically depressed, and a link is quite often seen between compulsive shopping and bulimia or kleptomania.

often mistaken for neuroses or personality disorders, are actually compulsions that manifest themselves as a tendency toward obsessive behavior and control, together with an inability to set limits on relationships, difficulty in expressing needs and feelings, and isolation, as well as physical, mental, and emotional deterioration.

Internet addiction

Internet addiction is a pathological compulsion that appears to be on the increase in proportion to the growing number of Internet users. Some of the symptoms of this addiction include spending hours in front of the computer screen, neglecting personal relationships and work, lack of sleep, or feelings of anxiety if unable to log onto the net.

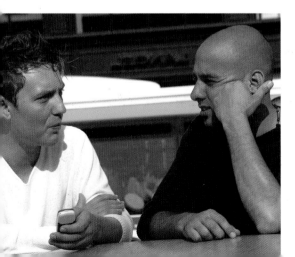

Every year, the number of people addicted to chat rooms, mobile phones, shopping and television increases.

smoking

Smoking is the most common avoidable cause of death. According to the most recent statistics, hundreds of thousands of people die prematurely each year as a result of smoking. Moreover, it should be remembered that thousands of nonsmokers die every year because of having been exposed to cigarette smoke. Despite these facts and the numerous public health warnings on the dangers of smoking, many people continue to smoke. Be that as it may, it should be noted that more people are quitting every day, and that is a positive sign.

Why do people smoke?

Smoking is not simply a bad habit; it is a form of drug addiction.

Smoking tobacco fulfills all the criteria that define addiction to a given substance: tolerance, dependency, withdrawal symptoms, and compulsive behavior patterns.

What do smokers inhale?

• Tobacco smoke consists of more than 4,000 chemical components, some of which are very damaging to health.
• Nicotine is only one of the molecules contained in tobacco smoke.
• Among other substances, tobacco smoke contains ammonia, benzopyrene, hydrogen cyanide, carbon dioxide, carbon monoxide, and traces of lead and arsenic.

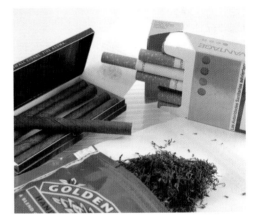

At present, tobacco continues to be the world's most commonly used psychoactive drug. Although the number of smokers has fallen in most industrialized countries of the developed world, the number has increased elsewhere.

▪ Smoking-related problems

• **Physical dependency** is caused directly by the nicotine, and this is responsible for the withdrawal symptoms.
• **Psychological dependency** refers to the propensity to associate smoking with a variety of situations: after eating meals, when drinking coffee, when with friends, at work… Many smokers convince themselves that it is impossible to disassociate these activities from smoking.
• **Social dependency** is when smoking is always part of a social activity or group event, during leisure moments, when meeting up with friends… Among adolescents, the habit continues to be thought of, mistakenly, as a sign of maturity and rebellion.

- Nicotine is the actively addictive component. Nicotine is absorbed through the mucous membranes of the respiratory airways and quickly reaches the brain via the bloodstream, where it is stored to be metabolized later by the liver and its waste removed by the kidneys.
- The brain has receptors that recognize nicotine, and when these receptors bond with nicotine molecules, they receive a "message" that is retained in their chemical structure. Therefore, when the receptors come into contact with this substance again at a later stage, the recognized message will be on display. It is because of this that nicotine is so highly addictive.
- Nicotine tar includes a range of substances capable of initiating the development of tumors. They are responsible for the various types of cancer attributed to smoking: cancer of the lungs, mouth, pharynx, larynx, esopha-

gus, bladder, etc. Benzopyrene is a major constituent of tar, and its carcinogenic effects have been amply demonstrated.
- Carbon monoxide is a toxic gas that derives from the combustion of tobacco and the paper holding it together in a cigarette. It is the same gas produced from the combustion of gasoline for automobiles. Carbon monoxide bonds with the hemoglobin in the blood making the transportation of oxygen to the cells more difficult or even impeding it altogether. The effects from a reduction of oxygen in the blood are felt by the body's most sensitive organs: the heart, brain, and other tissues, such as the skin.
- Other substances, such as ammonia or the phenols, are responsible for coughing and, after long-term smoking, chronic bronchitis and pulmonary emphysema because of the damage that they do to the mucous membranes of the respiratory system.

Cigarettes contain many harmful substances that scar the lungs when inhaled.

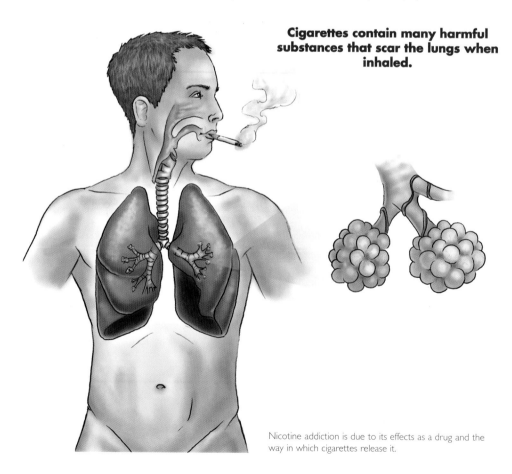

Nicotine addiction is due to its effects as a drug and the way in which cigarettes release it.

Effects of tobacco

- The combustion of a cigarette produces two types of smoke: the smoke given off when actively inhaled (the principal stream) and the smoke released when left to burn (secondary).

- The composition of these two streams is different. The principal stream involves combustion high in oxygen, because air is forced into the ignition zone when inhaling the smoke. Secondary smoke relies on incomplete, spontaneous combustion, which occurs at a lower temperature.

- These streams release particles and gases. The particles are composed of a mixture of hydrocarbons, nicotine, tar, and water. These molecules are small enough to reach the trachea, bronchial tubes, lungs, and very smallest airways.

- The gases produced in the greatest amounts are nitrosamines, hydrogen cyanide, acetaldehyde (ethanal), and nitrogen oxides. Many of these gases cause serious chemical harm to the body.

- In response to this aggression, the body increases the release of enzymes, oxidants, and free radicals that destroy the cells and lung tissue. Moreover, tobacco smoke also causes inflammation of the mucous membranes lining the respiratory system.

- Over time, the lungs lose their elasticity and their ability to function properly, and they fail to oxygenate the blood satisfactorily.

◗ Why should people quit smoking?

- Smoking has a destructive effect on all of the body's organs and systems.

- The risk of suffering from fatal illnesses as a direct consequence of smoking is extremely high.

- Smoking is responsible for nine out of ten cases of chronic respiratory illness and lung cancer, and more than half of all diseases affecting heart and lung function.

- Respiratory illnesses. Smoking destroys the natural defenses of the respiratory system, allowing serious damage to the lungs and consequent breathing problems.

- Cancer. 43 substances have been identified in tobacco smoke that are either a direct or indirect cause of cancer. Lung cancer is responsible for half of all cancer-related deaths, and the cause is smoking in 90 percent of cases. Smoking is also directly responsible for the appearance of cancerous tumors of the larynx, mouth, lips, tongue, pharynx, esophagus, and salivary glands.

- Furthermore, smoking is linked to the appearance of angina, embolisms, and heart attacks. Depending on its intensity, these can cause anything from permanent incapacity to sudden death. In addition, smoking aggravates circulatory problems.

- Diseases of the heart and the body's blood circulation system. The combination of nicotine and carbon monoxide from tobacco smoke has an extremely negative effect on the appearance of a variety of cardiovascular diseases that affect the heart, the blood vessels, and other organs of the body. Half of the deaths attributable to tobacco relate to cardiovascular problems.

- Obstruction of the blood vessels. The inhalation of nicotine and carbon monoxide weakens the walls of the arteries and causes atheromata (fatty deposits) to build up, which make it difficult for blood to circulate freely, causing high blood pressure and increased levels of cholesterol in the blood.

- Reduction in oxygenation of the blood. When carbon monoxide mixes with the hemoglobin in red blood cells it produces carboxyhemoglobin, which is incapable of carrying oxygen. This effect, added to the damage that tobacco causes directly to the heart, results in an inadequate supply of oxygen to the heart muscle, as well as increasing the need for oxygenated blood.

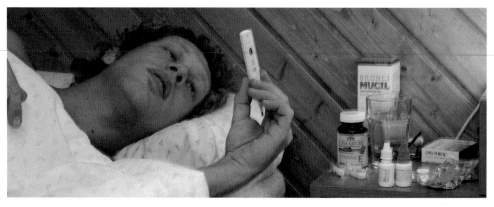

Some studies confirm that smokers spend, on average, 15 percent more days in bed due to illness than nonsmokers.

A smoker's face

- The skin is also exposed to the effects of tobacco smoke: directly, through contact with smoke in the atmosphere; and indirectly, through transmission via the bloodstream of the toxic substances within inhaled smoke.
- Tobacco causes alterations to facial skin. These changes produce a typical "smoker's face" and include fine lines on the upper lip and around the corners of the eyes (crows'-feet), deep wrinkles and narrower lines on the cheeks and jaw, sunken features,

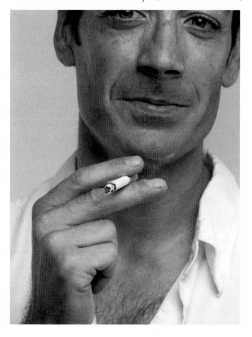

Smoking and dental disease

- Smokers develop characteristically discolored teeth and halitosis (bad breath).
- Many studies have linked smoking with the appearance of cavities, dental plaque, and oral fungal infections (candidiasis or oral thrush), although it has not been possible to establish a direct relationship between smoking and oral diseases such as gingivitis or periodontal disease.
- Smoking can also give rise to small whitish nodules located on the palate as a result of the irritant effect of smoke on body tissue (nicotine stomatitis).

and prominent cheekbones, coarser looking skin, as well as a pale, grayish complexion.

Quitting

The vast majority of smokers will reach a stage sooner or later in their lives when they will attempt to quit smoking, possibly for good.

Why is quitting so difficult?

Chronic exposure to nicotine results in addiction and the development of nicotine tolerance, or the need to increase the dosage of nicotine in order to produce the same level of stimulation.

- The body metabolizes nicotine quickly and eliminates it in only a few hours. Because of this, smokers lose part of that tolerance overnight and have the sensation that the first few cigarettes of the day are the strongest or most intense.
- Suspending the intake of nicotine leads to a withdrawal syndrome that can last for a month or more.

If you decide to quit smoking, your likelihood of success rises from 8 to 22 percent if you use nicotine patches or gum.

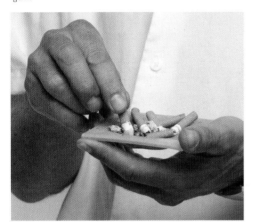

◢ **Withdrawal symptoms**

Nicotine simultaneously has a sedative effect and acts as a stimulant on the central nervous system. Quitting causes withdrawal symptoms. The most typical side effectside effect is headaches; however, the following withdrawal symptoms can also occur:

- Longing to smoke
- Giddiness and dizziness
- Irritability
- Lack of concentration
- Trembling hands
- Loss of appetite
- Eye pain
- Nausea
- Vomiting
- Changes to the sense of taste
- Anxiety about eating
- Muscular spasms
- Fatigue
- Weakness
- Sweating palms
- Pins and needles

Smoking phases

- **Smoker phase:** In the first phase, a smoker enjoys the habit, has no worries on the subject, and is sure that his health is fine. This phase typically includes smokers under 30 without diseases linked directly or otherwise to smoking. Almost half of all people who smoke are in this phase.
- **Revision or reconsideration phase:** The first doubts surface in the smoker, who has started to consider the possible negative effects on his health from smoking, as well as the positive effects of quitting the habit. He becomes a discontented smoker: i.e. he smokes, but he feels that it is bad to do it. 30 percent of smokers fall into this group.
- **Action phase:** The smoker feels obliged to quit smoking. His attitude changes, he knows that smoking is bad, and he quits. But he starts again and so reverts to the revision phase. This pattern can be repeated many times in a smoker's life. 20 percent of smokers are in this phase, having quit, but not for long enough to be able to say they have overcome the addiction.
- **Consolidation phase:** Smokers who manage to quit for six months without smoking are in this phase. A person cannot be considered to be a nonsmoker until at least one year has passed.
- **Relapse phase:** A variable percentage of smokers trying to quit will relapse, returning to the revision phase again. Relapses are usually accompanied by a loss of self-esteem.

Benefits of quitting

If you decide to quit smoking, remember that the benefits start from the moment that you stop.

- After 20 minutes, your blood pressure and pulse rate return to normal levels.
- After eight hours, the levels of carbon monoxide and oxygen in your blood return to normal.
- After a day, the risk of heart attack reduces.
- After 48 hours, your sense of smell and taste starts to return.
- After three weeks, blood flow through the circulatory system improves, and lung function improves by 30 percent.
- After nine months, coughs, fatigue, and breathing problems disappear.

- After a year, the likelihood of developing diseases of the heart and circulatory system starts to diminish, as does the risk of respiratory illnesses and cancer.
- After five years, the risk of developing heart disease is the same as that for a nonsmoker. Your risk of suffering from cancer of the lungs, larynx, and esophagus is reduced by half.
- After ten years, the risk of suffering from cancer of the lungs, mouth, pancreas, and esophagus is similar to that of non-smokers.
- After 15 years, the risk of suffering from a heart attack is the same as that for a nonsmoker.

▪ Advice about nicotine replacement therapy

- This is recommended only to patients with high physical dependency who wish to quit smoking.
- It is important to follow the daily course of treatment and gradually reduce the dosage.
- There are various types of nicotine replacement therapy. The most common are the nicotine patch and nicotine chewing gum. The patch provides the assurance of a constant release of nicotine, while the effect of the chewing gum is more like the fluctuations of nicotine in the bloodstream obtained through smoking cigarettes; for both, the possible side-effects and instructions should be considered carefully.
- It may sometimes be useful to combine both methods for smokers who, despite using patches, experience times during the day when they have an overwhelming urge to smoke.

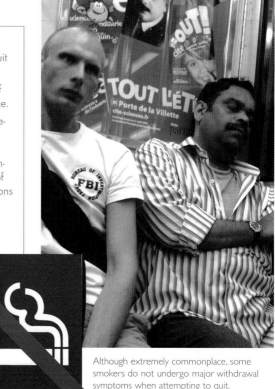

Although extremely commonplace, some smokers do not undergo major withdrawal symptoms when attempting to quit.

men's skin

A man's skin fulfills the same functions as a woman's; however, historically and culturally, men have not been in the habit of looking after their skin. Nevertheless, neglect is a mistake, because the skin is a vital bodily organ that performs a whole range of functions and also fulfills a significant role socially.

What is skin?

Skin is the largest organ in the human body: an adult has a surface area of skin measuring approximately 2 square yards, which is equivalent to a sixth of his body weight. Its principal functions are: to give the body its shape, to protect the muscles and internal organs, to regulate body temperature, to protect the body from external infections (fungal, bacterial, and viral), to prevent the penetration of ultraviolet rays, to establish sensory relationships with the environment, and to exhibit signs of systemic illnesses.

The skin is composed of three layers:

epidermis

The epidermis is the outermost layer of skin and is composes of various layers of keratinocytes (a tough, fibrous layer of cells) and its function is to protect and to regulate hydration (moisturizing) of the skin. At the base of this layer, another type of cells is interspersed among the keratinocytes: the melanocytes. Melanocytes are the cells responsible for producing pigment—melanin—which is the substance that filters out ultraviolet light and gives skin its color.

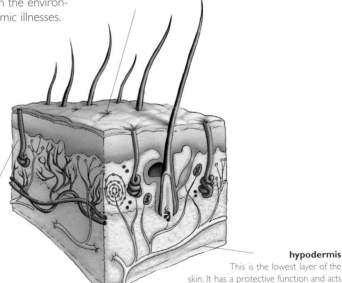

dermis

This is the connective tissue underlying the epidermis. Among other cells, it contains fibroblasts and collagen fibers, elastine, and reticulite. Also present in this layer are nerve endings, sebaceous glands, and hair follicles. It supports the epidermis by means of the elastic fibers and collagen that it contains. It is also responsible for hydrating and lubricating the skin by means of the sebaceous and sweat glands. Due to the high level of blood vessels, it is involved in regulating body temperature, and, because of its composition, it contains a significant reservoir of water.

hypodermis

This is the lowest layer of the skin. It has a protective function and acts as an energy reserve, being made up of a thick layer of fats. The hypodermis contains the sensory corpuscles, which are able to sense any changes in pressure and temperature exerted on the skin.

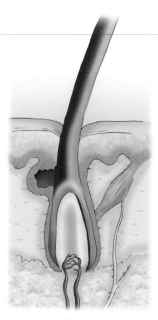

Hair follicle

Cutaneous annexes

- Cutaneous annexes include hair, nails, sweat glands, and sebaceous glands.
- The hair and nails are found in the dermis (the layer of skin immediately beneath the outer layer), but both structures are an extension of the epidermis (the outer layer of skin).
- The nails are hardened structures in the keratinous zone of the epidermis and are situated on the dorsal side (back) of the third joints of the toes and fingers.
- The sweat glands produce an acidic secretion that restricts the growth of bacteria on the skin as a form of defense.
- The sebaceous glands are located next to hair follicles where they open out and discharge their secretions—sebum: composed of lipids (fats) and cellular debris. The function of sebum is to lubricate the skin, which, together with the sweat gland secretions, creates an excellent layer of protection for the skin.
- The odor that skin gives off is caused by the free acids in the sebum secreted by the sebaceous glands and the bacterial decomposition of sweat. This odor has different characteristics for each individual and varies in intensity.

A hair is formed from a series of filaments toughened with keratin and firmly joined together. The hair follicle is the organ that produces the hair. It maintains a close relationship with the sebaceous gland to which it is attached in the dermis. Hairs fulfill a protective and sensory function.

What skin types are there?

Essentially, there are three types of skin:

Oily skin: shiny in appearance with dilated pores and very often blackheads.

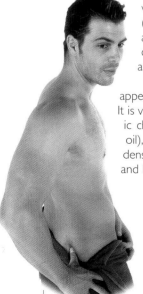

Combination skin: this is the most common skin type with a T-shaped oily zone (nose, forehead, and chin) and a dry zone on the cheeks, around the eyes, and neck.

Dry skin: has a dry, flaky appearance and often feels taut. It is very sensitive to atmospheric changes (due to the lack of oil), flakes away easily, and reddens when exposed to cold and low humidity.

How does skin alter over time?

Skin undergoes many physiological changes during the various stages of a person's life.

"Normal" skin is the skin we have in childhood. It is firm and healthy with a balance between its glandular secretions.

▪▪ Characteristics of men's skin

- **Greater number of hair follicles.** Many men decide to remove this hair, particularly on the face, through shaving.
- **Greater number of sebaceous glands.** Not only do men have more sebaceous glands, but they also secrete more sebum, which means that men's skin contains more sebum and is oilier than women's skin.
- **Greater skin thickness.** This is because men's skin has more collagen and elastic fibers, making it firmer, more resistant, and elastic.

The first changes begin in puberty: the balance is interrupted due to hormonal activity. Daily skin care is very important at this stage in order to avoid the appearance of acne and seborrheic dermatitis.

Another significant change occurs during adulthood, when internal processes and environmental factors (the sun, smoking, pollution, etc.) cause changes in the skin's appearance: spots and the first wrinkles appear.

Facial cleanliness

Cleanliness: Specific products should be used for facial cleansing in order to get rid of oiliness and bacteria. It should be done in the morning and at night.

Exfoliation: This gets rid of dead skin cells that block pores and close them off. This treatment is not a good idea if you have a skin infection of some kind, as it will spread the infection across the face.

Moisturizing: To avoid shininess, it is best to use a non-oily product that is pH-balanced with antimicrobial action.

Removing blackheads: It is not advisable to squeeze them, as you will only succeed in getting the pores infected. Many products are on the market to treat this condition.

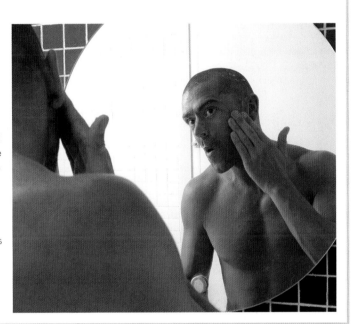

■ Why should men look after their skin?

- Men's skin is much more susceptible to irritation, because it is subjected to daily shaving and, moreover, because men show a greater genetic and hormonal predisposition to acne.
- At the same time, a man's skin is thicker than a woman's, and remains taut for longer. A man's skin may stay firm and elastic for a greater number of years, but, on the other hand, it can age drastically and less predictably than a woman's.
- A man's skin is much oilier than a woman's.

Oily skin in men

All skin is protected by a layer composed of water, lipids, and bacterial flora that hydrates and protects it. In the case of oily skin, the balance between these components has altered. This imbalance is due to the male hormone testosterone, which affects the production and distribution of sebum. An increase in the level of oils covering the epidermis disrupts the

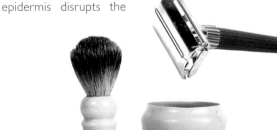

natural flora, secretes irritant fatty acids, and changes the pH level from 5 to 4.

The effect of the testosterone produced by the testicles is notable from the age of 14, and it becomes more obvious by the age of 25. In order to remove excess oil from the skin, it is necessary to follow a program of treatment based on cleansing and re-moisturizing. This should be gentle, as aggressive treatments will be counterproductive.

Hair care

Our hair is affected by a range of factors, such as illness, stress, seawater, the sun, the wind, hair dye products, hairspray, or other irritant hair products, as well as by inadequate personal hygiene. All these can cause hair to lose its strength, luster, and body, making it appear dull and unkempt. Similarly, poor diet and a sedentary lifestyle are also reflected in your hair, depriving it of health and vigor.

Every man has his own particular hair type (oily, dry, normal, coarse, fine, etc.), all of which are factors that should be borne in mind when looking after your hair.

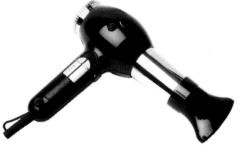

Shaving

- The best time of day to shave is soon after waking up when the muscles of the face are relaxed and after having showered when the warm water has softened your bristles and opened up your pores.

- If you are using an electric shaver, it is best to shave dry before showering.

- It is advisable to let your skin rest every so often and skip shaving. If any dermatitis or inflammation appears, it is better to give your skin some respite and time to recover. If there is no improvement, the best advice is to see a dermatologist.

- It is recommended to make regular use of a moisturizing cream, lotion, or balm to tone and soften the skin. These lotions give an immediate sense of freshness and rehydrate the skin.

■ Razor bumps

Razor bumps, known technically as pseudofolliculitis barbae, occur when bristles start to grow below the surface of the skin instead of out of a pore.

This condition occurs most commonly in the neck area, although it can also appear on the face.

One of the causes is cutting the bristles obliquely rather than at right angles, because this encourages the bristles to grow inward (and can lead later to inflammation and the appearance of pimples).

Razor bumps can also appear because of the skin's dryness or thickness.

Other factors that can give rise to this problem include frequent shaving, coarse or curly beard growth, the use of after shaves or eau de toilette, and changing the way that you shave.

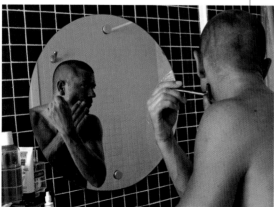

Hair types

- **Oily hair:** Oily hair looks shiny and sticks together in matted clumps. Frequently, people with oily hair also suffer from some type of sebaceous glands problem, because they secrete greater amounts of sebum than normal (this may be related to stress, hormonal changes, or the side effect of some medication). This hair type has to be washed using a shampoo created especially for oily hair and, if possible, should be rinsed using cold water in order to try to close the pores and reduce sebum secretion. Washing, combing, and brushing should be done gently so as not to over-stimulate the sebaceous glands.

- **Dry hair:** A dull, dry appearance is an indication of low sebaceous gland secretion. This hair is usually very fine and brittle, and it does not respond well to environmental factors (sun, wind), vigorous brushing, or hairdryers. It requires specialized shampoos and conditioners with natural humectants to improve its moisture-retaining properties. It is also advisable to use a moisturizing hair lotion at least once a week, as well as a head massage to stimulate sebaceous gland secretion. Combing and brushing should be done gently, and hairdryers should be used only at a low setting. Regular use of hair dyes, bleaching, and perms also contribute to dryness. As a rule, you should use dyes without ammonia or with natural pigments.

How much hair do you lose each day?

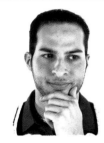

Hair falls out or dies at the rate of between 50 and 100 hairs a day, especially during the fall. Another new hair replaces each one that is lost within a natural cycle of regeneration. However, if you are suffering from excessive general hair loss, not just at a specific time of year, you should see a dermatologist.

The causes may be hereditary, although the reasons may also relate to hormonal changes, stress, illness, or the use of a particular sort of medication.

What is dandruff?

- Dandruff is a common problem and comes from a type of seborrheic dermatitis: pityriasis capitis.

- It is principally characterized by the presence of small whitish flakes of skin on the surface of the scalp, which may be localized or present throughout.

- It is a condition that affects adolescents and adults of both sexes, although it is more common among men.

- Its cause may depend on a number of factors, including hormones (androgen stimuli in the case of men), a genetic predisposition, stress, or a scalp infection.

- Treatment for dandruff is straightforward and results are usually rapid.

- Most of the time, using a specialized shampoo is all that is required.

- However, if the dandruff persists, or the dandruff seems to be linked to other symptoms, such as itching, psoriasis, scabs, or alopecia, it is necessary to take proper precautions and consult a specialist.

Skin conditions

Acne, warts, verrucas, and athlete's foot are some of the most common skin conditions.

Acne

Acne is a skin condition involving chronic inflammation of the sebaceous glands and it appears principally on the face and back.

The pimples that characterize acne are caused by the blockage and inflammation of the sebaceous glands and hair follicles, and a variety of types exist according to the degree that a person is affected (mild acne, acne cosmetica, acne vulgaris, cystic acne).

It originates with hormonal changes, which is why its highest incidence is in adolescents. In adolescence,

The causes of acne are varied. Genetics may play a role, but other factors can also come into play, such as climate, stress, or the use of certain cosmetic products that only aggravate the condition.

the production of sex hormones causes an increase in the production of sebum and also induces changes in the excretive behavior of the sebaceous glands. Affected follicles represent an ideal medium for bacterial growth. Bacteria multiply and contribute to inflammation.

Although it is teenagers above all who are affected by acne (in males the age at which it appears is generally between 15 and 19), it can in fact appear at any age.

Some medications, illnesses, or contact with certain substances (such as chlorine, for example) can be factors involved in its appearance later in life.

Treatment should take place as early as possible and needs to be appropriate for the grade and type of acne.

Retinoids (vitamin A-enriched topical treatments) are used to treat people suffering from acne with non-inflamed pimples—comedones or blackheads. They control the abnormal growth and death of cells in the follicles, thus eliminating blackheads and preventing their recurrence.

Topical antibiotics are used in cases of inflammation in order to suppress the bacterium *Propionibacterium acnes* and thus reduce the inflammatory process.

In cases of large pustules that do not respond to this treatment, medication such as oral antibiotic treatments Accutane (isotretinoin) or a synthetic derivative of vitamin A become necessary.

Practical advice for acne sufferers

- Wash the face and affected areas twice a day. If using soap, it must be pH-neutral or acidic. You must not rub excessively either when washing or drying to prevent stimulation of the follicles. Apply topical ointments prescribed by a physician once your face is clean.

- Consult your specialist on the most appropriate treatment for each individual case, as certain treatments commonly available from drugstores are not always suitable.

- Do not share face creams, soaps, or other types of treatment in order to avoid catching any infections.

- Apply a regime of hygiene to your whole body: shower daily, and wash your hair regularly.

- Always wear clean clothes and, above all, regularly change pillowcases.

- Avoid allowing your hair to come into contact with your face (insofar as is possible, keep your hair short, avoid bangs, etc.)

- Do not squeeze whiteheads, blackheads, or pustules. You

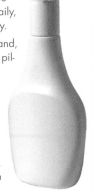

will only make the marks worse, and it may leave scars behind.

- Avoid resting your face in your hands to prevent facial irritation.

- Get enough direct sunshine: this is a natural source of vitamin D, which helps combat certain types of skin-dwelling bacteria and also has a naturally therapeutic effect on skin affected by acne. If your skin is exposed to the sun for long periods, you must use a non-oily UVA/UVB sunscreen (to prevent the pores from becoming blocked).

- There is no particular food that aggravates or causes acne, but you must eat a balanced diet. However, avoid food that takes a long time to digest, such as high-fat meats and nuts.

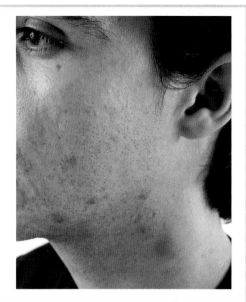

Warts

Warts or verrucas are small lesions of the skin, normally painless, that are caused by a virus and generally inoffensive. However, they can be unsightly, and occasionally itch or hurt (especially on the feet: plantar warts).

Common warts are not usually troublesome, unless they are in places that are constantly rubbed or subject to repeated pressure. Plantar warts, for example, can be extremely painful: if many of these appear on the soles of the feet, they can make walking or running difficult.

Whether treated or not, warts often reappear.

common warts
These frequently appear on the hands but can be found on any other part of the body.

genital warts
These are a type of wart that appear in the genital area and between the thighs, as well as around the anus.

flat warts
This type of wart usually appears on the face and hands. They are very common among children and adolescents and occasionally among adults.

subungual and periungual warts
These appear under and around the fingernails and toenails.

plantar warts
These are found on the soles of the feet.

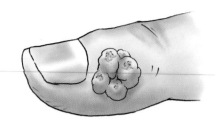

Genital warts are very contagious, while common warts, flat warts, and plantar warts are much less likely to be passed on. All warts can spread from one part of the body to another.

When treating warts, it is a very good idea to file them down while they are hydrated before applying any medication.

A whole range of dressings exists in the treatment of plantar warts that help to alleviate pressure or rubbing.

In the most extreme cases, warts may need to be physically removed. Various types of surgery are available: freezing (cryotherapy), cauterization (electrocauterization), or laser surgery.

There are many over-the-counter medications available from pharmacies that do not require a physician's prescription. These can be applied to warts every day over a course of weeks and are usually very effective. However, these preparations should not be used on the face or in the genital area.

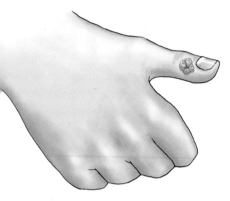

How to prevent the appearance of warts

- Avoid direct skin contact with someone who has warts.

- When filing down a wart, you must be careful to wash away any particles afterward so as not to spread the virus to other parts of the body.

- You should wash your hands properly after touching a wart.

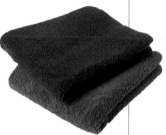

N.B.

- Whether treated or not, warts will often reappear.

- Genital warts are very contagious, while common warts, flat warts, and plantar warts are much less likely to be passed on. All warts can spread from one part of the body to another.

- When treating warts, it is a good idea to file them down while they are hydrated before applying any medication.

- A whole range of dressings exists for the treatment of plantar warts to help alleviate pressure or rubbing.

- In the most extreme cases, warts may need to be physically removed. Various types of surgery are available: freezing (cryotherapy), cauterization (electrocauterization), or laser surgery.

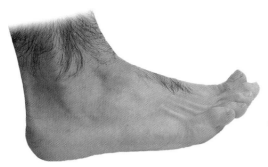

You should consult a doctor or pharmacist if a wart appears, and follow appropriate treatment. Under no circumstances should you try to scratch it, pull it off, burnt it away, or apply any other method of treatment.

Athlete's foot

- Athlete's foot is a fungal infection affecting the foot. Its medical name is tinea pedis.
- Athlete's foot is an infection that may be short-lived or persistent, or even recurrent, particularly if you are careless.
- The human body contains a great many microorganisms, including fungi and bacteria. Some of these are useful to the body, but others can multiply rapidly under suitable conditions and cause infections.
- Tinea pedis occurs when a particular type of parasitic fungus grows and multiplies, favoring the area in between the toes or, less commonly, on the hands.
- The fungal infection zone frequently appears reddened, and the skin becomes chapped and scabrous, flaking off in between the toes.
- In addition to the toes, the infection can appear on the heels, palms, and between the fingers. This fungal infection can spread to the nails, causing them to grow pale, swell up, and even drop out.

How to prevent athlete's foot

- Completely dry your feet after a bathing or swimming.
- Do not walk barefoot in bathhouses or public swimming pools.
- Frequently change your socks to keep your feet dry.
- Use antifungal talcum powder as a preventive measure if you are susceptible to this type of infection, or if you are constantly in contact with areas where you suspect this type of fungus may be lurking (gymnasiums or public swimming pools).
- Use well-ventilated shoes, preferably not made from man-made materials. It is advisable to change the shoes you wear from day to day to let them dry out completely before you use them again.

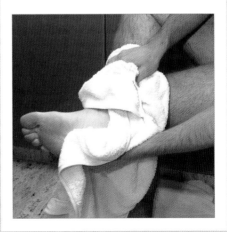

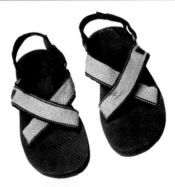

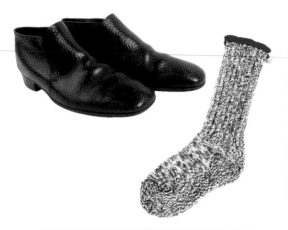

◢▪ **Very important**

- Keep your feet clean and dry, especially between the toes.
- Wash your feet properly with soap and water, and dry the area thoroughly and carefully at least twice a day.
- You should wear clean cotton socks and change them when you change your shoes, as frequently as possible to keep your feet dry.

How does athlete's foot develop?

This type of fungus usually proliferates in warm, humid parts of the body, and your risk of developing athlete's foot will increase if:

- You wear slip-on footwear that cannot breathe.
- Your feet are moist for long periods of time.
- You sweat a great deal.
- You injure your toenails or damage your skin.

To prevent children from developing athlete's foot in summer, it is important to ensure that their feet are completely dry after bathing or swimming and to prevent them from walking barefoot at public swimming pools and baths.

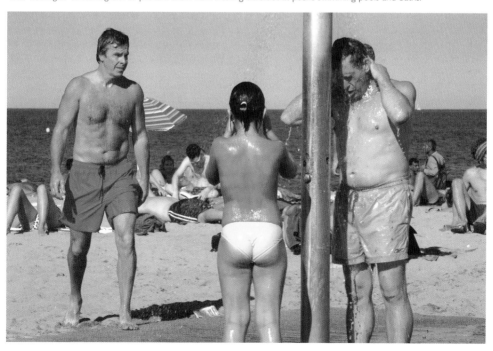

Marks on the skin. Different types of changes in skin pigmentation

- **Freckles:** These are completely harmless and do not usually grow. They are produced due to a localized increase in the synthesis of melanin in the epidermis. It is believed that heredity affects their development. Blonds and redheads usually get this freckling on areas of skin exposed to the sun, such as on the back of the arms and hands, the face, and the neck.
- **Liver spots:** These are freckles that are larger in size and with a more pronounced coloration. They usually appear as a part of the ageing process and are also referred to as senile lentigines.
- **Melasma:** Dark-colored shapeless marks usually on the upper lip, chin, cheeks, and forehead. They arise from exposure to the sun.
- **Vitiligo:** This is another type of skin condition in which lighter patches of skin appear where there is a loss of pigment due to a localized lack of melanin.

The sun and your skin

The arrival of summer tempts us to lie in the sun, take off our clothes, and enjoy more of our leisure time in the open air, exposed directly to the sun's rays. However, solar radiation becomes a risk to health when it exceeds certain limits.

Moderate exposure to the sun is beneficial to our bodies. The sun's rays encourage our bodies to synthesize vitamin D and strengthen our bones.

When we fail to take precautions while in the sun, the negative consequences that arise can be very serious, ranging from painful sunburn to skin cancer.

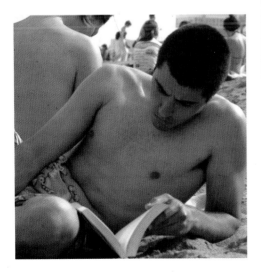

Physical properties of sunlight

- There are three different types of radiation which are classified according to their wavelengths:
- **Infrared radiation.** This has a wavelength of 800 nm and is what we feel as heat from the sun
- **Visible light.** The visible spectrum with a wavelength that ranges from 400 nm to 700 nm.
- **Ultraviolet radiation.** This is the truly dangerous form of radiation. It is divided into UVA light (380–315 nm) and UVB light (315–280 nm). Ultraviolet light causes skin to tan. However, it is also the principal cause of skin aging and skin cancers.

UVB rays are the most damaging. This ultraviolet radiation, once filtered through the atmosphere's ozone layer before reaching earth, is very important to life. However, the depletion of the ozone layer as a result of atmospheric pollution is causing a year-on-year increase in ultraviolet radiation and, consequently, an

The sun stimulates the circulatory system, increases calcium levels, encourages the production of vitamin D, balances the nervous system, and combats fatigue, depression, and stress.

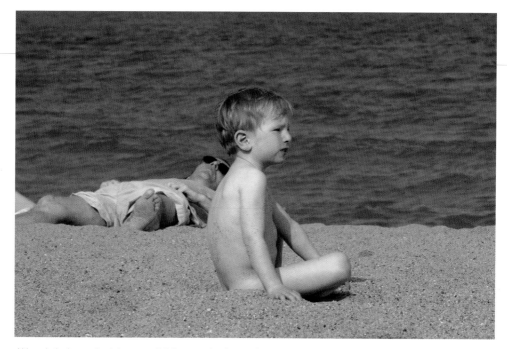

Although the human body has natural defense mechanisms against the sun (melanin production in the skin), if the skin is exposed repeatedly to the sun for long periods without protection these mechanisms tend to become exhausted. Consequently, a child who has been exposed to the sun without skin protection is at greater risk of developing skin cancer in adult life.

increase in the number of lesions that people are suffering.

Continued exposure of the skin to ultraviolet radiation can damage its genetic material and cause the incidence of diseases, such as skin cancer and cataracts, and can even weaken the immune system.

The intensity of ultraviolet rays depends on such things as the time of year. In other words, its intensity is greatest from the middle of spring until the middle of the fall, with the first part of summer being when it is at its height.

The fact that solar radiation can be damaging to health does not mean that we have to give up sunbathing altogether; but it does mean that we have to be sensible and attempt to prevent any negative effects resulting from extended exposure to it.

The risk from UVA rays

For many years, UVA rays were not considered to be a danger to health, because it was thought that they did not penetrate the outer layer of the skin. Nowadays, however, it is widely accepted that:

UVA rays can penetrate skin to the dermis (the layer below the epidermis, or outer layer);

the dosage of UVA rays is accumulative;

their effect is linked to that seen from UVB radiation;

they have a degenerative effect on skin collagen: the skin becomes prematurely wrinkled and aged.

For many years, the dictates of fashion have imposed on us the ideal of being bronzed and tanned. This has caused a proliferation in the use of UV tanning lamps and sunbeds: a situation that allows us to show off a year-round tan.

This equipment is found in many types of establishment, ranging from hairdressing salons and gymnasiums to beauty and tanning salons, and these often have no explicit standards to regulate their installation and operation.

Experts warn of the lack of controls that exist surrounding these appliances and recommend moderate, sensible use, as well as their operation by qualified personnel in officially approved centers.

When performing a self-examination, it is best to stand naked in front of a mirror to look at the whole body, because melanomas can also appear in areas of the body not exposed to the sun. Facing the mirror, inspect your frontal view (head, chest, stomach, arms, hands, and legs), and afterward inspect your rear view, for which you will need to use an additional hand-held mirror. Finally, inspect your sides, between your legs, your feet (including the soles), and your scalp. If you find any suspicious-looking lesions or moles, you should see your physician immediately.

Skin cancer

There are essentially three different types of skin cancer: basal cell carcinoma (BCC), squamous cell carcinoma (SCC), and melanoma.

BCC and SCC affect 95% of skin cancer sufferers. BCC appears from age 40 onward and SCC from age 50 onward in people who, because of where they live or the work they do (farmers, fishermen, etc.), spend a lot of time exposed to the effects of direct sunlight.

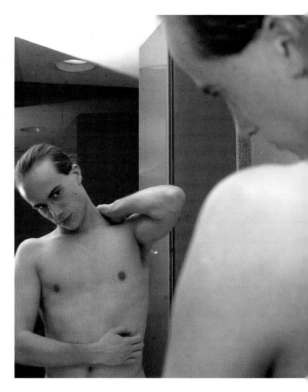

Precautions

If you use UV sunbeds or tanning lamps to get a tan:

- Make sure that they comply with safety standards.
- Do not overdo the time you spend under a UV lamp.
- Use protective products specifically made for UV lamp tanning.

Melanomas, although less common than the first two types, are much more aggressive. They are detected in only 5 percent of skin cancer cases; however, they are responsible for 65 percent of the deaths from this disease.

How to prevent skin cancer

- It is very important to take precautions at all times when sunbathing. You should not be exposed for too long to the sun when first sunbathing, and you should always use a good sunscreen, lotion, or cream with a high sun protection factor (SPF) that blocks both UVA and UVB rays. It should be reapplied several times, particularly after washing or swimming. Always have clothes at the ready so that you can cover up at some point. And do not forget to take sunglasses with you when you go to the beach.

- Melanomas are very aggressive cancers that can grow and spread cancerous cells throughout the body rapidly (metastasis); however,

one advantage of skin melanomas is that they can be seen externally from the very first, aiding early and fast diagnosis.

- Melanomas have the appearance of asymmetrically shaped spots or moles (with irregular, poorly defined edges). Signs of melanoma include changes in the size, shape, color, or elevation of a mole. A mole should be investigated if it appears to be growing and has a diameter greater than 1/2 inch.

- There is a 90 percent cure rate if melanomas are detected in the initial phase—early detection is vital. The best way to identify them in the initial phase is to perform a self-examination or have someone you trust do this for you.

▟ Sun exposure precautions

- You should start gradually when first exposing yourself to the sun. This should not exceed 20 minutes for the first few days. Afterward, you can progressively increase the amount of time you spend in the sun.
- Because of the altitude, less UV light is filtered out of the sun's rays in mountainous areas and these rays have a stronger effect on your skin as a result. On beaches, the sand and sea reflect and amplify the effect of the sun's rays. You need to protect yourself even on overcast days, because UV rays can pass through cloud.
- The best time of day for sun tanning without danger of sunburn is in the early morning and late afternoon. You should avoid exposure to the sun between 10 am and 4 pm.
- You should consult your physician if you are taking medication. Some drugs can cause skin reactions when combined with the action of the sun. When in the sun, you should not use after-shave, eau de toilette, or deodorants containing alcohol.
- You should apply sunscreens half an hour before going into the sun to give the agents in it time to start working at the cellular level. You should repeat applications every half-hour and after washing or swimming. Use sunscreens with a high sun protection factor for the most sensitive areas of the body: face, nose, lips, ears, etc. And increase your protection if you play outdoor sports.
- Skin needs to be protected with more care and exposed less to the sun if it is particularly sensitive. Redheads have delicate skin, as do young children, pregnant women, and older people.
- The appearance of cold sores (herpes simplex) on the lips increases in summer due to lack of sun protection. You should use a lip salve containing sunscreen.
- Protect your eyes and the area around them using polarized sunglasses.
- After sunbathing, or swimming in the ocean or pool, you should shower with freshwater to remove salt or chlorine, which is damaging to skin. After showering, apply a moisturizing or after-sun lotion, which will hydrate your skin, replacing the moisture lost through exposure to the sun.

Altering your skin: body piercing, tattoos, and hair removal

Whether following tradition or for purely esthetic reasons, some men like to have tattoos or have themselves pierced, and some also like to remove body hair.

Body piercing and tattoos

The fashion for body piercings and tattoos has grown markedly over the past few years and now includes even the very young among its fans.

Although people who have piercings and tattoos claim that they have been told all they need to know on the subject, this is not always the case. Many of the professionals in this market completely neglect to ask their clientele whether they suffer from any allergies or illnesses, nor do they inform them about the dangers of having recently drunk alcohol or drugs, or about the precautions or care required once a piercing or tattoo has been done.

It is essential that people performing piercings know how to clean the jewelry, which after-care treatments need to be used and for how long, the dangers of exposure to the sun, etc.

Different parts of the body respond differently to piercings. Only a professional is able to assess the proper site for a piercing and the size of jewelry that is most appropriate. You should be aware of the dangers that can arise depending on where you have a piercing on your body:

Earlobes. Earrings that put pressure on the earlobe can lead to infections.

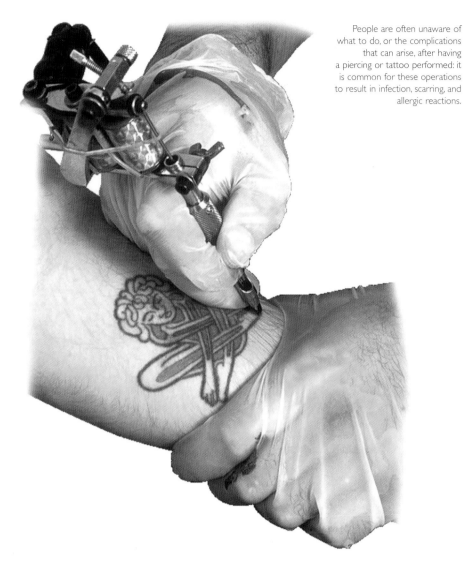

People are often unaware of what to do, or the complications that can arise, after having a piercing or tattoo performed: it is common for these operations to result in infection, scarring, and allergic reactions.

Ear cartilage. There is a greater risk of infection when piercing the ear's cartilage than there is with the earlobe, and even more so if the piercing is performed using a piercing gun.

Eyebrows. Lateral piercing is recommended for eyebrows, because other types of piercing can affect a nerve and even damage the tear duct.

Navel. The scar tissue can be jeopardized by clothing rubbing up against it. Moreover, people with prominent navels have to avoid catching their jewelry and tearing the piercing.

Nipples. This is a delicate area with a high risk of infection. It is important for women to avoid having nipple rings inserted during pregnancy.

Tongue. When the tongue is pierced, care needs to be taken not to damage the artery or lingual nerve. After piercing, the tip of the tongue may feel numb, and it may be difficult to speak. Long term, tongue piercings may cause gum lesions and damage to the teeth.

Penis. The penis, like the clitoris in women, is a very sensitive area with a high number of blood vessels. Piercings through this part of the body can cause bleeding, infections, and even reduce sensitivity.

Nose. There is a risk of infection in the nose, and damage can be caused to the cartilage if the septum is pierced.

Precautions before and after having a piercing or tattoo

- It is important to verify that you are not suffering from any illnesses or infections, because these weaken the immune system and can give rise to complications.

- It is important to be vaccinated against tetanus.

- People suffering from problems with blood clotting or to allergic reactions to metal should not undergo piercing or tattooing.

- Summer is the time least recommended to get a piercing or tattoo done. Additional perspiration, the beach, the sun, the ocean, and swimming pool water should all be taken into account, as they can make infection easier. After having a tattoo, you must avoid exposing it to the sun or UV rays for at least two months.

- In order to avoid infection or the transmission of viruses such as HIV or hepatitis, you should go to certified centers that adhere to approved standards of hygiene and health-risk prevention with regard to the cleanliness of the premises, the disposal of waste material, and the sterilization of equipment. Ideally, the tattooist will use sterilized disposable needles—so they will be used only on you.

- You should check that the inks used for tattooing are approved.

- You are advised to eat before having a tattoo done: having a tattoo done on an empty stomach can cause dizziness.

- You should not consume alcohol or drugs at least 48 hours before and after your session. Alcohol dilates the blood vessels, which can result in hemorrhaging when you have your tattoo done. Neither should you take aspirin two days prior to this, and coffee is best avoided as well.

- When paying for the service, it is essential that you always ask for a receipt in the event of any complaints afterward.

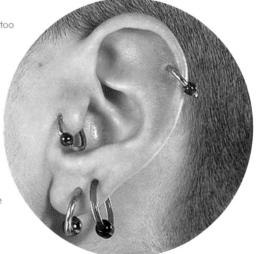

The scabs that form a crust over the design once the tattoo is completed must not be scratched or pulled off. If they are, this could cause the color to disappear from certain areas, thus requiring a greater number of return visits for retouching.

Neither should you sunbathe or swim in saltwater until the healing process is complete. At the same time, you need to ensure that the tattoo stays relatively dry.

Hair removal (Depilation)

Once, it was only men in the sporting world who used to remove their body hair. Athletes remove body hair because smooth skin offers less air or water resistance and is more comfortable and hygienic in a sporting environment.

Nowadays, many men remove their body hair whether involved in sports or not.

The favored areas for hair removal among men are from the back, shoulders, ears, face, and between the eyebrows. However, there are many who remove hair from the armpits, chest, legs, and even the arms.

Different methods exist for removing tattoos, although in some cases scarring or skin discoloration may be left behind. Success depends on the method employed, where the tattoo is on the body, its size, how it was done, the capacity of a particular individual to heal properly, and the age of the tattoo.

Hygiene while healing

Once a piercing has been performed, it is important to follow some rules of hygiene during the healing period.

- **Ear, nose, and eyebrow piercings:** It is a good idea to wash the area two to three times a day and to moisten any scar tissue that may have formed with warm water and a cleansing agent. In the weeks it takes for healing to complete, it is important not to use any moisturizers or other creams on the face. For cartilage, healing takes approximately eight to twelve weeks; earlobes take four to six weeks; eyebrows take six to eight weeks, as does the nose; and between the eyebrows takes six to twelve weeks.

- **Nipple and navel piercings:** Clean two to three times a day for six to eight weeks. Lather your hands with pH-neutral soap and carefully wash the piercing and the area around it. Moisten any scabs that may form. Gently turn the earring to allow the lather to enter, and repeat this action when rinsing to remove the soap. Apply the antiseptic treatment recommended by the practitioner who carried out the piercing, but for no longer than two weeks. It is advisable to use lukewarm saltwater for rinsing to lessen the risk of problems arising during the healing process.

- **Tongue or lip piercings:** For these types of piercing, you should avoid alcohol, spicy food, oral sex, prolonged kissing, and talking quickly. The piercing should be washed after every meal, smoking, and drinking for four to six weeks using an antibacterial mouthwash or with saltwater. External piercings should be washed two to three times a day for eight weeks. Remember that internal piercings can cause conditions such as bleeding gums, dental damage, increased salivation, inflammation of the tongue, problems with speaking, etc.

- **Genital piercings:** The cleanliness of these areas is very important: two to three times a day for four to six weeks. You must be very careful when using soap, as this can cause infections. The piercing must be cleaned before any sexual activity. Nevertheless, it is advisable to abstain from sex until healing is complete—and to use condoms as protection if you *are* going to have sex. You should avoid all oral contact and remember that spermicides and lubricants can cause irritation.

Methods most commonly used by men to remove hair

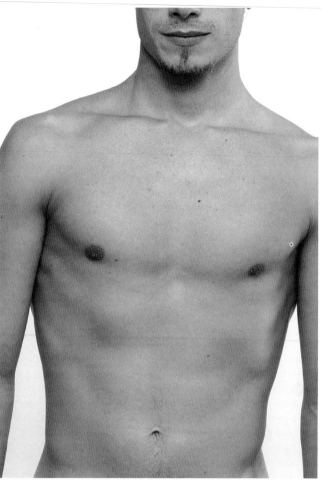

- **Laser:** This is a safe, fast, and effective type of hair removal and effective for all skin types and hair colors. Treatment usually starts off by gently wiping the zone to be treated and then applying an activating lotion that is left to penetrate the hair follicles. Next, the laser is passed slowly above the skin. The ray's energy passes through the lotion and is absorbed by the skin. The light is converted into heat, and the heat inhibits the follicle from growing a replacement hair. This technique needs to be repeated monthly, because not all hairs grow at the same rate or simultaneously. It is difficult to be exact about how many treatments any one person may need in order to achieve the hoped-for result, but between three and five sessions is usually sufficient.
- **Waxing:** Hair removal using wax is a system without any side effects, which is why it continues to be the most popular method. It involves a very simple technique, as the wax needs to be spread only on the area from which hair is to be removed and is then pulled away against the grain. Smoothness remains for three to four weeks, and the technique can be applied anywhere on the body.
- **Rotary epilators:** This is a relatively fast method, and involves using a device similar to an electric razor, except that it incorporates an anti-pain strip, the purpose of which is to perform a mini-massage on the area and so reduce the pain from plucking. The device grasps the hair and pulls it out by the root, allowing hair removal to last for three to four weeks. It can be applied to the whole body, except the face.

physical exercise and sport

While a sedentary lifestyle increases the risk of developing a range of chronic illnesses, prominent among which is heart disease, which represents one of the principal causes of death in the Western world, living a physically active life, on the other hand, brings with it a wealth of benefits to health, not only at the physical level but also psychologically.

The benefits of exercise

What do we mean by "physical activity" and "sedentary lifestyle"?

Physical activity means any bodily movement produced by the muscles that requires an expense of energy.

Physical exercise is defined as a type of physical activity that is programmed, structured, and repeated and which we perform to improve or maintain our state of physical fitness in one or more areas.

Conversely, a sedentary lifestyle is when the level of physical activity does not reach the minimum necessary to maintain healthy physical condition.

Numerous studies attest to the relationship that exists between physical activity and life expectancy, such that people who keep more physically active usually live longer than those who do not.

The human body is designed for movement and, therefore, it needs to be exercised regularly in order to remain operationally active and prevent illness.

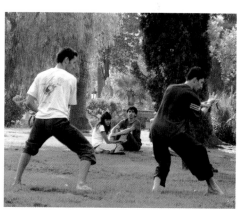

A good state of health is not defined solely as the absence of illness but also as being the state that allows a person to have a good quality of life physically, mentally, and emotionally. Conversely, poor health can mean more suffering from illnesses and even premature death.

What are the benefits to health from physical exercise?

During childhood and adolescence, most people maintain a higher level of physical activity through sport and team games. However, the amount of time we devote to sport diminishes considerably as the years go by. Furthermore, the number of people involved in physical activities that require some kind of effort, either at work or during leisure time, has been steadily decreasing over the last few decades.

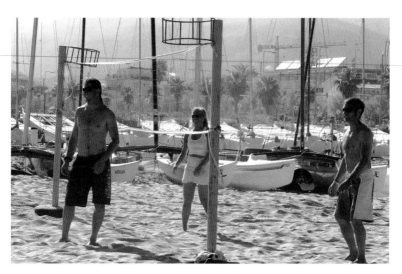

Taking part in physical exercise is clearly very good for your health: people who undertake some kind of physical activity feel better for it, both physically and mentally.

Our bodies adapt as a result of regular physical training. In other words, it transforms our various organs and bodily processes both physically and operationally. On the one hand, these changes allow us to prevent or delay the onset of illnesses and, on the other, they improve our ability to carry out physical tasks.

Moreover, from a mental point of view, regular physical exercise helps us face life with greater optimism and enthusiasm, as well as being a way in which to integrate within our communities and form social relationships.

◾ **Why do we need to exercise?**

- Because of the numerous physical and psychological benefits that come from undertaking regular physical activity compared with the risks posed by a sedentary lifestyle.
- Because it is not necessary to perform strenuous exercise for it to benefit your health.
- Because a minimum of 30 minutes of moderate intensity exercise every day, or almost every day, is adequate and can be easily achieved by anyone. Moreover, those 30 minutes can be divided up throughout the day into periods of physical activity, preferably lasting no less than 10 minutes each, and these exercise periods can be done at any time of day: walking at a fast pace, walking up stairs, gardening, or performing domestic chores.

Advice

Here are some suggestions for a program of physical activity:

- Start off gradually and gently.
- Vary your workout schedule: it is important to alternate days of intense, longer exercise with days of less intense, shorter exercise.
- Do not increase the level of intensity of your exercises unless the level of effort they require no longer tires you out.
- Do not perform the same exercise regime every day. You need to complement your principal activity with other ones to allow time for your muscles and joints to rest.
- Listen to your body. You need to be alert to how you feel to avoid entering into a state of chronic exhaustion. A good rule of thumb is to measure your heart rate in the morning when you get up: the heart rate falls as your physical condition improves. An increase in your base heart rate or persistent muscular pain can be signs of fatigue or injury.
- Exercise consistently.
- Set yourself objectives to reach a particular level of performance.
- Avoid exercise in very cold or hot weather.

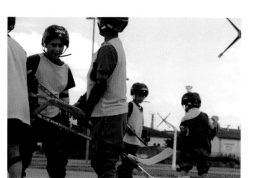

Teaching children about physical exercise and its benefits to health is vital in order to avoid the dangers of a sedentary lifestyle when adult.

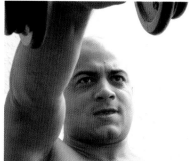

At present, statistics from the world's most developed countries are truly disheartening: people with a sedentary lifestyle account for 40 to 60 percent of the population, and only one in five people performs the minimum amount of physical exercise recommended for health.

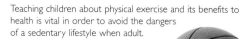

N.B.

Sports and physical exercise provide a range of health benefits:

- A reduction in the risk of mortality from cardiovascular disease in general and from coronary heart disease in particular.

- Prevention of and/or delaying the development of high blood pressure, and helping to reduce high blood pressure in those who suffer from it.

- Improvement in the level of lipids in your blood; i.e. reducing the level of triglycerides and increasing the level of HDL cholesterol in the bloodstream.

- Better regulation of glucose levels in the blood and a reduction in the risk of suffering from type 2 diabetes or insulin dependency.

- Improvement to digestion and the intestinal tract. Lessening your risk of suffering from certain types of cancer. There is much evidence for the benefits of preventive exercise in the case of bowel cancer.

- Increasing the burning of body fat and, therefore, helping control weight and avoid obesity.

- Helping to maintain and improve muscular strength and resistance, increasing your capacity to perform any physical activity in daily life.

- Helping to maintain the structure and function of the bones and joints. Physical activity not only causes no harm to the joints, but is also of great benefit in the case of diseases such as degenerative osteoarthritis or osteoporosis.

- Physical activity that requires lifting weights is essential for the normal development of bone during childhood and for achieving and maintaining correct bone density in young adults.

- Better quality of sleep.

- Helping you to give up habits such as smoking or drinking.

- Helping with your self-image and helps you to spend time involved in physical activity with your friends and family.

- Helping to relieve tension and improving your ability to deal with stress and anxiety.

- Fighting the symptoms of depression. Moreover, exercise generates feelings of enthusiasm and optimism.

- For children, physical activity helps to instill a lifetime habit of looking after your heart, and it prevents issues arising such as obesity, high blood pressure, etc., that would lead to the development of cardiovascular diseases in adulthood.

- For those in old age, an exercise regime reduces problems arising from falls, and helps to delay or prevent chronic illnesses, or even aging. Consequently, exercise both improves quality of life and increases personal independence.

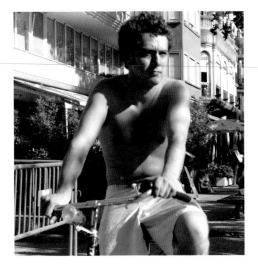

Everyone needs to consider why they want to work out and what their goals are before deciding on the type of exercise regime they intend to follow.

- Following the rules or standards required by your type of exercise or sport.
- Having health checks.
- Eating a proper diet and drinking enough water.
- Giving the parts of your body that you are exercising the most time to recuperate.

What is the reason for warm-ups?

Warm-up exercises are intended to prepare your body for physical exercise. They fulfill two very important functions: avoiding injury and improving the gains you can make from exercise.

At rest, blood flow to the muscles is relatively low and the smallest blood vessels are closed. When active, blood flow increases, such that the blood vessels start to dilate and prepare the muscles for the work they are expected to perform. As expended energy increases, so this physical activity causes muscular temperature to rise, reducing the likelihood of strain.

A warm-up should start off with movement of the major muscle groups in general to produce a general influx of blood. Next, you should concentrate on more specific muscle groups. The final phase in a warm-up targets specific movements involved in the exercise or sport that you are about to embark on.

Warm-ups should always be performed

The risks of physical exercise: sports injuries and fitness fanatics

The most common problem to arise from performing a physical activity of some sort is the risk of physical injury. It is an easily avoidable risk if you do not exercise beyond your limits and if your level of activity increases slowly and progressively until you reach your goals.

How to avoid sports injuries

Injuries can occur from time to time during any physical activity, whether recreational or at competition level.

They can happen as a result of accidents or due to the body being put under excessive strain (affecting bones, joints, and muscles) and are no different to comparable injuries that occur outside the context of sports or exercise.

Not only do these injuries need to be diagnosed correctly and treated properly, they also need to be prevented in the first place.

Preventing such injuries depends on a range of factors, such as:

- Proper physical preparation.
- Using appropriate equipment.

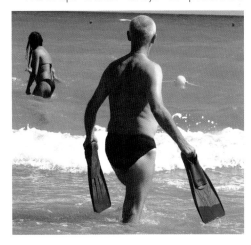

The intensity and degree of strain involved in exercise has to be assessed on an individual basis, taking a person's level of skill and physical condition into account.

before any exercise, sport, or competition, because they are the most obvious factor in preventing injury and for gaining the greatest benefit from your activity.

After your workout or sporting activity, you should also perform cool-down exercises allowing you to return to a state of rest gradually, to relax your muscles, and leave them ready for your next session.

What is flexibility?

Flexibility of the joints is a combination of joint mobility, strength, coordination, and the perception of movement and orientation which come from stimuli within the body itself and provide the ability to balance (proprioception).

Maintaining proper mobility (the range of articulated movement) and flexibility of the joints are very important for people about to do any physical exercise.

A number of points need to be considered with this in mind:
• The muscular temperature achieved through the warm-up.
• The degree of neuromuscular activity.
• The elasticity of the muscles, tendons, ligaments, and joints.
• Age.
• Mental attitude.

Joint flexibility is not the same for all joints. It decreases with age and is usually poorer in men than in women. It is very important to improve performance and avoid injury.

How do the various moving parts of the body respond during exercise?

A gradual warm-up of the body's various moving parts is very important, enabling them to deal with the increasing load placed upon them during physical exercise.

The bones are exercised through regular training and adjust to increased loads, making them stronger and more robust. These changes take place slowly and gradually.

Cartilage covers the surfaces of the joints and allows them to move in relation to each other smoothly and without friction. Physical exercise keeps cartilage strong, while inactivity weakens and thins its structure, making it easier for injury to occur. The best way to keep cartilage in good condition is through regular, gentle exercise.

The body beautiful

The "body beautiful" culture, in the sense of being interested in looking good rather than looking after your health, has led many young men to develop obsessive or compulsive behavior: bulimia, anorexia, and compulsive jogging syndrome are conditions typical of those who see themselves as needing to be thinner; and bigorexia is an addiction to physical exercise and the need to feel more muscular.

Exercise also modifies the structures formed by muscular and connective tissue (ligaments, joint capsules, tendons). Inactivity makes tendons and ligaments stiffer, which can cause them to be more easily strained.

Bigorexia (fitness fanaticism or exercise addiction)

Many young men are obsessed with working out, to the extent that they develop an addictive type of behavior: bigorexia, sometimes called "reverse anorexia."

While physical exercise is one of the great mainstays of health, because it boosts your physical condition in general and helps prevent many illnesses, excessive exercise that turns into an obsession can actually be damaging to health.

Bigorexia is a mental condition that leads a person to become obsessed about his muscle mass and to feel permanently dissatisfied with the state of his body.

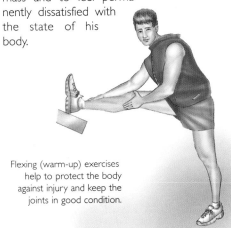

Flexing (warm-up) exercises help to protect the body against injury and keep the joints in good condition.

Young men with bigorexia, apart from spending hours in the gym, adopt special diets, weigh themselves several times a day, compare themselves with friends, athletes, or professional bodybuilders and, despite their physical achievements, continue to feel bad about themselves for not having acquired their ideal musculature.

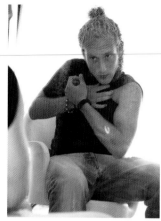

The problem with bigorexia is that it leads people to obsessive-compulsive behavior and causes anxiety and depression through feelings of failure in their attempts at self-improvement.

Many of these young men abandon their normal day-to-day activities so they can "imprison" themselves in gymnasiums day and night, while following strict dietary regimes that are low in fats and high in proteins and carbohydrates in order to gain muscle mass, and many start to misuse hormone supplements and anabolic steroids.

Anabolic steroids can cause irreversible damage to health. The metabolic changes that result have an impact on the liver and the cardiovascular system, raise cholesterol levels in the blood, and cause muscle cramps, kidney problems, and sterility.

The joints

The joint capsule is the sac that encloses a joint and is made up of a fibrous outer membrane to provide stability, lined within by a thin membrane that secretes synovial fluid. A greater amount of liquid is secreted if the joint is overloaded or if the synovial membrane is irritated, which is the cause of a swollen joint (joint effusion). Regular exercise maintains the strength of the connective tissue and delays its degeneration through aging. It also improves the mechanical and structural properties of the joints.

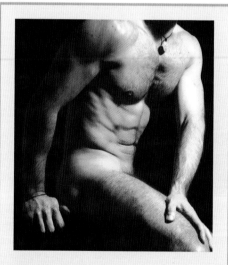

Perfect 10

Over the past few years, cases of bulimia and anorexia in men have increased by 20 percent. At the same time, other illnesses have appeared, such as the obsession with achieving a muscled body or compulsive jogging syndrome. The latter is a condition that requires a man to spend hours jogging whenever he feels that he has overeaten.

health at work

No type of work is without its risks to health, and that includes working in an office or in front of a computer. Some types of work present more obvious risks, of course. Being constantly subjected to noise, high temperatures, vibrations, or awkward postures, etc. is dangerous for health in the long term.

Work-related risks

Over the past few years, precautions to deal with work-related risks have undergone a major transformation. Until recently, security and, occasionally, hygiene were the only two basic areas that justified taking precautionary measures. Now other areas involving preventive measures against work-related risks are increasingly being recognized, such as medicine in the workplace, safety measures, ergonomics, and psychosociology—the latter being a field of knowledge that examines the psychological development of the individual worker in relation to his immediate working environment and the rest of the corporate organization.

Security or safety systems

Over the past few decades, measures to deal with health and security risks at work have been advancing steadily. Some types of work, such as construction or mining, involve obvious and implicit health risks. But whether you work outdoors or in a factory or office, there are always health risks and numer-

Preventive measures mean the collective actions or measures adopted or planned throughout all stages of work-related activity which have the aim of preventing or reducing the risks posed by that work.

ous ways to avoid these risks. For example, if about to expose yourself to the effects of a potentially toxic or carcinogenic substance, you should always make use of the safety system put in place by the company, and follow the instructions pertaining to safety.

Some companies are required to provide regular safety checks to identify any indications of ill-

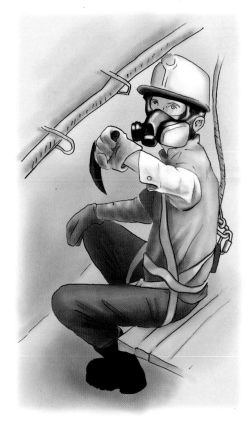

ness brought on by a particular type of job; for example, carrying out lung x-rays to show any signs of silicosis—a common medical condition in the mining industry. Many jobs involve risk of a higher than normal incidence of specific illnesses and medical conditions, particularly those

in the military, where of course there is a greater risk of becoming wounded or suffering burns.

Personal protection measures are any clothing or equipment used by an employee to protect him from one or more risks that might affect his safety or health at work.

■ What can have an effect on health?

Noise: In the long term, constant exposure to a high level of noise can cause deafness or ringing in the ears (tinnitus). This is why it is advisable to use earplugs or mufflers and reduce the amount of time spent exposed to the noise source.

Dust: Prolonged inhalation of mineral dust (asbestos, silica, coal, etc.) can reduce lung elasticity and cause fibrosis. The inhalation of organic particles (including fungal spores) can cause pneumonia.

Industrial solvents: If solvents are inhaled or come into contact with the skin, they can cause allergic reactions or cause damage to the liver and kidneys.

Radiation: The quality and quantity of spermatozoa can be affected in men exposed to radiation (like workers in nuclear power stations),

which may result in their offspring suffering from birth defects or leukemia.

Stress: All types of work involve situations and problems that cause tension, stress, and exhaustion. Long term, this may lead to stomach ulcers or irritable bowel syndrome.

Heat: Workers subjected to high temperatures run a greater risk of suffering muscular cramps, exhaustion, and even heart attacks.

Vibrations: The operation of manual machinery can affect the circulatory system in the fingertips, causing aches and pains.

Pesticides: Workers on agricultural land under intensive cultivation often suffer poisoning from treating crops with insecticides.

Sick Building Syndrome

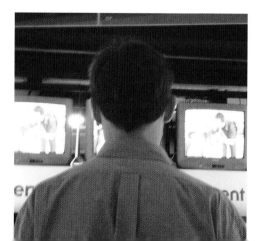

Nowadays, people spend a great amount of time in enclosed spaces that are contaminated in some way. These enclosed spaces can be our homes or our places of work. It is increasingly being recognized that poor air quality can have effects on health. Since the 1980s, these effects have been steadily increasing with the appearance of new modern structures that have a design and hermetically sealed type of construction, incorporating massive air-conditioning systems in which the recycling of air is very important for the purpose of ensuring energy saving.

The World Health Organization (WHO) has defined Sick Building Syndrome (SBS) as being a collection of problems and illnesses that

derive from poor ventilation, temperature disparities, the ionization of and electromagnetic charge in the atmosphere, particles in the air, gases and vapors from chemical sources, and aerosols, among other identified causative agents. The types of suffering that these situations produce vary: severe headaches, nausea, dizziness, persistent colds, and irritated airways,

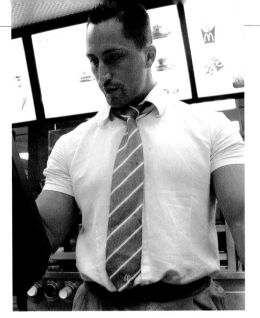

bial particles become airborne. One potential infection, although extremely rare, is caused by the *Legionella pneumophila* bacterium.

Contaminants can also come from outside of a building and penetrate via external air vents, or flow in through other openings when the quantity of air extracted from a building by its air-conditioning system is greater than the quantity of air supplied to it.

Poor air quality indoors occurs when ventilation is inadequate, which gives rise to a buildup of contaminants harmful to health. The air-conditioning system should not only control the level of contamination but should also provide a comfortable working environment: free of odors and dust, neither stuffy nor draughty, and with normal temperature and humidity levels.

skin, and eyes, etc. Allergies feature prominently among these problems.

Certain factors have a direct effect on employees' state of health: the ozone produced by photocopiers; the electromagnetic fields generated by computer terminals, artificial lighting, and other electrical equipment; toxic vapors from the adhesive used to fix wall-to-wall carpets and false ceilings and varnish, etc.

Health problems can originate from a variety of sources inside or outside a building. Chemical materials, bacteria, fungi, pollen, and dust can all contribute, as can factors that have nothing to do with air quality, such as temperature, humidity, light levels, noise, personal stress and job satisfaction, and a person's pre-existing state of health.

The potential sources of contamination in office buildings include: cigarette smoke, dust, inadequately maintained systems for central heating, ventilation, and air conditioning, cleaning products, pesticides, construction materials, furniture, the occupants' metabolic waste products (from breathing and perspiration), and cosmetics. These will be present to some degree in practically any building and cause serious problems regarding air quality only when found in excessive quantities. Dusty surfaces, stagnant water, and damp provide an ideal environment for the growth of bacteria. Some occupants of buildings may suffer allergic reactions when mold spores and other micro-

Certain factors have a direct effect on employees' state of health: the ozone produced by photocopiers; the electromagnetic field generated by computer terminals, artificial lighting, and other electrical equipment; toxic vapors from the adhesive used to fix wall-to-wall carpets and false ceilings; varnish, etc.

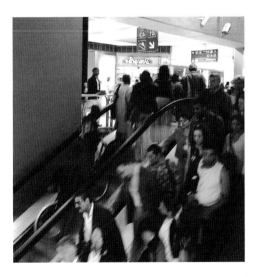

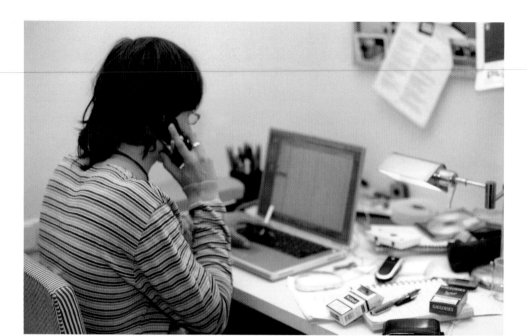

Work and health in the office

Modern offices are not usually very healthy places. The offices of the past with their filing cabinets, stacks of paper, and typewriters have made way for open-plan rooms with computers, photocopiers, fax machines, etc. These changes have brought with them a high degree of electromagnetic contamination, which has contributed in large measure toward making offices places of stress and tension.

After being sat down for many hours in the same position, muscle tone starts to diminish and the muscles become tense, stiffen, and ache.

This muscular tension can be reduced by performing simple relaxation exercises, such as flexing and extending certain groups of muscles.

No job is without its risks. Although some jobs involve more obvious types of risk, working at an office desk also has its problems: vision difficulties, back pain, varicose veins, constipation, cardiovascular conditions, headaches, etc.

Working for long periods in front of a computer screen can tire the eye muscles and make the eyes ache. In that situation, it is a good idea to fix your vision on a distant object from time to time. It is also important to ensure that your screen is not reflecting light.

Another type of injury comes from adopting the wrong posture when working, such as typing with a keyboard that is set at the incorrect height or overusing your computer's mouse. The typical symptoms include pains in your arms and wrists, as well as pins and needles or numbness in your hands.

Repetitive strain injury (RSI) refers to injuries that are caused by repeatedly moving certain joints in the same way, and it affects tendons, nerves, muscles, and other sensitive body tissues. It occurs in a variety of professions, ranging from secretaries and assembly line workers to musicians and athletes, as a result of the type of repetitive actions that they perform. Overuse of your computer's mouse and a poor sitting position can cause RSI in the wrist.

To avoid pain in the back, arms, and wrists, your hands and wrists should form a straight line when typing, i.e. at right angles to the keyboard and at the same level with your arms fully supported by the table. Your back should be resting against the back of your chair.

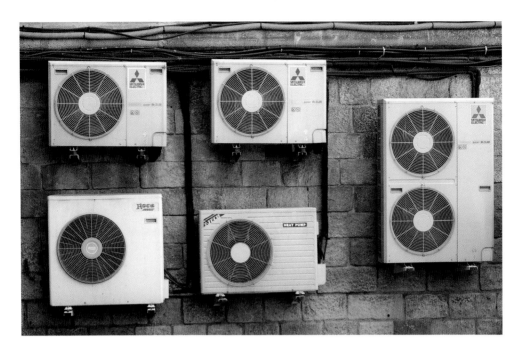

The right temperature is very important for feeling comfortable at work. You must adjust the air conditioning if you feel too hot or too cold. Having plants around the office raises the air's humidity level.

As far as your monitor is concerned, you should increase the viewing size of the text, even when using large screens, to avoid having to get too close to the monitor. One idea is to use colored text instead of the usual black on white. The ideal distance for viewing a screen is at least 25 inches, and the screen should be at eye level or just below to avoid neck strain or torsion.

■ Conditions affecting people in mostly sedentary occupations

- Back pain—24 percent
- Headaches—20 percent
- Spinal column injuries—16 percent
- Overweight—15 percent
- Aching joints—13 percent
- Circulation problems—11 percent
- Varicose veins and swollen ankles/legs—11 percent
- Constipation—6 percent
- Muscular tension and pain—6 percent

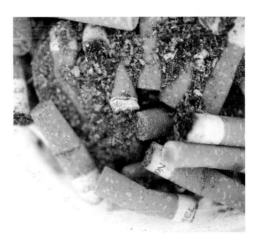

Breathing in cigarette smoke is one of the most serious risks possible in an office environment. Passive smokers have an increased risk of developing lung cancer, asthma, and emphysema.

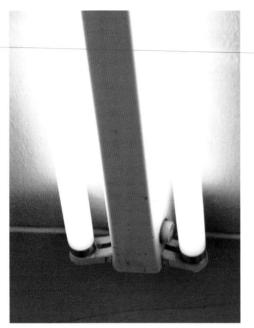

Fluorescent lighting should be filtered to eliminate the high frequency flickering that causes headaches and eye fatigue. It is better to use an adjustable desk lamp.

◢▪ How to sit in front of a computer screen

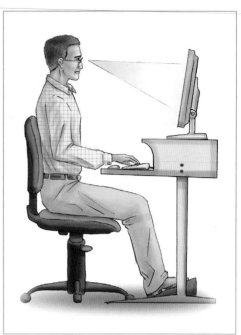

The mouse should be used gently without gripping it; to avoid excessive stretching, try to place it within easy reach and close to the keyboard. It is also recommended to use shortcut keys and commands on your keyboard as much as possible.

USING SHORTCUT KEYS INSTEAD OF THE MOUSE (FOR WINDOWS USERS)	
Command	**Function**
ALT + spacebar	Opens the menu (same as clicking onto the symbol at the top-left of the window)
Enter	Activates the highlighted item
CTRL+A	Highlights everything
CTRL+C	Copies selected text or object
CTRL+X	Cuts the selected text or object
CTRL+V	Pastes text or an object
CTRL+P	Prints the selected text or object
CTRL+S	Saves text or object
ALT+F4	Quits the active window
CTRL+Home	Takes you to the start of the text
CTRL+End	Takes you to the end of the text
ESC	Cancels or closes windows
TAB	Moves you from one icon or field to the next

▪ Position for hands on a keyboard

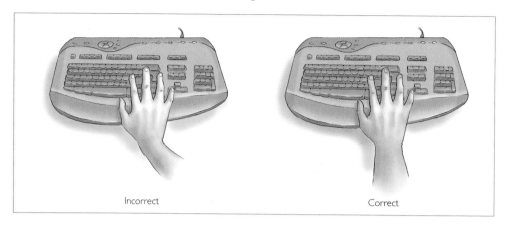

Incorrect   Correct

Back pain

Back problems can be caused by holding a static posture for long periods of time, or they may be due to intense physical activity or monotonous, repetitive strain, all of which can result in muscular imbalance. Back pain can come in many forms and affect us in different ways.

In many cases, back problems have a long history of development behind them, even if they appear to arise quite suddenly. Conditions such as lumbago, sciatica, or neck pain do not come about without a reason. Change of posture or awkward movement is responsible for 90 percent of all back pain. This worsens with time, resulting in problems with flexibility and our ability to function properly.

Habits to adopt

Pay attention to the way you sleep. We spend a third of our lives asleep. During that time, the spinal column should be kept straight. To ensure this happens, it is essential that your mattress is neither too hard nor too soft. Your pillow should act only as a means to

Poor back posture is very common. Much of our time is spent sat still, lifting and putting down heavy objects, or performing repetitive and monotonous movements. The muscular imbalance that results from this can cause discomfort and low back pain.

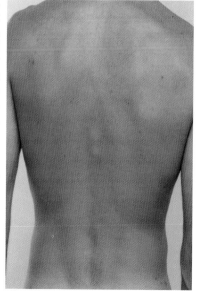

support the contours of your neck and head. Improper use can affect your cervical vertebrae. When sleeping on your back, the pillow should be supporting the back of your neck. If you are sleeping on your side, it should be supporting the hollow between your shoulders, neck, and head. And if you are sleeping face down, you should place the pillow at neck level, or not use it at all.

Getting out of bed. When you get up, you should avoid jerky or sudden movement, keeping muscular motion even and regular. Firstly, lower your feet to the floor. Once they are supported you can raise the rest of your body.

Sitting posture. When sitting, you must use the back of the chair to support your spinal column.

Common complaints

The spinal column runs down the center of the back and is divided into five segments: from top to bottom—the cervical segment (neck); the thoracic segment (shoulders to middle of the back); the lumbar region (lower back); the sacrum; and finally the coccyx (tailbone).

Pain can be felt in any of these segments, although complaints are most commonly located in the lumbar region. This part of the back is a principal focus of pain due to its pivotal and supportive function in the middle of the body.

The majority of back pain complaints are the result of common muscular strain, and only 1 in 200 cases has a serious reason underlying it, such as a tumor or spinal cord infection.

Wryneck (torticollis). Neck pain is felt when moving and is usually accompanied by an inability to turn or move the head. The pain and muscle spasm can spread to the shoulders or head.

Arthritis. This often occurs in the form of a continuous, non-acute aching that may extend to the buttocks and thighs, accompanied by rigidity of the back. This pain can surface in any part of the spinal column.

Slipped disk (prolapsed or herniated intervertebral disk). When an intervertebral disk is squeezed (herniated) against a nerve it produces intense pain—often localized in the lumbar region—which worsens when coughing, lifting weights, turning around, or bending down. If the pain shoots from the lower back and passes via the buttocks toward the feet, it can indicate that the sciatic nerve has been affected. In the most severe cases, it can affect control of the sphincter muscle.

Muscle strain. This is accompanied by aching, rigidity, and acute, periodic pain when moving in the "wrong" direction. The pain is usually located in the lumbar region. It may appear suddenly following an injury incurred from physical exercise, or it may develop gradually.

Low back pain. This refers to pain, generally accompanied by muscular tension, in the lumbar region, between the ribs, and the lower buttocks. It may be an acute or chronic pain (when it lasts longer than a month). It can extend to the calves (sciatica) or not (ordinary low back pain).

Pain in the neck (cervicalgia). This is a pain in the cervical vertebrae that radiates to the back of the neck, head, or arms. Sometimes it even leads to giddiness and nausea. This accounts for 30 percent of back pain. It is caused by poor posture or osteoarthritis.

Scoliosis. This refers to a spinal column deformity. Thoracic asymmetry results, depending on the degree of curvature. Consequently, this condition has a negative effect on a person's physical appearance. Moreover, it also gives rise to back pain, which can even result in the occurrence of respiratory disorders. The prevention and early diagnosis of this condition is very important, requiring regular checkups for schoolchildren.

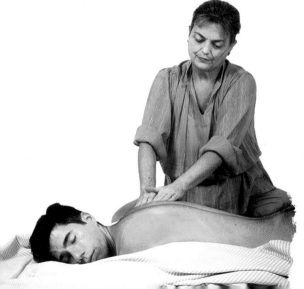

Lifting

When you are about to lift something heavy, you should always bend your knees, adopt a squatting posture with your back held as straight as possible, and, when standing up again, allow the muscles in your legs to take all the strain. Use the same technique in reverse when placing something heavy down on the ground.

If you bend over when lifting up or putting down a heavy object, you will be placing too much force on the muscles in your lower back.

Carrying

When carrying a heavy object, you must hold it as closely as possible to your body. If you hold it out, even at a short distance, your lower back muscles will be put under excessive strain. It is important to avoid twisting your torso around while carrying (or lifting).

How to protect your back

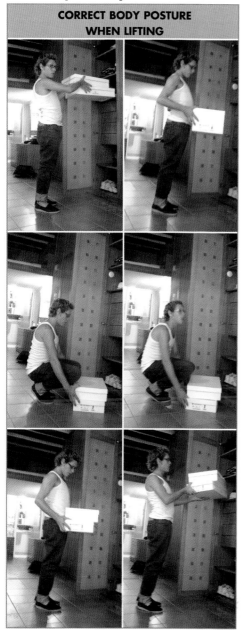

CORRECT BODY POSTURE WHEN LIFTING

Sitting

The idea is to be sitting comfortably. You must support your back using the back of the chair with your buttocks in place where the back of the chair meets the seat, and your feet should be resting firmly on the floor. Armrests are also a good idea, because they help to reduce the load borne by the lower section of your spinal column. Another good idea is to reinforce support for your lower back by placing a cushion at kidney level between you and the back of your seat. If you are using a computer, you should position your chair so that you are looking straight ahead (or just slightly down) at the screen without having to lower or twist your head.

Treating back pain

Typical ways of treating back pain usually consist of bed rest, muscular relaxants, painkillers, and even surgery.

- **Taking painkillers**, such as aspirin, acetaminophen (Tylenol), and ibuprofen.

- **Resting, but not too much.** If back pain occurs, you should give yourself some bed rest. Some studies have shown that, in the majority of cases, 48 hours of bed rest are better than a week, as spending too long in bed can interfere with recuperation because of the muscular weakness that it causes.

- **Cold compresses.** Ice is a very effective anti-inflammatory agent. Wrapping ice cubes in a towel and applying it to the point of pain can reduce muscular spasms and alleviate pain.

- **Applying warmth.** Warmth can help to reduce feelings of pain; but it does not have an anti-inflammatory effect. It is better to use a cold compress first and apply warmth afterward.

- **Activity.** Once the pain has gone, it is best to do some gentle exercises to increase your flexibility and strengthen your back muscles.

Headaches

One of the most common medical complaints at any age is that of headaches (cephalgia). The reasons for them vary widely: neck disorders, stress, anxiety, or agitation cause the muscles in the back and neck to contract, altering the flow of blood to the head and thus causing headaches.

As a general rule, headaches simply involve acute pain without presenting any underlying problems. Sometimes, however, the root of the problem lies in an illness of some kind. For example, meningitis causes a headache, together with fever, nausea, stiffness in the back of the neck, and hypersensitivity to light.

Headaches not linked to diseases can be divided into: tension headaches, migraines, and cluster headaches.

Tension headaches

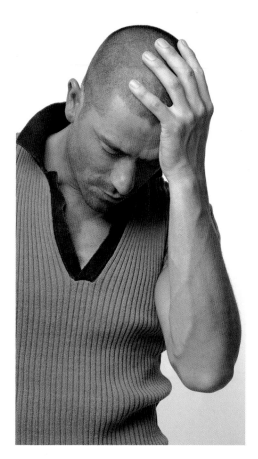

Squinting, emotional upset, poor posture when seated in front of the computer, grinding the teeth (bruxism), and even chewing gum can cause tension headaches.

These are the familiar headaches caused by stress, fatigue, or muscular tension, and they are the most common. They represent 70 percent of all headaches and affect almost all of us at some time or another in our lives.

They typically involve a dull pain that ranges from light to moderate. The pain is continuous but not pounding and can last from between quarter of an hour to a week.

It usually affects both sides of the head and it is not easy to specify an exact point of pain. Sufferers commonly experience a sensation of tension in the jaw, the upper back, and neck muscles.

Migraines

Migraines account for a quarter of all headaches, although they are more common among women.

They involve intense and incapacitating pain on one side of the head.

They are usually described as throbbing or pounding, and they can even be accompanied by feelings of nausea, vomiting, swelling of one side of the face, and cold hands, as well as hypersensitivity to light, noise, and movement.

Migraines can last for hours or days and are recurrent.

Although migraines can occur suddenly, some sufferers experience a change to their vision prior in an attack referred to as "migraine aura." The aura generally involves flashing lights, wavy lines or zigzag patterns, blind spots, temporary loss of peripheral vision, or colored spots. These signs usually appear between 10 and 30 minutes before the pain begins.

Cluster headaches

This type of headache usually occurs quite suddenly at night, and the pain is usually very intense and located to one side of the head, generally at the temple or in the orbit of the eye.

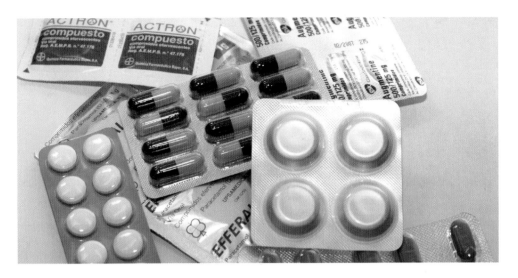

The pain is acute, nagging, and continuous. Usually this type of headache appears intermittently over long periods of time.

The best treatment

Drugs. Headaches are usually treated using painkillers (analgesics), which can be purchased without a medical prescription, with a particular emphasis on anti-inflammatory drugs such as aspirin or ibuprofen. If they fail to work, the headache becomes chronic, or a migraine ensues, it is best to consult a specialist and have him or her recommend you appropriate prescription drugs. You should remember that you can develop a tolerance to painkillers over time and, with continual use, higher dosages will be needed to produce the same effect.

Exercise. Exercise causes the body to release endorphins; these are naturally produced chemical substances that act as painkillers.

Relaxation. A good strategy for alleviating headaches is to change whatever it is you are doing, calm your breathing, practice relaxation techniques, and eliminate causes of stress around you.

Ice. Applying an ice-cube compress to the part of your head that hurts is very effective at reducing pain.

Massage. When your headache is the result of stress and muscular tension, it is

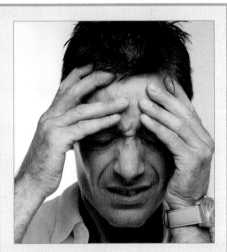

Migraines

One of the most common types of headache is the infamous migraine—different than the rest, because the pain affects only one half of a person's head. It involves acute, penetrating pain that "comes and goes." Furthermore, it is accompanied by nausea, vomiting, dizziness, general feelings of discomfort, etc.

a very good idea to massage the base of the skull for at least ten minutes. Then move on to massaging the temples, the base of the neck, and the shoulders.

Causes of headaches

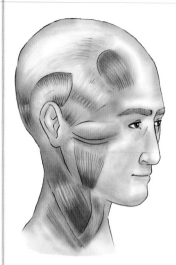 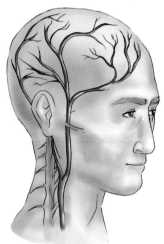

In general, headaches are caused by muscular tension, vascular problems, or a combination of these simultaneously. The majority of headaches can be remedied with over-the-counter painkillers.

Types of headache

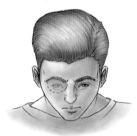 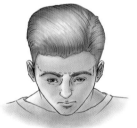 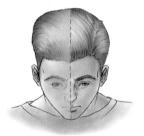

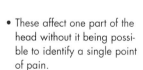

Tension headaches

- These affect one part of the head without it being possible to identify a single point of pain.
- Sometimes, they are caused by tension, pain, and stiffness in the jaw, the upper back, neck, and scalp.
- The pain is felt as pressure.

Migraines

- These involve a very intense pain on one side of the head, from the orbit of the eye upward.
- The pain is usually pulsating and coincides with the heartbeat. Swelling of one half of the face can also appear.
- Some people are able to predict the onset of a migraine as a result of changes to their vision referred to as "migraine aura."

Cluster headaches

- This condition usually causes pain on one side of the head, particularly behind an eye or the temple.
- The pain is continuous.

cosmetic and plastic surgery

Men are becoming more and more concerned about their physical appearance. Every day, more beauty and skin-care products come onto the market for men's faces and bodies, and increasing numbers of men are also attending cosmetic surgery clinics in search of solutions for the complexes that they have about their bodies.

Men and cosmetic surgery

Men are becoming increasingly concerned about their physical appearance, and many do not think twice about surgical intervention to sort out minor defects and deal with their complexes. They usually turn to specialist cosmetic surgery centers for hair transplantation, nose operations, and the reduction of bags under the eyes. However, men are also resorting to lipo-suction and breast-reduction surgery to get rid of those extra pounds.

In general, there is no specific age at which women decide to have surgery, while men usually do it at three particular points in their lives. The first of these stages is in adolescence, when the majority of those who decide to put themselves in the hands of a plastic surgeon opt to have work done on their noses (rhinoplasty) or ears. Men in their thirties tend to want to cor-

Men may have jumped on the bandwagon of fashion and body consciousness, but they still feel it is something of a taboo area: while they do not fear an operation in itself, they do worry about scarring that might give them away afterward.

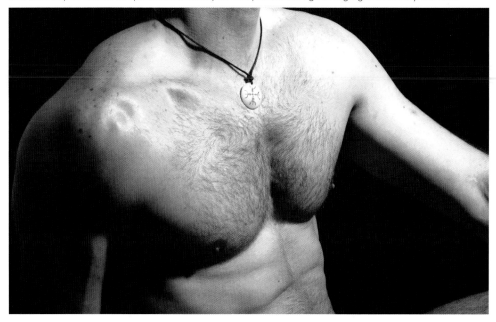

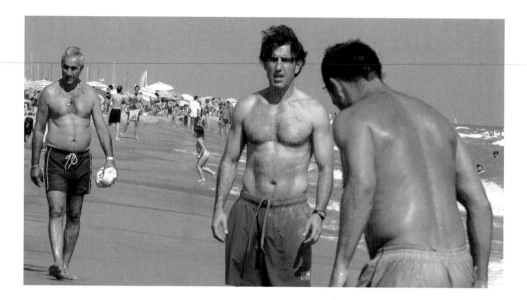

rect the buildup of excess body fat, especially around the waist. And from the age of 40 onward, men typically want the removal of bags under the eyes, a double chin, or crows'-feet.

Nevertheless, despite the increase in the number of men taking advantage of plastic surgery, it still remains very much a taboo area, with cosmetic and beauty treatments still regarded as being essentially in the female domain. For that reason, many men prefer to keep quiet about having undergone cosmetic surgery.

Liposuction

Liposuction refers to the surgical removal from the body of excess or unwanted fat found below the surface of the skin.

Over the past few decades, liposuction has become the most popular surgical procedure.

When undergoing liposuction, the patient's general physical condition is more important than his age.

If you decide to undergo cosmetic surgery, you should visit a registered center, where your treatment will be performed by surgeons who specialize in plastic and cosmetic procedures. Discuss and clarify all your concerns with the surgeon before agreeing to any type of procedure.

Liposuction is advised for men who have followed dietary and/or exercise regimes but who retain deposits of body fat. Overweight patients can benefit from this procedure, which, while not generally being regarded as a way to lose weight, does produce satisfactory results. However, it is much better if a man's weight is close to normal if he is intending to undergo this type of surgery.

This surgical intervention involves making a small incision wide enough to allow the insertion of a suction tube or cannula. One end of the tube is connected to a suction machine.

Almost any area of the body can be subjected to a liposuction procedure, ranging from the jowls, nape of the neck, cheeks, arms, and stomach to the thighs, buttocks, and hips.

After surgery, the treated area has to be wrapped up in an elasticized bandage, which needs to be worn for several weeks post-operatively.

You cannot expect to see immediate results following liposuction. At first, the areas treated will be swollen and leave the patient with a burning sensation. Analgesics are used to dull any pain, and a course of antibiotics is usually advised to prevent infection.

Surgical intervention of any kind involves a certain element of risk. In some cases, this procedure can lead to a trauma or complication of some kind, especially if surgery is performed on a large area in one operation. Although uncom-

Liposuction

Fat tends to get deposited in particular areas, depending on a person's sex. Fat deposition in men locates predominantly around the belly and waist. A person should not resort to liposuction to treat obesity. Liposuction is recommended for individuals who are near to their ideal weight and have persistent, localized fatty deposits.

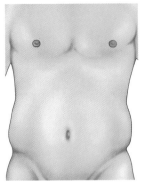
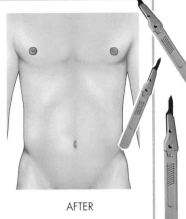

BEFORE   AFTER

mon, other difficulties can also arise: an infection or excessive loss of bodily fluids.

This notwithstanding, liposuction is a highly safe procedure when performed under the proper conditions and by a team of specialists. It is a very effective technique, and its results can be permanent if you follow an appropriate dietary and healthy exercise regime.

Breast-tissue reduction (reduction mammaplasty)

Gynecomastia, or the abnormal growth of breast tissue in men, is a common condition that affects 40 to 60 percent of the male population.

It has been linked to certain medications or medical conditions; however, in the majority of cases, no single reason can be identified for its appearance among men.

For men concerned about their physical appearance, breast-tissue reduction can be a godsend.

The procedure involves extracting the fat and glandular tissue from the breast area and, in extreme cases, the removal of excess skin as well.

Men who smoke, are regular drinkers of alcohol, or take certain drugs, such as marijuana, are not good candidates for this operation, as these substances can cause the condition. In such cases, patients are advised to give up these habits to see first whether their breast tissue decreases naturally as a result before undergoing any kind of surgical intervention.

Before deciding on breast-tissue reduction, it is important for the physician to perform an examination in order to assess what the possi-

ble causes of breast growth might be (liver conditions, ingestion of drugs containing estrogen or anabolic steroids, etc.). The surgeon will perform a mammogram or a mammary ultrasound scan, the aim of which is to obtain an overview of the breast tissue's composition. The appropriate surgical technique is decided on once the amount of fatty and glandular tissue has been ascertained.

In most cases, this is an elective type of surgical procedure that is performed under general anesthesia. Swelling and discomfort occur following an operation; however, these symptoms disappear after a few days. The final results will be seen approximately three months after the procedure.

Following the operation, it is important to avoid sunburn, as this impedes the healing process, and to avoid physical activities or exercise.

Neck lifting

Lifting techniques allow skin to be stretched wherever wrinkles appear or wherever, with the passage of time, the skin has lost its elasticity and is sagging. Neck lifting assists in helping the skin to regain its original contours.

It is a technique that is recommended to adults with sagging skin at the throat that forms a "turkey neck."

Although complications are extremely uncommon if a specialist performs the operation, small red scars can be left behind the ears, the facial nerve can be affected, and infections can occur, as well as hematomas (bruises), irritation, and minor hemorrhaging.

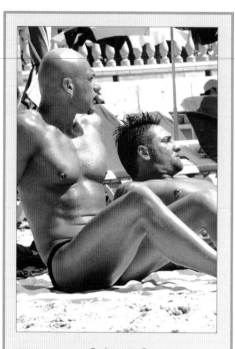

Pectoral implants

Men can also increase the size of their pectoral muscles. Many men, particularly bodybuilders and sportsmen, fail to develop pectoral muscle mass to the extent that they would like, despite training and routine workouts. In such cases, men may resort to assistance via implants or pectoral prostheses. These implants are made from silicone. Unlike breast implants for women, pectoral implants are made of solid silicone and are not filled with gel. However, their consistency is smooth and supple, giving the impression of firm, well-developed muscle tissue.

As with liposuction, the treated area is bandaged to prevent swelling and the formation of hematomas.

In order to avoid possible discomfort, it is advisable not to move the neck during the first few hours after the operation and to refrain from physical activity, sleeping on your side, and talking too much, for the first few days.

Upper or lower eyelid surgery (blepharoplasty)

Men turn to plastic surgeons to correct fatty deposits that form "bags" under the lower eyelid, or to remove excess skin from the upper eyelid.

This technique makes adjustments to the amount of skin that surrounds the eyes, reducing wrinkles and correcting the effects brought on by aging.

Two methods of surgical intervention are employed for eyelids: upper blepharoplasty, or correction of the upper eyelids to improve appearance; and lower blepharoplasty, or correction of the lower eyelids to eliminate fatty deposits, excess volume of the orbital muscle, or bags under the eyes.

In men, signs of these effects start to appear from the age of 30 and are usually hereditary. However, other factors also exist, such as anorexia, hormonal and emotional imbalance, overexposure to the sun, and the consumption of tobacco, alcohol, or drugs.

Some of the complications that can arise include hematomas and swelling, asymmetry of the eyes, conjunctivitis, lumps and irregularity, tiny white bumps produced by the temporary blockage of sebaceous gland pores, scarring, and a downward displacement of the lower eyelid (which usually resolves itself).

Nasal surgery (rhinoplasty)

Rhinoplasty, or surgery to reshape the nose, is one of the most common of all plastic surgery procedures.

Rhinoplasty can reduce or increase the size of the nose, change the shape of the bridge or tip of the nose, narrow the nostrils, or change the angle made between the nose and the upper lip.

Birth defects and facial wounds can also be corrected; and it can also be of assistance in helping those with breathing problems.

In all these cases, the final result depends on the original nose, and the surgeon needs to make sure he achieves a harmonious effect in relation to the rest of the face.

Following surgery, a plaster cast splint is placed around the nose and kept in place for a week and plugs are inserted into the nostrils for 48 to 72 hours to prevent any post-operative bleeding.

Some bruising and swelling is normal, and this usually disappears within 15 to 20 days.

▪ Otoplasty

Cosmetic ear surgery or otoplasty is performed to bring abnormally large or prominent ears closer to the head.

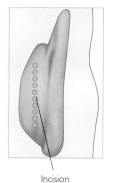
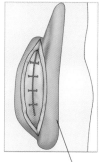

Incision

The cartilage is sutured behind the ear

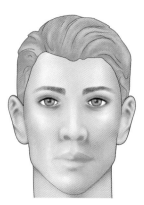

BEFORE

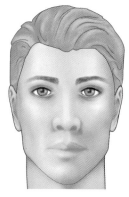

AFTER

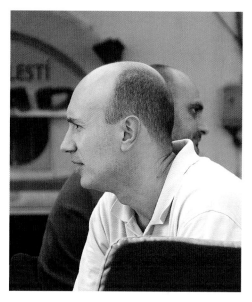

In micrografting (follicular unit transplantation), the area from which the hair is extracted is usually the back of the head, where there is a greater density of hair, and from there it is transplanted to the sides and front.

Hair transplantation

When hair transplantation procedures were in their infancy, the results were often poor as well as being painful. The "plugs" of hair implanted lacked a natural appearance, and the scars on the scalp were much too noticeable. Thanks to modern technological advances and new drug treatments, micrografting (or follicular unit transplantation) is now a better option for fighting baldness.

The process involves grafting single hairs or small groups of two or three hairs, follicle by follicle. By means of a needle, a microscopic puncture is made in the scalp into which the hair root is inserted.

The results are very natural-looking and, moreover, constitute a lasting solution, because the grafted hair is the patient's own and continues its lifecycle as normal, only on a different part of the scalp.

The treatment is simple and relatively free of pain, but it should be borne in mind that it cannot produce miracles. It cannot achieve a complete repopulation of the area that has under-

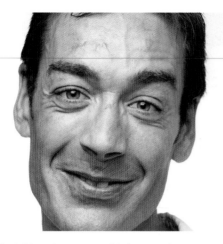

The facial muscles are responsible for expressing our emotions (anger, happiness, sadness, etc.). These muscles are located just below the skin and are in charge of distinct facial movements. However, their continual use causes these areas of the face to become marked with lines, even when at rest, the most typical of which are frown lines on the forehead, lines between the eyebrows, and lines at the corners of the eyes (crows'-feet).

gone hair loss; although it certainly succeeds in making a major improvement from an aesthetic point of view.

Botox®

The type A botulin toxin is a highly toxic compound produced by the bacterium *Clostridium botulinum* and has been reproduced synthetically in laboratories for medical use.

Application of this toxin causes temporary paralysis of the muscle tissue into which it is injected. It has been in use for many years, particularly in ophthalmology for the treatment of strabismus and blepharospasm and in neurology for a variety of conditions relating to Parkinson's disease.

The toxin is injected into the muscle that causes the wrinkles. This is done using a very fine needle. The dosage is extremely low and does not constitute any major risk.

The toxin acts on the motor endplate, which is the connection between the nerve and the muscle tissue. It prevents the release of acetylcholine, which is the substance that transmits impulses from the nervous system to the muscle.

Its effect is not permanent, as the nerve protects itself by producing new nerve endings and new connections with the muscle. This means

that the muscle will start to reactivate some three months after the injection. The injection starts to take effect after four to five days and lasts for three to six months, after which the treatment has to be repeated.

However, it appears that, following repeated injections, the muscle begins to weaken and requires lower dosages to achieve the same effect, thus producing a more lasting result.

It is important that the treatment is used in moderation and only ever performed by qualified professionals.

Used incorrectly, the toxin can result in awkward facial expressions, particularly if anatomical features and motorial functions unique to the patient are not taken into account. For example, frowning may be necessary for some people in order to open and close their eyes properly, as well as to keep their eyebrows at a certain level. For such patients, the incorrect injection of the toxin could interfere with how they are able to look at things and also with their appearance, through lowering their eyebrows to an unacceptable degree.

Recently, another use for botulin toxin has been identified: reducing excessive perspiration from the hands and armpits. The toxin blocks the release of acetylcholine, a medium for the neurotransmission of signals from the sympathetic nervous system located in the sweat glands, thus reducing excessive perspiration. While this is an effective treatment, it is not permanent and needs to be repeated.

▪ Nasal surgery or rhinoplasty

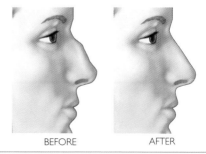

Reduction rhinoplasty, performed either under general anesthesia or under local anesthesia and sedation, typically attempts to refine nasal bone structure or remodel the end of the nose.

BEFORE   AFTER

erection, ejaculation, and orgasm

Human beings have their own particular way of responding to each other sexually, distinguished only by the specifics of their anatomy, whether male or female. Sexual response in both men and women is composed of five phases that are manifested differently according to their sex: desire, arousal, plateau, orgasm, and resolution. In general terms, men's sexual mechanism is more complex than women's, which makes men more prone to experiencing a range of problems related to their sexual response.

Sexual arousal

Sexual arousal can be triggered by a multitude of mechanisms that stimulate any of the senses, and this arousal provokes a physiological response.

Motivation and stimulation play essential roles in the act of sex, as it should not be reduced to the mere satisfaction of a biological urge but should involve the existence of a bond with the other person: feeling desired, loved, secure, united—these being the factors that cause one partner to feel sexual desire for the other.

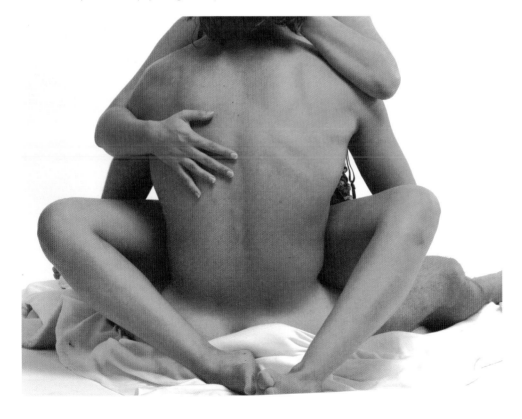

Male sexual response

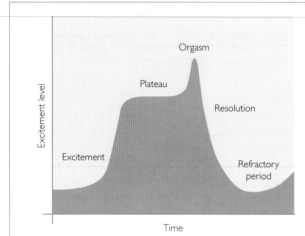

Excitement level

Orgasm

Plateau

Resolution

Excitement

Refractory period

Time

Male sexual response consists of five stages: sexual desire, excitement, plateau, orgasm, and resolution. For men, the resolution period includes a span of time referred to as the "refractory period" in which an ejaculation cannot be produced regardless of any sexual stimulation.

In men, it produces a clearly visible signal: the erection of the penis. The rapidity with which an erection is achieved varies from individual to individual, but men tend to become erect less quickly as they grow older, older men requiring greater stimulation to become aroused.

During erotic play, an erection may diminish or even disappear completely, but this is all part of the body's normal physiological response. However, if a loss of erection occurs frequently, making it impossible to sustain an active and sat-

isfactory sex life, a medical condition requiring treatment may underlie the problem.

During arousal, and in addition to an erection, a man also experiences contraction of the scrotal muscle, causing the testicles to be drawn toward the body, and an increase in heart rate, blood pressure, and neuromuscular tone in general.

Physiology of an erection

An erection is one of the responses to occur as a result of stimulation or sexual arousal. It is produced due to the capacity of the penis to become engorged with blood, which is then deposited in two special tubular structures in the penis referred to as the "corpora cavernosa." In its flaccid state, blood circulates through the corpora cavernosa without accumulating; but during an erection, the caliber of the arteries that supply blood to the penis increases, while the veins close up due to the effect of pressure from the buildup of blood.

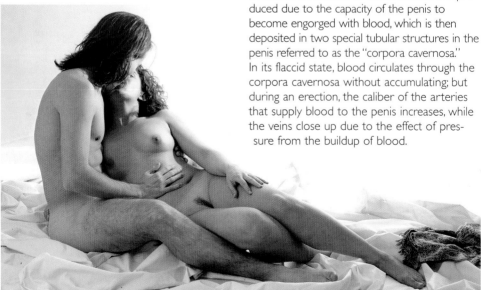

This engorgement with blood is what enables the penis to become rigid and increase in size—the definition of an erection—but in order for this to occur, it is necessary for blood flow to the organ to be working properly and for there to be no medical conditions or anomalies.

Apart from the physiology of the penis needing to be in working order, regulatory neurological mechanisms also intervene when an erection occurs. The stimulation of the blood vessels of the penis is caused through the action of nervous impulses that can have a variety of origins, such as through direct contact; via the sensory organs—sight, sound, touch, taste, and smell intervene directly in the sexual process; and mental factors, since psychological stimuli, originating in the cerebral cortex in the form of memories, fantasies, desires, or thoughts, play an integral role in male sexual response.

All of the neurological stimuli converge in the spinal medulla either separately or combined, and from there they send signals to the corpora cavernosa of the penis via the parasympathetic nervous system; thus caresses, fantasies, dreams, odors, or tastes stimulate the sexual response, which is manifested firstly as an erection.

Once ejaculation has finished, or the arousal phase has ended, the penis empties itself of blood, returning to its flaccid, dormant state.

An erection can also occur without any apparent cause: this often happens in puberty/adolescence, but many men past this stage of their development experience involuntary erection, particularly during sleep or on waking. Techniques have been developed to monitor erections while asleep for the purpose of assessing the mechanics and physiology of the penis, and it has been confirmed that a man may have between four and six erections during the night. They are produced throughout a man's lifetime, although they diminish with age. The purpose of this type of erection would appear to be to oxygenate the tissue of the penis. Morning erections can occur due to the stimulating effect of a full bladder.

Diminishment of sexual desire

The diminishment of sexual desire is a persistent deficiency or absence of sexual fantasies and of the urge to perform sexual activities. The diminishment of desire occurs as much in men as it does in women. Some people feel a lack of sexual desire or interest in sex throughout their lives. This condition may be related to traumatic experiences during childhood or adolescence, to the absence of sexual thoughts, fantasies, or dreams, or, occasionally, to abnormally low hormone levels. However, the problem develops more commonly following years of normal sexual desire and is usually a result of boredom in a relationship, depression, hormonal imbalances, or because of the use of sedatives, tranquillizers, certain types of medication to treat high blood pressure, and drug abuse.

The orgasm

Men's orgasms can be divided into two stages:

- The first stage involves the emission of semen as far as the prostatic urethra. This first expulsion is produced by rhythmic contractions of the prostate gland and the seminal vesicles, which puts pressure on the prostatic urethra, causing a sensation of imminent ejaculation that cannot be curbed once these reflexive mechanisms have been activated.

- The second stage is ejaculation itself, which involves the rhythmic contraction of the urethra's musculature, the prostate gland, the seminal vesicles, and the muscles at the base of the penis, as well as a series of sensations throughout the body.

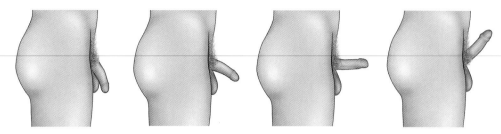

Certain medical conditions inhibit erections.

A continuous, high level of sexual excitement is present during the plateau phase, which is short in duration. In this phase, the rigidity of the penis and the size of the glans increase, the testicles are retracted to their maximum extent, and pre-ejaculatory fluid is secreted in order to lubricate the duct (urethra) and thus ease the way for subsequent ejaculation. Although this pre-ejaculatory fluid precedes the issue of semen and has a low sperm count, it should be remembered that it still contains sufficient sperm to fertilize an egg. As stimulation increases, the pelvic muscles start to spasm, accelerating the moment of ejaculation.

The erect penis

When erect, the penis becomes rigid, hard, and centered in relation to the abdomen. The penis inclines to an erect position corresponding to the angle of the vagina (approximately 45° from the body), which, in combination with its increased rigidity, facilitates penetration. The normal length of a flaccid penis is between 3¼ and 4¼ inches with a circumference of between 1½ and 2¼ inches. During erection, a penis normally increases in length and girth by 30 percent, so that on average the erect organ will attain a final length of between 5 and 6¼ inches, with variations of

■ Transverse cross sections of the penis

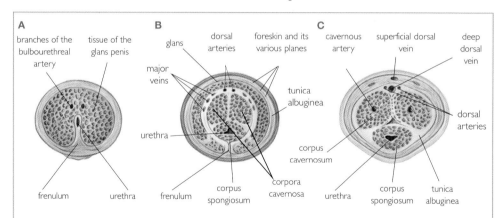

A — branches of the bulbourethreal artery; tissue of the glans penis; frenulum; urethra

B — glans; major veins; dorsal arteries; foreskin and its various planes; tunica albuginea; urethra; frenulum; corpus spongiosum; corpora cavernosa

C — cavernous artery; superficial dorsal vein; deep dorsal vein; dorsal arteries; corpus cavernosum; urethra; corpus spongiosum; tunica albuginea

The penis contains two cylindrical chambers that run its whole length. These are the corpora cavernosa. They are formed of a sponge-like tissue comprised of irregular cavities through which blood can flow, and muscle tissue, and separated by connective tissue. The corpus spongiosum—another cylindrical structure—is located between the two corpora cavernosa and contains within it the urethra. An erection starts following physical or mental stimulation, which translates into a relaxation of the muscles found in the corpora cavernosa. This relaxation allows blood to enter and fill the spaces (caverns) in the corpora cavernosa. The blood puts pressure on the corpora cavernosa, causing them to dilate and become rigid. When the muscles of the corpora cavernosa contract, blood flow is stopped, and the penis returns to its flaccid state. The failure of any of these mechanisms will make it impossible to achieve an erection.

between 4 and 9 inches (10 and 23 cm) in length, and a circumference of 4½ to 5½ inches.

As sexual stimulation increases, very high levels of sexual excitement are reached that lead to the threshold of orgasm, triggering a series of reflexes that together constitute the sensation of orgasm itself.

The resolution period consists of the phase in which the changes generated by sexual stimulation return to their starting point. For men, the initial part of this phase is called the refractory period in which a fresh ejaculation cannot be produced even if there is sexual stimulation. This period is very brief in young men, but it lengthens progressively with age. It has also been shown that the more ejaculations produced over the course of a day, the longer the refractory period.

Dysfunction relating to ejaculation and orgasm

Physiologically, orgasms are a reflex mechanism in the case of male sexual response, a series of nerve processes are triggered bringing about ejaculation if the glans penis is sufficiently stimulated. However, sexual pleasure is not necessarily defined by whether or not a man ejaculates. As for women, it is the brain that governs the sensation of satisfaction.

When sexual activity is not linked either to feelings or emotions, the orgasm ends up being reduced to a mechanical reflex—a mere release of tension.

For this reason, it is important to be aware of the role that sexuality plays, the genuine experience of pleasure, and knowing when and how to achieve it. Culturally, men are often brought up to reduce sexual gratification, almost exclusively, to their own genital-based

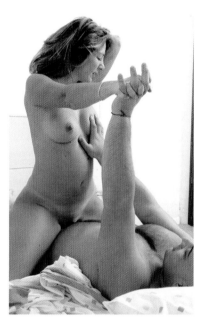

Normally, behavioral therapy to overcome delayed ejaculation requires partners to make a number of behavioral changes in the privacy of the home which will engage them in sexual activities that minimize the pressure to perform and concentrate principally on enjoyment.

needs. And, indeed, erection and ejaculation can all be over in a matter of minutes.

Delayed ejaculation

This is a condition in which ejaculation is retarded.

There are different degrees of this: in the most extreme cases, ejaculation is completely absent (see "Anejaculation" below), but mostly it involves a reduced response so that intense, prolonged stimulation is necessary to produce an ejaculation.

Medical conditions can be among the physical causes for this, such as diabetes, neurological damage, or congenital abnormalities; it may also be the result of prostate or urinary tract surgery, or due to drug abuse or prescription medication (e.g. drugs to reduce blood pressure, or antidepressants).

Psychological reasons may include a restrictive upbringing, traumatic events, fear of pregnancy, fear of vaginal penetration or of ejaculating in the presence of a partner, or emotional problems with that partner.

Treatment firstly involves ruling out physiological causes and treating them if they exist. Behavioral therapy attempts to lessen anxiety and teach techniques for controlling the moment of ejaculation.

Anejaculation

This is an extremely rare condition that makes it impossible to achieve ejaculation and, in most cases, is psychological in origin.

Apart from psychological reasons, this inability to ejaculate can also be attributed to physiological causes (prostate surgery, neurological conditions, the side effects of some drugs, or neurological complications as a side effect of diabetes, etc.).

Anejaculation may be total or partial—some men are able to ejaculate through erotic dreams or masturbation, or in casual sexual relationships. In such cases, the source of the problem is usually psychological.

Feelings of guilt, relationship problems, the discovery of a partner's infidelity, and a strict sexual upbringing are some of the most common causes.

Treatment involves discounting possible physical causes, treating them if they exist, and, if the cause is psychological, undergoing a course of behavioral therapy that teaches a man to enjoy and feel comfortable about his sexuality.

Retrograde ejaculation

In ejaculations of this type, the semen is redirected toward the urinary bladder instead of exiting via the urethra.

In retrograde ejaculations, semen mixes with urine in the bladder and is eliminated from the body during urination without causing damage to the bladder. A man can tell if he is suffering from retrograde ejaculation by the very slight amount of semen that he produces. A couple's inability to conceive may also point to this. His urine will have a whitish appearance, and a urine sample taken after ejaculation will reveal the presence of semen.

A prostate operation may cause a man to lose the ability to expel semen via the urethra. However, in such cases men retain the sensation of orgasm, because their muscular spasms continue unabated, and it is these that the brain translates into feelings of pleasure.

In addition to surgery, retrograde ejaculation may be caused by usually neurological disorders or congenital abnormalities.

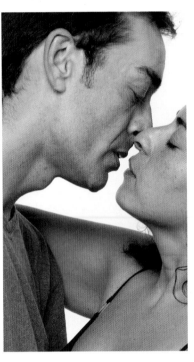

Painful ejaculation

Pain on ejaculation can be caused by prostatitis, urethritis, and any other infection of the urogenital system, although it may also be due to an over-tight foreskin or other physical abnormalities.

In some cases, the reason for it is psychological; in such cases, it usually involves a psychosomatic condition.

Treatment consists of verifying the patient's reason for complaint, and treating it if it has a physical cause, or having the patient undergo a course of behavioral therapy if the cause is psychological.

Male dyspareunia

In dyspareunia, coitus becomes very painful. The pain is generally experienced during penetration or when thrusting.

The cause may be due to a fibrous degeneration of the corpora cavernosa in the penis (Peyronie's disease).

Testicular pain can also arise following very vigorous intercourse.

All infections of the prostate and seminal vesicles can give rise to pain during intercourse. Pain can also occur because of problems with the foreskin and/or glans.

Anorgasmia

This condition is typified by an absence of any pleasure sensation on ejaculation. A man has normal erections, is able to penetrate without difficulty, and eventvally ejaculates, but he gets no pleasure from it.

Its cause may be neurological, but it is more commonly psychological in origin.

masturbation

From the eighteenth century and well into the twentieth century, masturbation was considered as something perverse, immoral, dirty, and damaging to health. It was even linked to illnesses, such as tuberculosis, insanity, paralysis, hair loss, and blindness. As a result of all these beliefs, all activities relating to masturbation were condemned, with devices and methods even being conceived that would prevent the young—male or female—from indulging in the practice. In the twentieth century, medicine, psychiatry, and psychology have attempted to undermine such beliefs. Masturbation is normal and even healthy; it does not cause any physical or psychological harm. However, despite the change in attitude of present-day society, myths still persist about this form of sexual expression.

Masturbation

Masturbation refers typically to genital stimulation to produce orgasm that is performed manually, although it can be done by other means.

Boys play with their sexual organs from a very young age, and many of them achieve orgasm from masturbation, even before being able to ejaculate.

The first instance of masturbation proper usually occurs during the final years of childhood or at the onset of puberty.

Many men discover masturbation by accident. Rubbing against something or, perhaps absent-mindedly, fondling the penis or stroking the testicles feels pleasurable and may encourage taking self-stimulation to the point of orgasm.

With time, masturbation can become more enjoyable with greater experience and progressive understanding of your body.

Some men like to masturbate with something acting as a lubricant between hand and penis.

A common type of lubrication is saliva, but this can become tiresome and inadequate if good lubrication is wanted.

Masturbation is another form of sexual expression and is a normal, healthy activity for anyone, young or old, male or female.

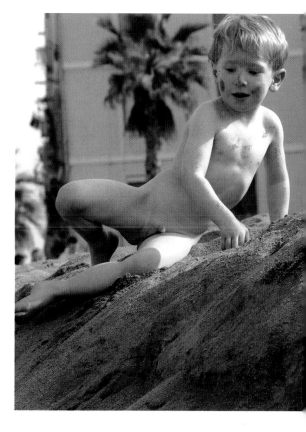

Boys play with their sexual organs from a very young age. The first experience usually involves a mixture of feelings: pleasure, excitement, curiosity, and anxiety.

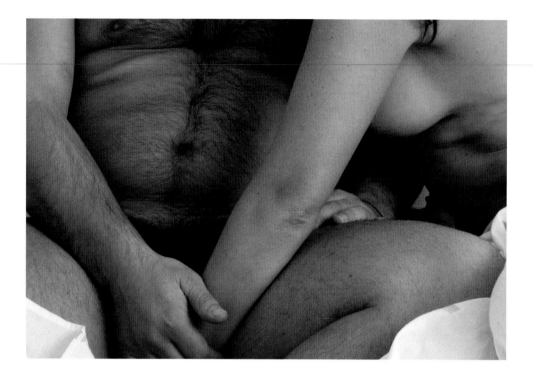

▪ Positive aspects of masturbation

- Masturbation is an act of self-discovery.
- It allows you to learn about what excites you, about your genitals, and to enjoy auto-eroticism.
- It keeps your sexual machinery in good working order: in the case of men, the reflexes for erection and ejaculation.
- It is a valuable means by which to feel sexually independent and is an excellent preparation for subsequent sexual relationships with others.
- It allows you to understand your own sexual needs better and thus enables you to tell your partner what you like, so avoiding awkwardness and feelings of frustration.
- It helps you to relax and alleviate sexual, physical, and mental tension.
- Alone, it is a way of practicing safe sex: i.e. there is no possibility of transmitting diseases or unplanned pregnancies.

Another method is to masturbate with soap or shampoo while showering or in the bathtub. Although it may feel enjoyable, it can have its disadvantages. Soap or shampoo can irritate the skin when applied too vigorously, and they can cause the skin to dry out if used over a period of time, causing rashes and even flaking. Soap can cause a burning sensation or irritation if it penetrates the urethra.

There are alternatives, such as body oils, body moisturizers, or water-based lubricants that can be obtained in drugstores.

Masturbation for two

While masturbation certainly refers to self-stimulation, masturbation between partners can be a variant in the erotic foreplay enjoyed prior to intercourse. This involves stimulating each other's most sensitive (erogenous) zones. Mutual masturbation can be an alternative if you do not want to reach orgasm by means of penetrative sex, whether because of an illness or pregnancy, or for any other reason. Mutual masturbation is the direct stimulation of your partner's most erogenous zones using the hands or other parts of the body to achieve effective results. Whether spontaneous or part of normal sexual activity, it can be used to play out and describe each person's desires and preferences and those of the couple as a unit.

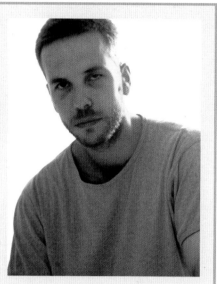

Men's indulgence in masturbation is such a universal phenomenon that sexologists or specialists dealing with male-specific conditions consider its absence to be abnormal and an indication that "something, somewhere, has gone wrong."

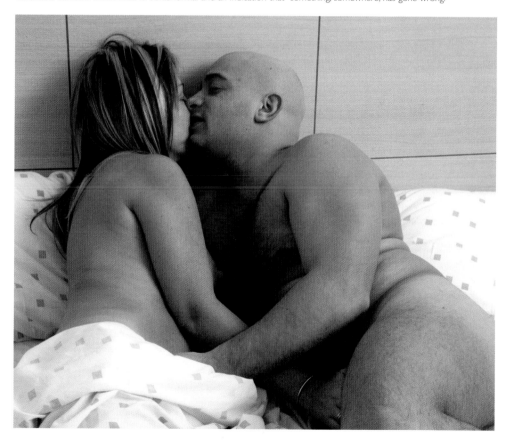

Myths and reality

- **Masturbation causes physical harm.**
This is a completely false assertion.
Masturbation is a normal, healthy human activity and does not cause any physical disorder.
It does not cause acne, nor does it cause blindness or hair loss, loss of mental faculties, loss of sexual potency, impotence, or infertility, and it does not affect penis size.

- **Masturbation causes psychological damage.** This is completely untrue.
Masturbation is a normal, healthy human activity, and it is not the cause of personality disorders, nor does it result in personality changes or alter mental health. Masturbation is psychologically harmful only when it becomes compulsive as a means of escaping relationship problems or when it is used as an escape without attempting to solve problems in some other way (see below).

- **Only people without a sexual partner masturbate.** This is not true. According to statistics, 95 percent of men masturbate and have achieved orgasm at least once through masturbation. Masturbation is only one form of sexual expression, and indulging in it does not mean that a man is dissatisfied with his sex life within a couple. Furthermore, masturbation can help a couple learn to identify the stimuli each of them needs to achieve orgasm, thus improving the quality of their lovemaking.

- **Only young, immature people masturbate.** This is untrue. While it is certainly the case that masturbation is extremely typical of adolescence, it continues to be practiced throughout adulthood.

- **Only men masturbate.** Untrue. Women masturbate as well. Different statistical studies show that 54 percent of women have masturbated at some time in their lives. There is evidence of a consistent increase in masturbation among Western women.

- **Masturbation is harmful, particularly when done to excess.** Masturbation is not harmful, but it can have some negative effects if:

  – it interferes with or substitutes for sexual activity enjoyed between partners. In other words, if a person would rather masturbate than have sexual intercourse, or if a person masturbates after intercourse, because he or she does not feel that their desired level of sexual excitement has been reached;

  – or it turns into an obsession, or it is done compulsively: i.e. when someone feels that masturbation is the only way to alleviate tension or escape, or when it interferes with his social life or causes feelings of remorse, guilt, or worry.

safer sex

The two fundamental goals of sex as a human activity are procreation and pleasurable communication at an intimate, interpersonal level. Therefore, it should be a source of satisfaction and development for a couple. However, if a person fails to be responsible and take heed of the information available on sex, it can become a route for transmitting diseases and risking unwanted pregnancy. The diseases that are transmitted from one person to another via the mucous membranes of the genitalia are referred to as "sexually transmitted diseases" (STDs).

Safer sex

Safer sex means taking precautions when participating in sexual activity so as to avoid acquiring sexually transmitted diseases (STDs) or transmitting them to your partner. These diseases range from genital herpes, genital warts, chlamydia, gonorrhea, and syphilis, to the life-threatening HIV and hepatitis B and C, but include many others besides.

Sexual abstinence is the most effective method, although this is not easy to sustain either biologically or psychologically. Maintaining a sexual relationship with one steady partner who you know to be STD-free is also wholly safe.

Taking into account that the transmission of diseases is caused through genital contact, some specialists have proposed calling STDs "genitally transmitted diseases," reserving the word "sexual" to describe a much broader and extensive range of human practices—such as kissing, embracing, caressing, etc.

Unsafe sex not only implies the transmission of disease but also the possibility of unwanted pregnancy. Unplanned conception, especially outside the context of a stable relationship, or in the case of a teenage pregnancy, can be the source of many significant complications.

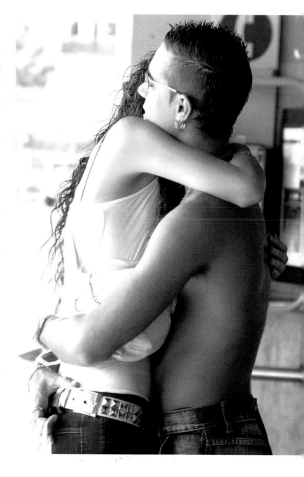

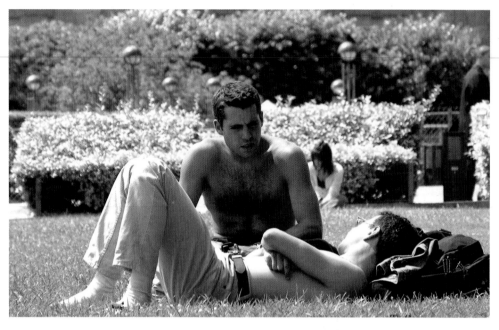

Risky sex

Risky sex includes any sexual activity that increases the risk of acquiring a sexually transmitted disease (STD). High-risk behavior includes:

- Having multiple sexual partners.
- Having had an STD or your sexual partner having had one in the past.
- Not knowing your partner. Being unaware of whether they have or have had an STD.
- The use of drugs or alcohol in situations or environments where sexual relations are likely.

- Being with a partner who injects drugs.
- Being sexually promiscuous.
- Practicing anal sex without a condom.

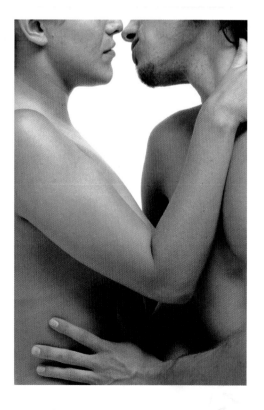

Among the diseases caused by bacteria are syphilis, gonorrhea, chancroid, donovanosis (*Granuloma inguinale*), and LGV (*lymphogranuloma venereum*). Trichomoniasis, a parasitic infection, is one of the most common sexually transmitted diseases. Included among the viral STDs are HIV (the virus that can lead to AIDS), genital herpes, genital warts (*Condyloma acuminata*), and hepatitis B. Some of these infections can be acquired by other means—for example, intravenously (blood transfusions, sharing needles, etc.)—and can then be passed on through genital contact.

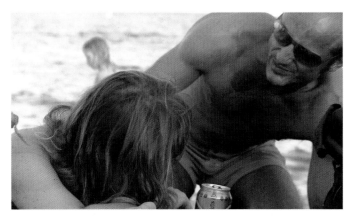

When one partner in a relationship breaks a commitment to be faithful, that person should be aware that unfaithful sexual activity needs to be "safe" in order to protect his or her usual partner.

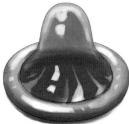

Latex condom before unrolling

Details to bear in mind for safe condom use

- Condoms must be officially approved by the FDA.
- You need to check their use-by date.
- It is advisable to buy them in pharmacies and not from places that cannot guarantee a proper storage environment: the effect of heat on latex can be damaging.
- Just as heat can damage latex, neither should you ever carry condoms close to your body or store them in warm places, such as your car's glove compartment or your billfold.
- The wrapper should be intact at the time that you want to use the condom.
- The condom should be used from the very start of sexual intercourse through to the end.
- Condoms should not be reused.
- Using a lubricant helps, because it minimizes the possibility of the condom splitting. It is recommended to use water-based lubricants only, as oil-based lubricants, lubricants made from petroleum derivatives, or Vaseline® can weaken the latex and cause it to rupture.
- It is recommended to use latex condoms for anal, vaginal, and oral sex. You should bear in mind that STDs can still be passed on even if you use a condom, because a condom does not protect the surrounding areas. However, condom use definitely reduces that risk.

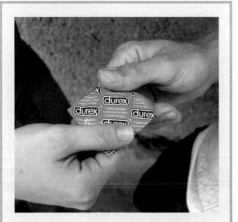

Condoms

The condom offers the greatest security to anyone choosing to maintain an active sex life, either within or outside of a stable relationship. Great strides have been made in the manufacture of condoms, and nowadays they are of better quality, more comfortable, and more effective than before. Although the most widely available versions are made for men, female condoms (femidoms) also exist. Whichever type is used, they afford protection to both partners equally.

N.B.

- **Get to know your partner:** This may seem obvious, but many people embark on sexual activity without first establishing a committed relationship that might give them trust and allow for open communication. It is important to ask your partner about past sexual history, whether they have or have had any STDs, whether they have taken drugs intravenously or shared needles, as well as their present state of health.

- **Avoid contact with semen, vaginal fluid, or blood:** It is essential that you always use a condom and do so correctly. Using additional lubricants can reduce the barrier effect. It is recommended to use condoms for anal and oral sex as well as for vaginal sex.

- **Avoid the excesses of alcohol and drugs:** Using alcohol or drugs can diminish your capacity to communicate properly with your partner and can lead to a lack of conscientiousness about using protection. Alcohol and drugs can lead to inappropriate decision-making and high-risk activities.

- **Be responsible:** People infected with HIV (HIV-positive) may not donate blood, plasma, organs, or semen. From a moral, ethical, and legal perspective, HIV-positive people should alert any prospective sexual partner to their status. They should not exchange body fluids during sexual activity and should use condoms to protect their partners.

- **Maximize precautions if your partner is trying to conceive:** Women with an STD should seek advice before becoming pregnant, because the child runs the risk of being born with serious complications. An expectant mother with an STD will need to ask for medical attention to prevent infection of the fetus.

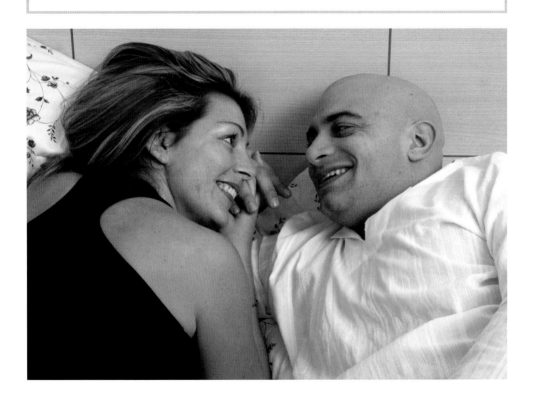

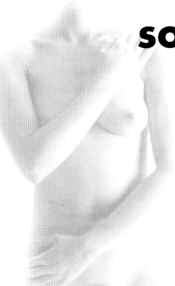

some things men should know about women

Women respond to sex in a different way than men. Social issues and physical aptitude mean that how a man experiences sex is distinct from how a woman does. A woman's capacity for stimulation is motivated as much by internal factors as it is by external ones and is far more accentuated than a man's. Understanding the female anatomy and talking to your partner about her sexual tastes can improve how you relate to each other sexually and help achieve greater sexual satisfaction as a couple.

Female anatomy

The external structure of the female reproductive system centers on the vulva, which is the location of the labia majora and labia minora, the entrance to the vagina, and the clitoris. The internal components are the vagina, the cervix, the uterus, the Fallopian tubes, and the ovaries.

The labia majora and minora are expansions of skin that cover and protect the entrance to the vagina. The labia majora are covered in pubic hair.

The clitoris is an erectile organ located in the upper part of the vulva near the anterior junction of where the labia minora meet. It is an organ that is very sensitive to sexual stimulation, equivalent to the male penis.

The hymen is a thin, elastic tissue situated at the entrance to the vagina. This membrane yields and tears during the first experiences of penetrative sex, which need not be uncomfortable if penetration is gentle. In some cases, a small amount of bleeding may occur as a result of such intercourse. The hymen can even break simply through physical exercise or dissolve of its own accord.

The ovaries are a woman's reproductive glands, which produce eggs (ova) and female sex hormones.

The Fallopian tubes are ducts that link the ovaries to the uterus, and it is in these that fertilization occurs.

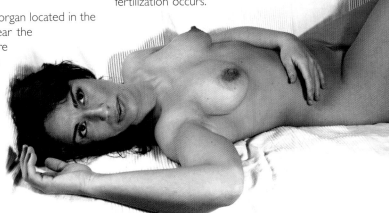

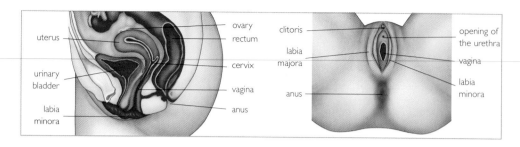

uterus · ovary · rectum · cervix · vagina · anus · urinary bladder · labia minora · clitoris · labia majora · anus · opening of the urethra · vagina · labia minora

---

The menstrual cycle

- A woman's menstrual cycle is the period of time taken from the first day of a period to the first day of the next one.

- Each woman has her own particular cycle; in general terms, however, this cycle takes 28 to 30 days.

- Female sex cells or gametes (the ova or eggs) are stored in both ovaries.

- Each month, during the menstrual cycle, an egg matures and leaves the ovary, entering into the Fallopian tube (ovulation) on the way to the uterus.

- If the egg is fertilized by a sperm while on its way, it implants itself in the lining of the uterus; and, if no fertilization takes place, it is eliminated and expelled together with the uterine lining (menstruation).

The uterus (womb) is a muscular organ covered in a mucous lining that, in the event of pregnancy, accommodates the fertilized egg (ovum) so that it can develop into an embryo. If no fertilization occurs, this lining is shed at the end of the menstrual cycle (menstruation).

The vagina is the elastic channel that runs from the vulva to the cervix (neck of the uterus or womb). The vagina is capable of dilation: it is perfectly adapted to accommodating the penis during intercourse—whatever its size—and to accommodating a baby's head at the time of giving birth.

Female sexual response

Women exhibit a cycle of sexual response just as men do.

Desire phase. Desire is triggered differently in men and women.

Men's desire is projected more directly toward the physical, whereas women appear to be aroused more by emotions and feelings.

Whatever the case, each woman is an individual, and many factors can be involved: cultural, upbringing, environment, social, psychological, etc.

Excitement phase. Lubrication of the vagina in women equates to erection of the penis in men. The vagina's lubrication is a direct result of the increase in blood flow to the pelvic region, which causes dilation of the blood vessels (vasodilation) in the walls of the vagina, thus producing greater lubrication. Women also undergo an expansion of the labia majora and minora, and the clitoris becomes progressively erect.

Women experience what is referred to as an "orgasmic platform," that is, an increase in the volume of the outer third of the vagina due to the increased vasodilation of this area. It causes a reduction in the diameter of the opening to the vagina and thus greater contact between the genitals of the man and the woman—which explodes the myths relating to the importance

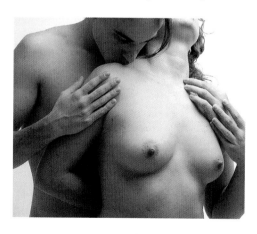

The clitoris

- The clitoris is not as small as it might appear; it is filled with nerve endings and branches and is bigger and more complex than what you can see or touch.
- The external view of the clitoris is merely the visible part of a larger structure: extending beyond what is visible is the glans clitoris, which is about ¾ inch in length, and beyond that are the clitoral corpora cavernosa, which are ligaments 2–2¼ inches in length that extend along either side of the pelvis.
- During sexual stimulation, these tissues fill will blood and the whole system develops an erection similar to that of the penis in men.
- The clitoris glans is the most sensitive part of the genital area.
- In women, orgasm is caused by direct or indirect stimulation of the clitoris.
- Unlike the penis, the sole function of the clitoris is to provide a woman with feelings of pleasure.

of penis size, given that the vagina adapts to fit. At the same time, the upper two-thirds of the vagina increase in width and depth;, there are fewer nerve endings here, which means that depth of penetration does not translate into an increase in pleasurable sensations, which also disproves the need for a larger penis in order to obtain greater sexual enjoyment.

▪ The G-spot

Not everyone agrees about the existence of the Gräfenberg or G-spot. The G-spot is a female zone of stimulation that is separate from the clitoris and located in the anterior, inner wall of the vagina at the point of the pubic bone (pubis): i.e. some 2 inches from the vulva orifice.

▪ Stimulating the clitoris

The clitoris is a very erogenous organ; however, the majority of women do not find it pleasurable to have it played with if sexual foreplay is not already in progress—embraces, caresses, and kissing (petting). Extremely vigorous stimulation of the clitoris can even cause a woman pain; therefore, it is advisable to stimulate the clitoris indirectly, i.e. the area enveloping and surrounding it.

Plateau phase. For both sexes, this phase involves a high and sustained level of sexual excitement.

Orgasm phase. Orgasm is the phase that marks the climactic point of sexual pleasure. Female orgasm does not involve a sensation analogous to a man's imminent moment of ejaculation.

Instead, a sudden burst of warmth and pleasure is felt in the clitoral area and the orgasmic platform, which then spreads throughout the body; in addition, a series of involuntary muscular spasms is triggered in distinct areas of the body, with these being most acutely felt in the orgasmic platform, the uterus, and the anal sphincter.

For some women, the sensation of orgasm may be repeated several times after the initial experience if sexual stimulation is continued.

Resolution phase. This is characterized by the return of the clitoris to its flaccid state and, similarly, by the return of the labia majora and minora to their initial size, the disappearance of areolar tumescence (engorgement and erection of the nipples), the lowering of blood pressure, and a slower heart rate.

Female sexual problems

Unlike men, whose sexuality is much more genitally focused, a woman's is more complex and all encompassing; a woman's sexuality combines the physical and corporeal with the emotional and mental. Although it is a generalization, when a woman "entrusts her body" to a man, it is normal that her motivation for doing so is due to an emotional bond with him of some kind and not simply a means to obtain physical pleasure.

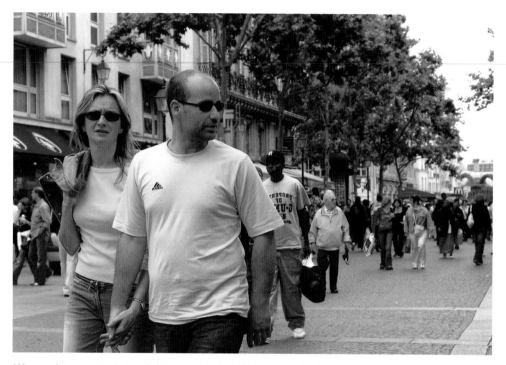

Women rely to a great extent on their hormonal cycles, which cause mood swings, unpredictability, and general changeability—as much a problem for women themselves as for their partners. Women are subject to a multitude of physical and psychological changes during the menstrual cycle, pregnancy, and the menopause.

Women should enjoy sex too

Whatever sexual dysfunction a woman may be suffering from, she needs to know that she, too, has a right to enjoy sex and that solutions exist for the great majority of these conditions. She should not hesitate to consult a gynecologist first to rule out any physical causes and, with her partner if necessary, visit a therapist or sexologist to treat and resolve the problem.

Female sexuality incorporates a variety of factors that condition a woman's sexual behavior:

Biological factors, including genital response, hormonal cycles, and procreation.

Psychological factors, which are as much to do with mood, as to do with emotions, to which it is important to add a socio-cultural factor, such as upbringing and ethical and moral values.

During sexual intercourse, women are less stimulated than men by visual triggers; however, stimulation does come about more strongly through auditory and tactile sensations.

Women become aroused more gradually than men and need an atmosphere of tenderness and gentleness. They have highly erogenous zones

The enjoyment that women get from their sex lives can be impaired by a number of factors, including the pressurized and competitive lifestyle of today, a poorly balanced diet, sexual roles and stereotyping, stress, addiction, depression, low self-esteem, and exaggerated personal expectations. A couple's relationship that can be described as monotonous and routine or, at its most serious, damaging and including psychological and physical abuse will doubtless have very negative repercussions on a woman's sexuality. As a general rule, once a relationship has gone downhill and there is neither communication nor respect, sexual activity ceases.

that produce enormous gratification if stimulated pleasurably. However, hurriedness, a demanding attitude, or an inexpert lover who concentrates more on himself than on his partner can result, for the woman's part, in dissatisfaction, frigidity, or failure to achieve orgasm, and can even make a woman wish to avoid sexual contact.

Female sexual dysfunction

Female sexual response is profoundly conditioned by psychological and emotional factors, which explains why, up until now, the efforts made to produce a female version of Viagra® have not been very profitable.

Female sexual dysfunction is a type of psychosomatic disorder that can manifest itself as a permanent or temporary condition in a woman's sex life and affect any of the phases of sexual response (desire, excitement, orgasm). Emotional and communication-related factors arising from the attitude of a woman's partner play a significant role in this.

In its most serious form, a very damaging relationship marked by denigration and verbal or physical aggression can cause a woman to become sexually dysfunctional, whereas, under different circumstances, she might enjoy a normal sexual response.

In general, women complain about their partners lacking romance, sensuality, and passion.

Faced with a male chauvinist attitude combined with a fear of losing their partner, some women feel obliged to fake orgasms.

The concept of frigidity, often employed contemptuously, has been used to generalize all types of female sexual dysfunction; however, the main types of dysfunction are inhibited sexual desire, anorgasmia, dyspareunia, and vaginismus.

Inhibited sexual desire: the general inhibition of desire and feeling of sexual excitement.

A woman suffering from this dysfunction sees lovemaking as a punishment.

A lack of communication with her partner and her own lack of interest result in a situation in which she invents excuses to avoid lovemaking, at the same time as feeling great dissatisfaction and fearing infidelity by her partner and abandonment.

The causes of this are essentially psychological in origin: boredom or routine, relationship disputes, fear of pleasure, anxiety, stress, depression, low physical self-esteem, etc.

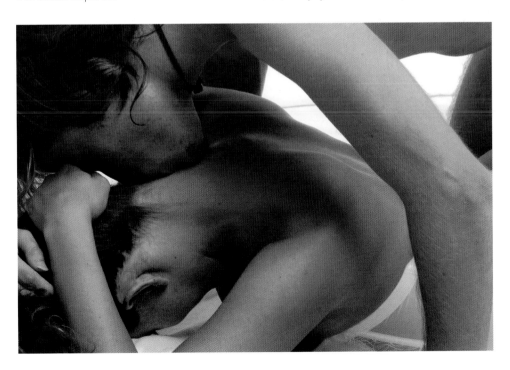

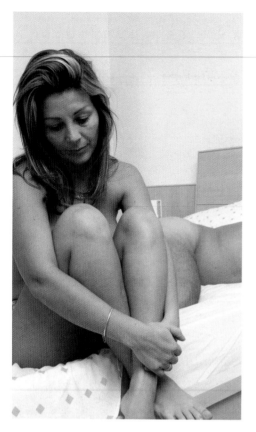

Causes of female sexual dysfunction

- Communication problems in a relationship.
- Anxiety or depression.
- Feelings of guilt and shame about sex.
- Fear of pain, catching a disease, or becoming pregnant.
- Lack of proper stimulation.
- Absence of lubrication.
- Changes relating to the menopause.
- Nerve damage due to surgery or traumatic injury.
- Medication.
- Infection or gynecological illness.
- Previous sexual abuse.

Dyspareunia refers to the pain that some women experience during intercourse that prevents them from enjoying sex. Apart from possible physical causes, such as infections or injury, the pain may be linked to psychological factors, such as a traumatic episode in the past, fear of pregnancy, or lack of sexual desire.

Anorgasmia: the inability to achieve orgasm despite feeling sexual excitement.

Different types of anorgasmia exist: primary anorgasmia, in which a woman has never experienced orgasm in her life; secondary anorgasmia, when she used to have orgasms but can no longer achieve them; absolute anorgasmia, when she is unable to achieve orgasm under any circumstances; situational anorgasmia, when she only achieves orgasm under certain circumstances; and random anorgasmia, when a woman can achieve orgasm but not as frequently as she feels is appropriate.

The main causes are psychological: traumatic sexual experiences, stress, depression, lack of information about sex, etc. Only five percent of cases have a physical cause due to some type of traumatic injury or drug use.

Dyspareunia: pain or discomfort felt by a woman during intercourse, often making it difficult or impossible. This ranges from a minor vaginal complaint or irritation to extreme pain.

The causes may be physical in origin, such as an infection, genitourinary diseases, allergies to barrier contraceptives (condoms, diaphragms, intrauterine devices (IUDs), spermicidal agents), vaginal dryness, and, in old age, senile vaginitis.

Psychological causes include loss of interest in a partner or past sexual trauma, and these can mean a lack of excitement at the time of penetration and insufficient vaginal lubrication.

Vaginismus: the inability to have sexual intercourse due to the reflex contraction of the pubococcygeus muscle affecting the lower third of the vagina.

Women suffering from vaginismus can sometimes benefit from the use of sex toys and even reach orgasm, as long as it does not involve penetration.

In most cases, the causes are psychological: lack of information about sex, traumatic experiences, rape, sexual abuse, fear of pregnancy, or fear of contracting a sexually transmitted disease (STD).

family planning and contraception

Sex involves much more than the capacity to procreate: it is through sex that a man enjoys, loves, communicates, and shares with his partner. But the capacity to procreate is an intrinsic aspect of life as a couple, even if you decide that you do not want to have children. In today's society, it is becoming increasingly necessary to plan for the arrival of a child in order to engage in and enjoy the responsibility of parenthood. Contraception is becoming more and more accepted and practiced by couples who are not ready to start a family. Experience shows that family planning and contraceptive methods are the best way to avoid the incidence of unwanted pregnancies. Abortions are one of the most significant causes of illness and death in women from deprived social and economic backgrounds and in countries with restrictive abortion laws.

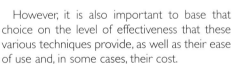

Many types of contraception have been developed in recent years in an attempt to meet the needs of most, if not all, couples.

Every couple is able to choose from one or more types of contraception, with health always uppermost in mind.

Contraception, whether for men or women, involves a collection of techniques intended to prevent conception and thus avoid pregnancy. Birth control techniques have been practiced for over 3,000 years.

However, it is also important to base that choice on the level of effectiveness that these various techniques provide, as well as their ease of use and, in some cases, their cost.

Couples may also decide to postpone pregnancy when medical conditions, such as diabetes, high blood pressure, cardiovascular problems, HIV, congenital illnesses, etc. threaten the health of the mother and/or the future baby. There is a best choice and more appropriate type of con-

Being able to plan to have a baby makes a couple more responsible.

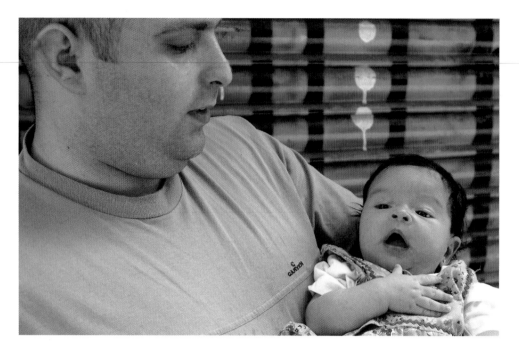

traception in each case, depending on the reason for not wishing to have a child. In such cases, it is very important to consult a doctor on the best method of contraception to use.

Types of contraceptive technique

Natural methods: These are not usually very effective, because the body and its physiology do not comply rigidly with a mathematical approach to a woman's cycle.

Coitus interruptus: Suddenly interrupting sexual intercourse as soon as a man feels that he is about to ejaculate.

Basal body temperature method: This involves consulting tables relating to body temperature throughout the menstrual cycle in order to spot the peak in temperature produced by ovulation. This method has a low level of reliability.

The Billings ovulation method: This attempts to verify when a woman is ovulating by observing the amount of cervical mucus in the vagina.

Vaginal douching: This is not recommended because it usually cannot be done quickly enough to flush out the sperm, and in fact may even force the sperm further up into the uterus.

Sexual abstinence.

Until very recently, birth control was considered to be a women's responsibility. Family planning had been regarded as a task exclusive to women, given that it was women who experienced maternity in a direct sense. Nowadays, having a child is seen as the concern of both parties and, in fact, men have accepted an increasingly important role in avoiding pregnancy.

Barrier methods: These prevent sperm from entering the vagina.
Male and female condoms.
Diaphragm.

Chemical and hormonal methods:
Spermicides.
Hormonal contraception can be taken in a variety of forms and also exists to suppress ovulation for months at a time:
Orally – "The Pill".
Subcutaneous contraception (injections).
Contraceptive vaginal ring.
Contraceptive patches.
Intrauterine device (IUD).

Irreversible (or partially reversible) contraceptive methods:

Tubal ligation for women (tying off the Fallopian tubes).

Vasectomy for men.

Emergency methods:

Morning-after pill: Only to be used in an emergency, as it has many side effects.

▪ Factors to bear in mind when deciding on a form of birth control

- **Availability:** It is important to consider the availability of any given type of contraception. For example, can it be obtained without prescription, without the need to consult a specialist, or, in the case of minors, without parental consent?

- **Cost:** This is another matter to bear in mind when assessing whether using a type of contraception is feasible for a couple. In order to raise awareness in young people or those less predisposed to use contraception, it may be practical to compare the cost to them of birth control with the cost and consequences that follow from an unplanned pregnancy.

- **Effectiveness:** How effective is a particular form of birth control? How well does it prevent conception? It is important to be aware of the level of effectiveness of a given technique, both statistically and in relation to the individual characteristics of each person, in order to assess what the most effective method for a couple to use really is.

- **Health risks:** Health and safety must always come first for everyone. For that reason, you should weigh up the potential safety aspect of

particular contraceptive methods from an individual perspective. Some birth control methods may not be good choices because of the potential risks that they pose to health—as can happen in some cases with oral contraceptives.

- **Unplanned pregnancy:** When choosing a method of contraception, an individual or couple must keep in mind the possibility that an unplanned pregnancy might still occur despite their best efforts. If having a child would have disastrous consequences, you must choose the most effective method possible. On the other hand, if a couple are simply trying to postpone a pregnancy but feel that if pregnancy occurred sooner than expected it would not be entirely unwelcome, they will be less concerned with effectiveness than with other aspects, such as comfort or cost.

- **Commitment of both partners:** The commitment and willingness of both partners is very important in order for any method of contraception to work properly and thus to avoid unplanned pregnancies.

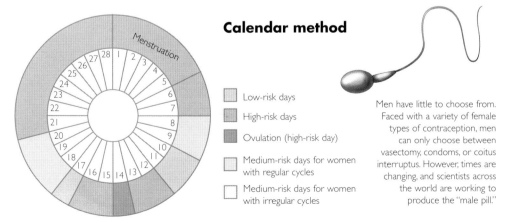

Calendar method

▢ Low-risk days

▣ High-risk days

▣ Ovulation (high-risk day)

▢ Medium-risk days for women with regular cycles

▢ Medium-risk days for women with irregular cycles

Men have little to choose from. Faced with a variety of female types of contraception, men can only choose between vasectomy, condoms, or coitus interruptus. However, times are changing, and scientists across the world are working to produce the "male pill."

◼ The ideal male contraceptive would be one that satisfies the following conditions:

- Provides maximum safety.
- Does not produce side effects.
- Is acceptable to the partner.
- Does not affect libido, virility, sexual potency, or the possibility of pregnancy at some point in the future.
- Does not interfere with the spontaneity of lovemaking.

Male contraceptives

The condom

The condom, prophylactic, or rubber, among other names, is a thin, cylindrical sheath, both pliable and elastic, that is placed over the erect penis before penetrative sex, whether vaginal, anal, or oral.

It acts as a barrier and prevents semen from entering the vagina, stopping sperm from reaching the cervix.

What to do if a condom gets lodged inside the vagina

After ejaculation, the penis generally loses its volume and firmness, resulting in the condom becoming too big for its contents. Therefore, it can slip off and be left behind in the vagina if a man does not pull out immediately. Consequently, when withdrawing, you should hold the base of the condom firmly to prevent it from slipping. If a condom has been left inside and you are unable to remove it with your fingers, you should visit a medical center immediately where staff can extract it and supply any medication necessary to prevent a possible unwanted pregnancy.

For condoms to be effective it is very important to use them properly:

Always use approved condoms made of quality latex with a small teat or reservoir at the end. If a condom does not have that feature, put it on in such a way that you leave some room

ADVANTAGES	DISADVANTAGES
Easy to use and obtain.	Lack spontaneity.
Do not require medical assessment.	Reduce sensitivity.
Reduce the risk of cervical cancer in women.	There is a risk of rupture (approximately 2 percent for vaginal sex and 10 percent for anal sex).
High safety. Condoms are very effective if used correctly, especially if used in combination with spermicides or other contraceptive agents.	They can engender a sense of emotional or psychological rejection, as they prevent direct genital contact between partners.
They offer protection against sexually transmitted diseases, especially HIV, although protection is not total in all cases.	For men who find it difficult to achieve or maintain an erection, using a condom can exacerbate their problem or anxieties.

at the end into which to ejaculate.

Always check the use-by date.

A condom can be used once only.

Do not try out a condom in advance. Do not inflate or stretch it before putting it on.

A condom should be put on when your penis is erect.

You should open a condom wrapper on one side using your fingers, and you should never use your teeth, scissors, or other sharp-edged implements, as the condom can be torn as a result.

Wearing two condoms at once is not safer. Using two condoms at a time creates greater friction between the latex surfaces, which can make tearing more likely. Using one condom at a time is perfectly adequate.

Only use water-based lubricants. Products that are petroleum- or oil-based are inappropriate, because they damage the latex and

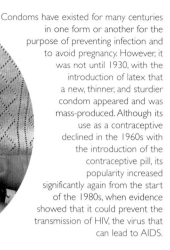

Condoms have existed for many centuries in one form or another for the purpose of preventing infection and to avoid pregnancy. However, it was not until 1930, with the introduction of latex that a new, thinner, and sturdier condom appeared and was mass-produced. Although its use as a contraceptive declined in the 1960s with the introduction of the contraceptive pill, its popularity increased significantly again from the start of the 1980s, when evidence showed that it could prevent the transmission of HIV, the virus that can lead to AIDS.

◾ What to do if a condom becomes ruptured

In such an instance, the best solution is to visit a medical center (hospital emergency room or family planning center) as soon as possible—within 48 hours following intercourse—so that the gynecologist can prescribe the woman with the morning-after pill and thus avoid a possible unwanted pregnancy.

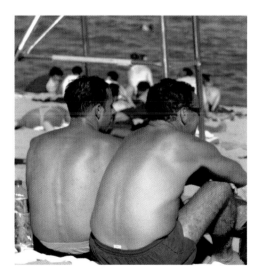

The transmission of HIV and other STDs during sexual intercourse can be effectively prevented if quality condoms are used correctly and consistently.

increase the likelihood that the condom will tear.

Coitus interruptus

Also referred to as the "withdrawal method." This is a traditional method of birth control and, despite what you might think, is very widespread. It is a technique that requires the man to withdraw his penis from the vagina before he reaches orgasm and ejaculates. Consequently, his sperm does not reach the vagina and there is no possibility of conception. However, this method requires considerable skill on the part of the man. It is unreliable compared with other methods of birth control. Some couples are sufficiently self-disciplined that they use this as a form of contraception, but it needs a lot of practice and skill to perfect it. Pregnancy can occur with this method, because:

Withdrawal may be incomplete, or because the man may be unable to withdraw in time;

Pre-ejaculatory fluid can contain sperm that may be left in the vagina prior to orgasm and withdrawal of the penis;

Ejaculating on a part of the body close to the vagina can result in sperm finding a way inside despite withdrawal and thus going on to fertilize an egg.

This method is also blamed for problems in sexual relationships due to the difficulty the woman then has in achieving orgasm, which can create dissatisfaction and even pelvic congestion. It also affects a man, because he has the worry of ejaculating and has less time to think about lovemaking and pleasure.

How to use a condom

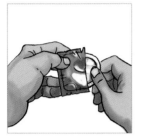

1: Open the wrapper by tearing off one side, and remove the condom using your fingers. Never use teeth, scissors, or other sharp implements, which could damage the condom. Check that you have it the right way up so that it rolls down correctly.

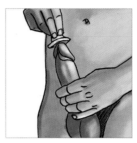

2: Hold the condom tightly by the reservoir teat using your thumb and index finger. This prevents air from entering the reservoir. Your partner can take part in this as part of the foreplay prior to penetration.

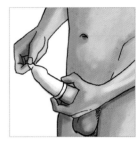

3: Place the condom on the head of the penis and, without letting go of the reservoir, unroll the condom along the length of the penis.

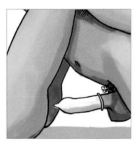

4: The condom should be rolled onto the penis when it is erect and prior to penetration, whether vaginal, anal, or oral.

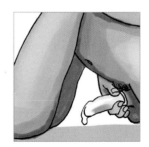

5: After ejaculation, withdraw the penis before losing your erection. You should hold the condom at its base when withdrawing to avoid the condom being left inside or spilling its contents inside the vagina or anus.

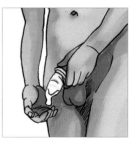

6: Once you have withdrawn the condom, you should check it for any tearing, then tie a knot in it to prevent it from leaking, and dispose of it in the garbage.

The femidom

- The femidom (female condom) consists of a kind of cylinder-shaped polyurethane bag that is inserted into the vagina to protect its walls and is supported outside by a ring that also covers the clitoris and the vulva's labia minora.

- Being made from a strong and resistant material, it is not very flexible, which is why it is usually used together with lubricants and spermicides.

- As with the male condom, it should never be reused; a new one should be used for every fresh act of intercourse.

What happens to the sperm?

The testicles continue to produce sperm, but, they die, in the absence of any exit, and the body eliminates them by itself.

A vasectomy can be reversed through microsurgical techniques called "vasovasostomy," although the re-establishment of fertility as a result cannot be guaranteed.

Vasectomy

Vasectomy is the most radical method of male birth control, but it is also the most effective: after treatment, pregnancies are rare—at less than 1 percent. This technique, which has become increasingly straightforward, consists of cutting and interrupting both of the vas deferens tubes through which sperm passes from the testicles to the penis. This technique produces a complete absence of spermatozoa in a man's semen. Although vasectomy is widely thought of as an irreversible intervention, the possibility of a reverse procedure certainly exists by means of microsurgery, referred to as "vasovasostomy." This procedure is expensive, complex, and not always successful. Rejoining the vas deferens ducts can take up to four hours of surgery under general anesthesia.

A vasectomy is a simple, effective, and safe operation that stops a man from fathering children.

Given that the procedure is irreversible in most cases, taking this decision is a major step for both partners. It is therefore very important for couples to be fully aware of all the facts relating to this type of surgery and their implications.

A man and his partner must be certain about this decision and not want to have children or any more children than they already have. It is important to bear all options in mind. You should not forget that circumstances arise in life—such as a divorce, separation, or remarriage—that might make you want to have children after all. Consequently, a man must be absolutely sure about his decision.

Reasons for a vasectomy

- You already have all the children that you want.
- You are unable to maintain and raise any future children.
- You want to enjoy sexual relations without worrying about unwanted pregnancies.
- Both you and your partner do not like or cannot use other methods of birth control.
- Vasectomy is simpler and less expensive than female sterilization (tubal ligation).
- You want to avoid pregnancies that would be high risk to mother and/or baby due to health problems or congenital diseases.

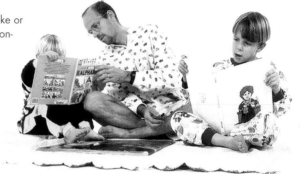

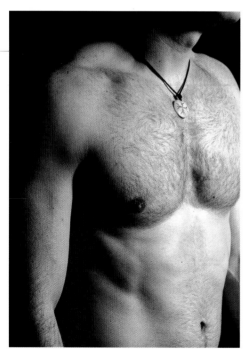

A vasectomy takes about 15 minutes, does not require hospitalization, and is performed under local anesthesia. However, it is not fully effective for some three months afterward, or until a man has ejaculated roughly 20 times. The risks and side effects are minimal, and in no case has a vasectomy affected either a man's sex drive or his capacity to get an erection. Men continue to ejaculate the same as before; the sole difference is that their semen does not contain any sperm.

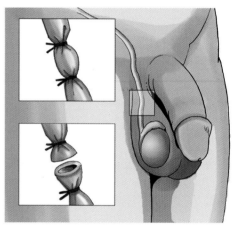

A vasectomy is a means of contraception, i.e. it prevents pregnancies. However, vasectomy cannot under any circumstances provide protection against STDs or venereal diseases. To be protected against such infections, it is necessary to keep on using other prophylactic methods, such as condoms.

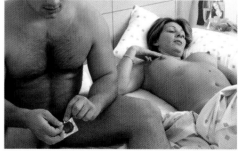

ADVANTAGES	DISADVANTAGES
Permanent method of birth control.	Requires a surgical procedure under local anesthesia.
Does not interfere with sexual relations, neither does it affect a man's sexual potency.	It does not offer protection against STDs.
Safer and less expensive than female sterilization.	Regrets after the operation.
There are no serious risks or long-term side effects.	There is no guarantee that fertility can ever be restored.

After a vasectomy, you are recommended to...

Rest for one or two days.

Apply ice to the scrotum to prevent swelling.

Take anti-inflammatory or painkiller medication if you feel discomfort.

Wear an athletic supporter or jockstrap or, if you do not have one, tight-fitting underwear.

Use some form of contraception until your physician confirms that sperm are no longer detectable in your semen. Sperm usually disappear after 4 to 8 weeks and after 20 to 30 ejaculations.

Continue as normal with your sex life after a week, or whenever you feel comfortable, depending on the advice of your physician.

◾ What does vasectomy involve?

Vasectomy is performed with the man lying face up and with the penis and scrotum uncovered.

Local anesthesia is used, meaning that the man is awake and fully conscious but feels no pain. The anesthetic is injected into the scrotum, the groin, and the adjacent areas. A man will notice that he is being touched, but it will not be painful.

Using a fine scalpel, a small incision or cut is then made in the skin where the vas deferens is located.

Since the reproductive organs consist of two testicles and thus two vas deferens ducts, two incisions will have to be made for each duct in the majority of cases.

(Some surgeons use a technique in which only one incision is made, but this is rare.)

Part of the vas deferens is pulled out of each incision and a cut is then made through it. The two cut ends of the duct are sewn up and remain separate without any link that might allow sperm to pass from one end to the other. Finally, the incision is closed.

A vasectomy does not affect a man's sex life in any way. He will continue to have the same erections that he had before the operation and will continue to ejaculate the semen produced by secretions from the prostate gland and the seminal vesicles. The sole difference is that the semen will not contain any sperm.

Vasectomy does not affect a man's sex drive. The hormones that regulate sex drive continue to be produced in the testicles and are absorbed directly into the bloodstream. Consequently, there is no adverse effect on a man's libido.

As with any surgical procedure, however minor, complications can occur, albeit infrequently. Although uncommon, after a vasectomy the side effects can include:

Infection of the wound. Aches, fever, and a general feeling of illness occur when the area operated on becomes infected.

Epididymitis. If you feel testicular swelling, discomfort, and pain, it may be that the epididymis has become infected.

Bleeding in the scrotum with a hematoma.

Female contraception methods

Women have many more ways to prevent conceptionavailable to them than men —although that does not mean that contraception is consequently a woman's sole responsibility. Pregnancy is a matter for two people and, if it is not wanted, preventing it should be a shared responsibility.

Diaphragm

This is a barrier method of contraception. It consists of a flexible rubberized or plastic container that is inserted into the vagina before sexual intercourse such that it surrounds the cervix. It is filled with a spermicidal agent to ensure that sperm cannot pass into the uterus beyond. It is put in place a few hours before sex and should be removed six to seven hours afterward. Diaphragms can be obtained with a medical prescription with the advice of a doctor and are more expensive than other contraceptives, such as condoms.

Contraceptive sponge

These are synthetic sponges impregnated with spermicide. The sponge is soaked before sexual intercourse, inserted into the vagina, and placed over the cervix. After intercourse, the sponge must be left in place for six to eight hours. This method is similar to the diaphragm.

IUD (intrauterine device)

This is a small device that is inserted into the uterus and prevents a fertilized egg from attaching to the uterine lining. There are different types available, made from a variety of materials: plastic, copper, and silver. The most recent designs have reduced the risk of infection and are usually tolerated better than before. IUDs are one of the most popular contraception

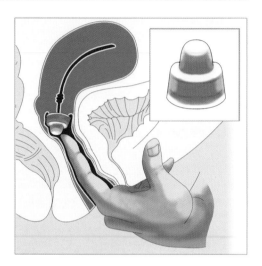

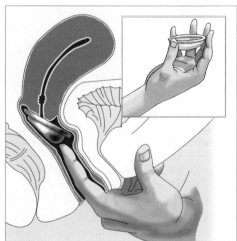

methods among women, because they do not interfere with intercourse and do not affect fertility once removed. The insertion of an IUD must be done by a gynecologist, and it must be changed regularly every 3 years and checked every 6 months.

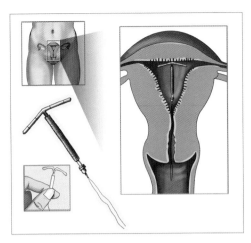

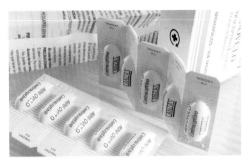

a range of healthy effects, such as reducing acne and the incidence of certain types of ovarian and endometrial cancer. Furthermore, it regulates the cycle and reduces menstrual pain and bleeding.

Cervical cap

This method of contraception is very similar to the diaphragm, the only difference being its thimble-shaped appearance.

Tubal ligation

This refers to surgical sterilization and is the female equivalent of a vasectomy. It involves a permanent procedure that prevents eggs from being transported to the uterus by sealing the Fallopian tubes. This operation can be performed through laparoscopy or once a baby has been removed from the womb in the event of a Caesarian section. Although tubal ligation is treated as a permanent procedure, there have been some instances in which it has been reversed.

Spermicides

These are foams, creams, or suppositories that act by killing spermatozoa and are inserted into the vagina before sexual intercourse. They are easily obtained from the majority of pharmacies. Spermicides are not very effective if used on their own, but if they are used in combination with a condom or diaphragm, they are very good at preventing pregnancy.

Contraceptive pill

The pill is based on a group of hormones that prevent pregnancy in different ways: it overrides ovulation so that the ovaries fail to release an egg and it also causes changes to the cervical mucus, making it thicker and thus making it more difficult for spermatozoa to swim toward the uterus. The pill also prevents the uterine lining from developing enough to accommodate and nourish a fertilized egg. The pill has side effects for women over 35 who smoke, are obese, or have high blood pressure, as it increases their risk of being affected by cardiovascular diseases. Taking the pill does not reduce fertility and is linked to

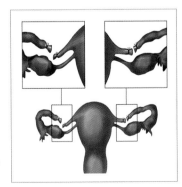

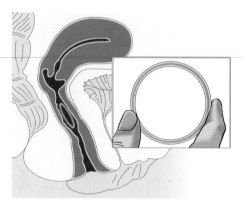

Tubal ligation refers to surgical sterilization and is the female equivalent of a vasectomy.

Subcutaneous implant

This involves a matchstick-sized plastic rod impregnated with a hormone being placed under the skin. Once under the skin, a constant dose of hormone is released for a period of three years. Its mechanism inhibits ovulation. Its main advantage is convenience, as a woman does not have to worry while it is fully functional. Its drawbacks are essentially the minor surgical procedure required to insert and extract the rod and a lack of control over the menstrual cycle.

Contraceptive patches

This method has some similarity to the contraceptive ring as it also frees a woman from the daily responsibility of taking oral contraceptives. It provides the body with the hormones necessary to prevent an unplanned pregnancy. In the case of patches, the hormones are absorbed through the skin. Each patch lasts for a week, and so three different patches are used over the course of one cycle (one a week); no patch is use in the fourth week, when the period occurs, as with all types of hormonal contraceptive.

Contraceptive vaginal ring

This is a flexible ring measuring approximately 2 inches in diameter. It is inserted into the vagina, where it releases the hormones progestogen and estrogen to prevent pregnancy. A woman can insert the device herself and leave it in the vagina for three weeks, removing it every fourth week for the week when she has her period. Hormonal contraception requires a medical prescription and regular assessment.

Emergency contraception

The post-coital pill is not a method of contraception but an emergency measure. It consists of a combination of hormones that alters the female reproductive cycle, thus preventing pregnancy from becoming established. The "morning-after pill" acts by suppressing ovulation, preventing fertilization, or, if an egg has been fertilized, preventing it from implanting in the uterine lining. It has an almost 100 percent rate of success when taken in the 24 hours immediately following an episode of risky intercourse. It can be administered only with a medical prescription.

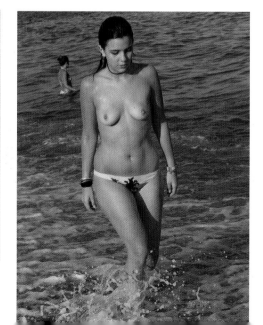

men and pregnancy

Deciding to be a father is one of the most important decisions in a man's life. One thing is for certain, regardless of a man's age, circumstances, or marital status, the arrival of a new being will affect his life in a whole multitude of ways. In particular, his relationship with his partner deepens, and a much stronger, lifelong bond is created—even if partners split up or divorce. The journey into fatherhood can be a very productive time in a man's life, providing new social, emotional, and even financial challenges. Despite the problems and difficulties that can arise, being a father can be one of the most enriching experiences in a man's life.

Conception

From the very moment of conception, a woman's body starts to undergo changes and the first signs of pregnancy begin to show.

The first step is to visit the gynecologist, who will confirm whether a woman is indeed pregnant and order tests and controls to be done.

The development of the fetus varies greatly in the three trimesters of pregnancy: its major organs form in the first trimester; in the second, development continues and the baby's various organs become more complex; while in the third trimester, the fetus increases in size, readying itself for birth.

This process produces major physical and psychological changes in the mother. In the first trimester, it is common for her to feel tired, drowsy, and nauseous. During the second trimester, a woman generally feels very active and positive. In the third trimester, it is normal for her to feel anxious and suffer some discomfort and tiredness faced with the imminence of childbirth.

All women experience some discomfort during pregnancy. These episodes of discomfort are not usually signs of something more serious and normally disappear after the birth. However, more serious complications requiring medical intervention can arise. For that reason, it is necessary for a pregnant woman to have regular checkups, and she should consult her gynecologist in the event of any symptoms that appear out of the ordinary.

Exercising and maintaining a balanced diet are essential to a healthy pregnancy, as they assist the fetus in developing properly, reduce discomfort for the woman, and help make labor easier.

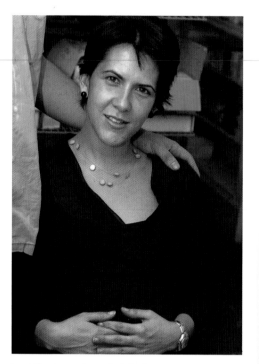

In addition to regular medical checkups, once a woman suspects she is pregnant, she must adopt a variety of elementary precautions, avoiding exposure to harmful substances and sources of infection to safeguard the baby's development.

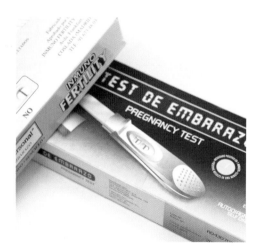

The first symptoms

The clearest sign for the majority of women is that their periods cease. Before this, some women also notice other changes, such as more sensitive, swollen breasts, nausea, dizziness, vomiting, fatigue, and the need to urinate more often.

It is not uncommon, particularly during the first trimester, for a woman to feel repelled by certain foods, odors, and tastes that she once liked. Moreover, she may experience sudden mood swings and increased sensitivity, which can affect relationships with her partner and those closest to her.

If confronted with these initial symptoms, it is advisable to have them confirmed as signaling pregnancy—the existence of one or more of these signs does not necessarily mean that a woman is definitely pregnant.

Initially, many women resort to using the pregnancy test kits typically available from pharmacies. These simple urine-testing kits detect the presence of the hormone human chorionic gonadotropin (hCG), the role of which is to separate estrogen and progesterone at the start of pregnancy in order to form the placenta. The manufacturers of these kits guarantee that they are virtually 100 percent reliable.

A more precise urine analysis to detect the presence of this hormone can be done in a laboratory. However, the definitive test for pregnancy is diagnostic ultrasound, which leaves no possible room for doubt.

Whatever the case, visits to the gynecologist are mandatory. From this time onward, the gynecologist is the one who will establish the guidelines to follow over the next nine months, as each pregnancy is different.

In most urine-testing kits, all that you need to do is place the reagent in contact with the urine sample and read the results after 3 minutes (the time required depends on the brand). A change in color shows the presence of hCG. A control window allows you to verify whether the test has been done correctly. If a mistake has been made when using the kit, the window remains blank.

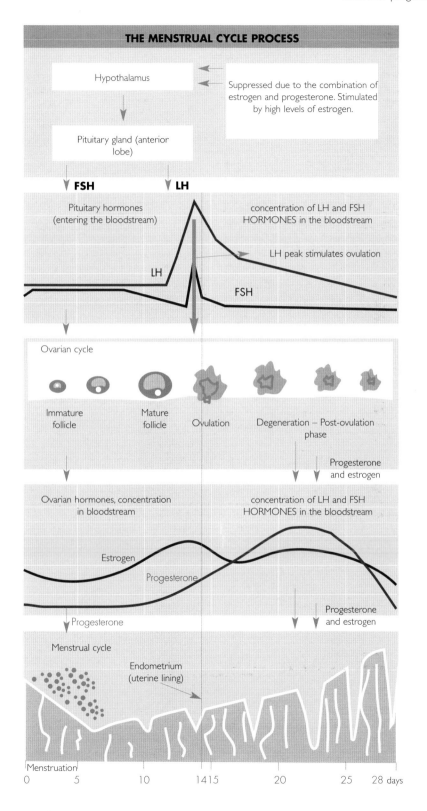

THE MENSTRUAL CYCLE PROCESS

Hypothalamus

Suppressed due to the combination of estrogen and progesterone. Stimulated by high levels of estrogen.

Pituitary gland (anterior lobe)

FSH   **LH**

Pituitary hormones (entering the bloodstream)

concentration of LH and FSH HORMONES in the bloodstream

LH peak stimulates ovulation

LH

FSH

Ovarian cycle

Immature follicle

Mature follicle

Ovulation

Degeneration – Post-ovulation phase

Progesterone and estrogen

Ovarian hormones, concentration in bloodstream

concentration of LH and FSH HORMONES in the bloodstream

Estrogen

Progesterone

Progesterone and estrogen

Progesterone

Menstrual cycle

Endometrium (uterine lining)

Menstruation

0   5   10   1415   20   25   28 days

Pregnancy step-by-step

The news that you are to be a father can spark a host of emotions, often contradictory: happiness on one hand, concern and fear on the other. Worries are normal and commonplace for all fathers during pregnancy. The future baby is not only the mother's. Although a man can-not participate physically in gestation, he can be closely involved in the whole process and can take part in all the medical checkups and preparations for birth. Moreover, he can help and support his partner at a time of so many major physical and emotional changes so that her pregnancy culminates in a joyful birth and a healthy baby.

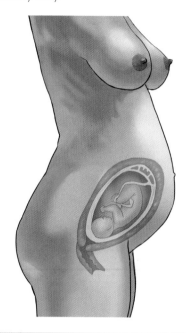

First trimester

Some women do not show any outward signs of being pregnant in the first trimester of gestation. However, it is at this time that a woman's body adjusts to the pregnancy and undergoes major hormonal changes.

- Absence of menstruation.
- Increased volume and sensitivity of the breasts.
- Darker pigmentation of the nipples.
- Feeling of fatigue and drowsiness.
- Possible nausea and dizziness, especially in the morning.
- Increase in weight by between 2¼ to 4½ lbs.
- Increase in size of the uterus.
- Increased vaginal secretions.
- Slight discomfort in the pelvic region.
- Frequent need to urinate.
- Rapid mood swings.
- Insecurity and anxiety.

Second trimester

Generally speaking, women feel much better in this period, as some of the discomfort and initial irritations disappear.

- Increase of 8¾ lbs in weight.
- In some cases, the breasts start to secrete colostrum (breast milk).
- The belly starts to bulge.
- The fetus makes its first detectable movements.
- The line between the navel and pubic hair darkens.
- Chloasma or the "mask of pregnancy" appears—facial marks or patches of freckles
- Physical discomfort may appear, such as heartburn or a blocked nose.
- A woman feels more positive and secure and experiences fewer mood swings.

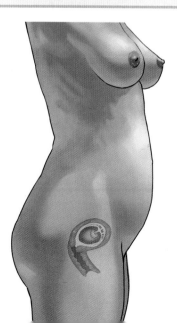

Third trimester

Women begin to feel increasingly impatient about seeing the baby and going into labor.

- Increase of between 6½ and 11 lbs in weight.
- Appearance of fatigue and back pain.
- Frequent need to urinate.
- Increased perspiration.
- Uterine contractions.
- Worries and fears about the imminent birth.

from the first week, and the heart begins to beat almost at the end of the month. The placenta starts to form around the embryo, which measures approximately ¼ inch.

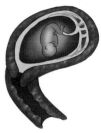

Third month: The fetus is already fully formed and moves its legs and arms. It has eyelids and measures about 4 inches. It weighs about 1½ oz.

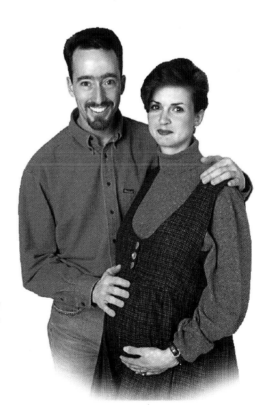

What are the stages of pregnancy?

First month: The embryo's appearance is similar to a disk. The head starts to develop

Fourth month: The fetus is covered in fine, transparent skin. Its body is completely enveloped in a covering of fine hair referred to as "lanugo." Its intestines start to fill will a greenish substance called "meconium." The fetus weighs about 6½ oz and measures just under 6 inches.

Sixth month: The fetus spends between 18 and 20 hours asleep and moves a lot when awake. Its face is complete and it can already open its eyes. The lungs are developing. It measures about 10 inches and weighs almost 2 lbs 3 oz.

Ninth month: The fetus receives antibodies from its mother, and its lungs are now ready to work outside the womb. The skin is no longer wrinkled, and the lanugo is shed almost completely. The fetus weighs close to 6 lbs 10 oz and measures about 20 inches.

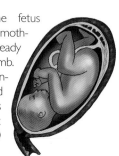

You and your child

The relationship with your child can begin much earlier than at its birth, while it is still in the womb:

- From the second trimester, you can connect with the fetus by feeling it kicking or feeling the movements it makes in response to the sounds that it hears.

- In the final stage of pregnancy, parts of the baby's anatomy become identifiable, and you can start to caress the child.

- You can also listen to its heartbeats by placing your ear to your partner's belly just below the navel. The heartbeat will sound very fast.

Couvade syndrome (Sympathetic pregnancy)

- Couvade syndrome is a name that derives from the French word couver meaning to "incubate" or "hatch" and affects some fathers during their partner's pregnancy.

- When the syndrome occurs in men, they experience pregnancy symptoms normally associated with women.

- According to various studies, this syndrome occurs in 10 to 65 percent of fathers-to-be, and it is estimated that 1 in 4 men consult a doctor with some of its symptoms.

- As a rule, symptoms start after the third month of gestation or at the time approaching birth and mimic the typical symptoms of pregnancy.

- Men may also experience mood swings, nausea, vomiting, fatigue, low blood pressure, leg cramps, and abdominal pains similar to uterine contractions.

- Various theories exist to attempt to explain these symptoms. Some studies relate these symptoms to the hormonal changes that arise in pregnant women. According to these studies, women might be emanating chemical signals that their partners are picking up. These generate in the man a protective state of mind toward his partner, and at the same time cause the symptoms of sympathetic pregnancy tso that, to some extent, he shares them with her throughout the whole of the gestation period.

- Other studies indicate that men undergo hormonal changes during their partner's pregnancy. An increase in the level of prolactin and cortisol in men is said to generate the symptoms and behavior exhibited by most fathers and those fathers-to-be who are already submerged in the world of babies.

The role of the father

One way in which a man can participates actively in his partner's pregnancy is by trying to be involved in everything that is to happen, keeping himself well informed and going with his partner to antenatal checkups, getting to know the medical staff who will be monitoring and assisting with the pregnancy, taking part in pre-birth parenting classes leading up to the birth, and being present at the birth itself.

Antenatal checkups are routine office visits made in order to monitor the progress of a pregnancy and the development of the child, as well as to prepare properly for the birth.

Checkups during pregnancy are usually at walk-in clinics. In the majority of cases, they do not require the involvement of expensive or complex equipment. The objectives are:

To detect any illness in the mother.

To prevent, make early diagnosis of, and treat any complications that might arise during pregnancy.

To monitor the normal growth and health of the child. Nowadays, highly advanced technolo-

Monitoring the future mother's weight gain is another of the routine antenatal checks. Both being underweight and being overweight can present risks to mother and baby. Maternal malnutrition can result in: a baby with a low birth weight, premature birth, premature rupture of the amniotic sac, etc. A woman should be examined if her weight increases suddenly and dramatically, as it may be the result of conditions such as high blood pressure, diabetes, hyperthyroidism, increased amniotic fluid, etc.

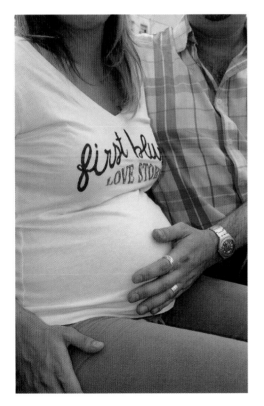

gy exists capable of dealing with any medical conditions that the baby might present before its birth (fetal surgery).

To reduce the symptoms and discomfort associated with pregnancy.

To prepare the mother and father both physically and mentally for labor.

To provide support and education on the subject of family health and childcare.

After it has been confirmed that a women is expecting a baby, the first checkups usually assess the signs and symptoms during the first trimester of pregnancy:

Cessation of menstruation.
Enlargement and sensitivity of the breasts.
Intolerance to certain odors and foods.
Dizziness, nausea, vomiting.
Increased need for sleep.
Emotional changes, etc.

During this first stage, it is very important to take iron to prevent anemia and folic acid to prevent fetal abnormalities (hydrocephalus, spina bifida, etc.).

The mother undergoes profound changes during pregnancy, and these need to be monitored carefully.

The baby also has to be assessed throughout its gestation. It should be remembered that the first trimester is fundamental to its development.

A complete screening of the mother to detect anemia and infections, such as toxoplasmosis, and STDs, such as syphilis, HIV, hepatitis B, etc.

Determining the mother and baby's blood group and Rh factor to identify any possible conflict.

Performing a first-trimester ultrasound scan in which an assessment is made of the position of the gestational sac and fetal health, and the number of weeks that the woman has been pregnant is confirmed.

After the first 17–18 weeks of pregnancy, it is possible to hear the fetus's heartbeats via an amplifying instrument. The normal cardiac frequency should be between 120 and 160 beats a minute.

What is a genetic assessment?

All couples want their baby to be normal and healthy and, as a result, one of the greatest concerns of future parents is, whether the baby has Down's syndrome or any other congenital abnormality of some sort.

There are various types of diagnostic procedure. Some do not compromise the health of the fetus at all; others may include an element of risk.

Tests that present no risk to the baby are ultrasound scans and the analysis of blood samples taken from the mother to assess fetal proteins and hormones.

Amniocentesis (amniotic fluid testing) and chorionic villus (placental tissue) sampling can present a risk to the baby, although only in very few cases.

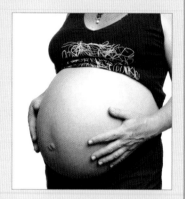

▪ Ultrasonography

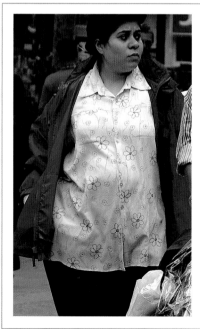

Ultrasonography is a diagnostic tool that uses ultrasound to monitor the fetus as well as the placenta, amniotic fluid, wall of the uterus, etc. The World Health Organization (WHO) recommends taking three ultrasound scans during pregnancy, but the actual number will depend on each individual case.

What can you see from an ultrasound scan?

• Between week 8 and 12: the gestational age of the fetus, whether the egg is normal, and whether it is a multiple pregnancy.

• Between week 12 and 15: the scan confirms the gestational age of the future baby and reveals any sign of embryonic anomalies that require subsequent confirmation (e.g. Down's syndrome).

• Between week 20 and 22: checks for malformations, fetal growth, location of the placenta, sex, fetal activity.

• Between week 34 and 36: growth of the fetus, any abnormalities with the placenta or amniotic fluid, malformations, sex, chronic fetal distress, femur length, biparietal diameter (measurements across the head forward and sideways), abdominal circumference, position, and approximate weight.

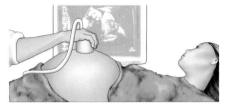

- When performing an ultrasound scan, the woman lies on a gurney, and a transparent conductor gel is applied to her abdomen and pelvis, which helps transmit the sound waves. Next, the physician moves the transducer over the abdomen and the image obtained of the baby appears on a monitor.
- Another method is to place the transducer in the patient's vagina (transvaginal ultrasound scan).

- This technique complements conventional ultrasound technology, as it provides better detail.

Biochemical markers

Various biochemical markers found in the mother's blood serum can reveal information about the unborn child, particularly chromosomal abnormality that can be an indication of Down's syndrome. Examining the serum for such abnormalities is not conclusive, and can only point to "increased risk" of the child having some form of abnormality. Other conditions that may be indicated are neural tube defects like spina bifida and anencephaly. Conversely, biochemical markers may reveal little risk of such conditions, whereas the conditions do exist—a false negative. For this reason, either of the tests below is preferable to give clear information, although they do present some risks of causing a miscarriage.

Amniocentesis

This procedure can be performed from week 16 under local anesthesia. A needle is inserted through the abdominal wall and wall of the uterus until it reaches the uterine cavity. A small amount of amniotic fluid is then obtained for analysis. This procedure is monitored using a constant ultrasound display to avoid injury to either the baby or the placenta.

The fluid and its cells are analyzed and the results returned within three weeks.

Chorionic biopsy

An abdominal puncture can be performed after the ninth week of gestation. It is performed under a local anesthetic, and an ultrasound display is used to monitor the procedure. A small quantity of chorionic cells (placental tissue) is extracted. Results from the biopsy can be obtained in four days.

Couples and pregnancy

A couple's personal relationship usually alters during pregnancy, as the changes and feelings that this new situation brings are many and varied. And, more importantly, there is a new member of the family who has to be included in the relationship. A man can sometimes feel abandoned by his partner who is now devoting a lot of attention to the changes that she is undergoing and the new emotions that the arrival of a child produces. Furthermore, thanks to the hormonal revolution that pregnancy brings, a woman's moods often become highly changeable, causing her to

Amniocentesis and chorionic biopsy are techniques used to obtain information on certain matters relating to the baby's genetic makeup. Small samples of placental cells or amniotic fluid are extracted, which are then used to analyze chromosomes, biochemical content, cellular function, or to determine gender in the event of illnesses relating to one particular sex. These studies may be advised if the mother is considered to be at an "at risk" age or if there is any suspicion that the baby is suffering from a medical condition following an ultrasound scan or analysis of biochemical markers. The risk from either procedure is roughly the same. They are linked to subsequent miscarriage in 0.5% of cases (1 in 200 women).

feel at first sad and depressed only to feel later sudden contentment and to burst spontaneously into laughter. Trying to understand these ups and downs, maintaining open communication, and becoming closely involved in the pregnancy are some of the key points for strengthening a couple's relationship and getting through the temporary craziness that pregnancy can induce.

■ Changes experienced by the woman

- During pregnancy, a woman's body undergoes rapid physiological changes, which are also accompanied by psychological and emotional symptoms.

- She has to cope with a phase of great emotional instability: she feels vulnerable and needs attention and sympathy. Within only a few minutes, her moods can change significantly, ranging from misery to joy and everything in between. She may go from crying one moment to laughing the next, and then feel infuriated or sad, only to feel elated soon after.

- This vulnerability translates into behavior or attitudes that extend to her partner, family, and friends. A man may respond to all this with confusion or impatience; however, it all comes down to a woman's need to readjust herself to the changes that she is experiencing, and her partner has an important role to play in this: to lend his emotional support and be the person with whom she can share her feelings.

Feelings during pregnancy

- News of the pregnancy. Fatherhood affects a man on a very deep emotional level. If the pregnancy is welcome, news of it creates feelings of happiness, self-confidence, and pride, both as a father-to-be and as a man.

- The first months of pregnancy. During the first months of the gestation, the changes that a woman undergoes become increasingly obvious, making the concept of fatherhood much more real. At first, it may be hard to get to grips with the idea of incorporating a new person in the family, but bit by bit a man starts to become more aware of the new situation. Sometimes it may be something of a shock to have to absorb all the changes going on all around, and

this can even turn into a feeling of fear. But these are normal feelings when a man is confronted with such important changes in his life.

- Feeling of abandonment. Sometimes, the transition to fatherhood can be difficult and can even be accompanied by a man feeling unhappy or feeling that he has been "abandoned" by his partner. It is common in such cases for him to bury himself in his work or to devote himself excessively to activities away from home in an attempt to avoid this new life. It is rare for this emotional condition to be extreme, but in the instances where it does occur, a man should see a specialist or psychologist who can help him overcome these fears.

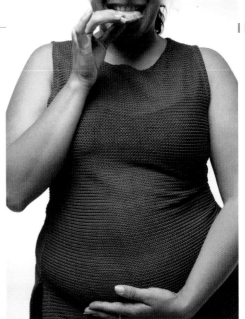

From a psychological perspective, cravings may be related to anxiety and a regression to a woman's oral stage of psychological development. Wanting to eat only particular things may stem from the need to obtain particular nutrients and thus compensate for any deficiencies in the body. A woman often feels the need to supply her body with anything it demands. But these caprices may also be a woman's way of expressing certain emotional needs and seeking attention from the people around her.

Fear of miscarriage can fuel anxiety and increase the need for support and sympathy.

Pregnancy and sex

A couple's sex life during pregnancy is often a cause of concern for many couples from the moment it is confirmed that they are to be parents. Both mother and father-to-be often worry or even fear that sexual intercourse could be detrimental to the health of the mother or baby. Sex during pregnancy is a matter that should be discussed openly with the gynecologist who is monitoring the pregnancy, and his or her recommendations should be followed accordingly.

- There is no reason why sexual relations during pregnancy should pose any danger to either mother or baby.

- Only in the case of pregnancies where there is a possibility of miscarriage are sexual relations discouraged, particularly if penetration is involved. It should also be borne in mind that contractions are produced in the uterus during orgasm and that semen contains prostaglandin, which can also cause uterine contractions; and although no risk is posed under the circumstances of a normal pregnancy, this might have an adverse reaction in cases of pregnancy where there is a high risk of miscarriage.

- Sexual relations are also advised against in the event of blood loss, or spotting, during pregnancy. In any event, the gynecologist is the person who should decide whether or not to disallow penetrative sex during pregnancy.

- Logically enough, with all of the hormonal changes going on inside a woman during pregnancy, it can also affect her sex drive. Some women experience a general reduction in their libido, while for others it increases. Most typically, however, women do not show any appreciable change in their sexual needs.

- Apart from hormonal changes, the physical changes that a woman undergoes through the various stages of pregnancy can also affect her sexual appetite. Speaking in very general terms, during the first trimester pregnant women experience a reduction in sex drive, followed by an increased sex drive in the second, which usually diminishes again in the final trimester the nearer that birth approaches.

- Bearing the physical side of sex in mind, sexual relations could potentially affect the pregnancy. At no time should a woman ever feel physical pressure, pain, or discomfort during any sexual activity.

- Gentleness, tenderness, and communication are essential if a couple are to continue enjoying sex during this period.

- The positions most recommended when continuing with sexual intercourse so as to cause no harm to mother or baby are: the man positioned behind the woman; both partners lying on their sides with the woman's back supported by the man's chest; or with the woman astride the man.

Advice on this new stage in life

Despite all the elation and pride men feel about the arrival of a child, many of them wonder how this new stage in life might affect them. You need to be realistic and recognize that a new being is going to be part of the family and that this will mean less personal freedom for some years and that many decisions will have to be adapted to the needs of the future baby.

- **Accept the changes:** The first step toward fatherhood is to accept that you are entering into a time of change that may involve conflicts and intense confrontational emotions; however, it is vital to understand that this period in a person's life is an extremely important one.

- **Be open with your partner:** It is very important to share your feelings and any of your thoughts openly with your partner.

- **Be involved in the pregnancy, the birth, and caring for the child:** There have been changes in attitude in recent years, undermining stereotypical views of the father's role and degree of participation in pregnancy, labor, and caring for his child in infancy. Men have ceased being mere observers, and are becoming more actively involved in prenatal care, being present when their partner goes into labor, and lending her emotional support.

- **Avoid self-indulgence:** Becoming a father encourages a man to make lifestyle changes, giving him the opportunity to re-evaluate decisions and question some of his values. He may be seized by doubts, but he must try to put these into proportion and not allow them to create tensions, anxiety, or even depression. It is very important to see things from a realistic perspective to avoid getting into extreme situations.

A man's role during labor

The presence of the father during labor not only helps the mother, who feels safer and calmer as a result, but is also a good way to start to bond with the baby that is about to be born. Moreover, it has been shown that fathers who are present at the birth of their children are much more involved in caring for the baby and enjoy a much closer relationship with the child during the first years of its life.

- Involvement of the father during labor is as beneficial to the baby and father himself as it is to the mother.

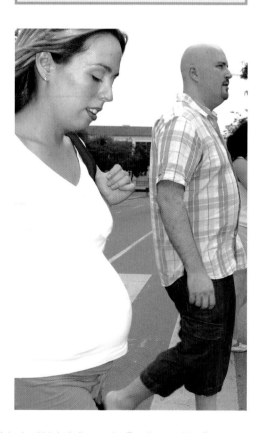

Pregnancy causes radical hormonal changes to a woman's body, which, logically enough, affects her sex drive. Since every pregnancy is different, it is not possible to define fixed standards of behavior, but, in general, approximately 40 percent of pregnant women feel a reduction in desire, 50 percent do not experience any noticeable change, and 10 percent notice an increase in their libido.

- It affords the father the opportunity to live through highly intense emotions that can help him to get in touch with and release his feelings as well as reinforce the bond with his partner and child. It benefits the mother, because being able to depend on a partner who is responsible and conscious of his role as a father makes her feel calmer, supported, and understood, and gives her more time to look after herself and nurture the relationship with her partner, which otherwise may be relegated to second place once the child has arrived.

- However, if a woman prefers not to be accompanied by her partner, or if the man feels uneasy about it, it is better for him not to be present at the birth. He can still follow events closely from behind the delivery room doors.

- Most men who have accompanied their partners at pre-birth parenting classes are more greatly motivated to have an active presence when their partners go into labor, as they will have had the opportunity to dispel their fears and mentally prepare for the event. This focus binds a man and his partner more closely together, creating a solid foundation on which to base their new role as parents.

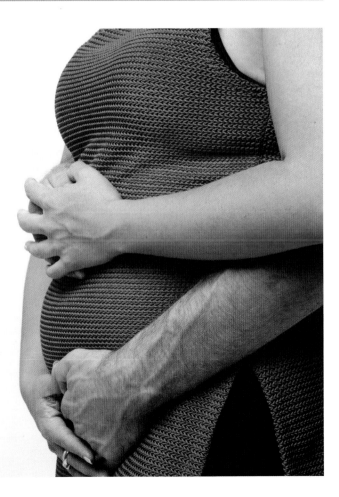

If possible, a man should help with relaxation and breathing exercises both in pre-birth parenting classes and during labor. Being a part of the whole process makes for a smoother transition into fatherhood. Being present during labor makes a man empathize more with his partner's emotional ups and downs. As a result, his perception and understanding of a woman's particular state of mind will increase during pregnancy, her labor, and afterward.

Pre-birth parenting classes

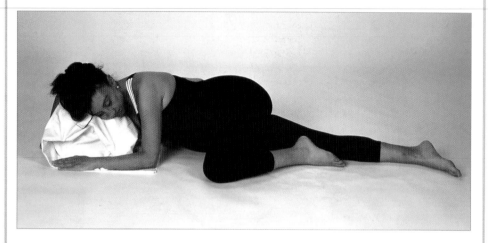

Pre-birth classes help to provide a better experience of the whole process of pregnancy, labor itself and the new phase that ensues after the baby's arrival. It is a good idea to attend such classes if they are available for couples, so as to create a greater bond between the parents and child. Moreover, these sessions will equip both parents with the information necessary to prevent complications arising during pregnancy and during labor and birth. Contact with other pregnant women also helps an expectant mother to lessen her anxieties and share common concerns about maternity. These classes usually consist of theoretical and practical elements.

- The theory provides all the information you need relating to birth, clarifies uncertainties, and discusses the different options available for giving birth. In addition, it deals with the reasons for the various exercises that are performed in the practical part of the session.
- The practical session includes learning about relaxation and breathing techniques that help reduce labor pains and mentally prepare the parents for labor.

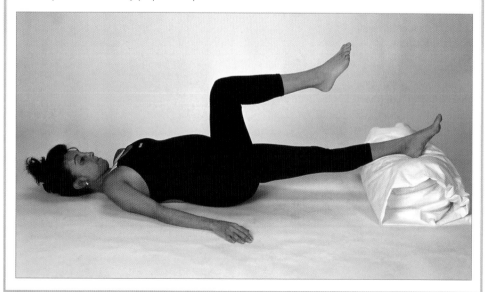

Going into labor

- When a woman first goes into labor, the upper part of her uterus contracts at regular and closer intervals, while the membrane of the lower uterus stretches and becomes thinner as her cervix dilates to enable the passage of the fetus through the vaginal birth canal. Subsequently, the woman's abdominal muscles also start to contract in a downward motion.

- The whole process is referred to as "labor" and can take less than 3 hours or stretch out for over a day. For first-time mothers, the average time is 13 to 15 hours. Subsequent births take considerably less time.

- First stage of labor. This period lasts until the full dilation of the cervix. It usually commences with minor contractions that increase in frequency and intensity.

- Second stage of labor. The baby starts to move its head through the vaginal birth canal until it is born. After it has been delivered, the first thing that the midwife does is to clean its nostrils and mouth to help it breathe. Subsequently, the umbilical cord is clamped and cut.

- Final stage of labor. The contractions of the uterus expel the placenta, its membranes, and the rest of the umbilical cord. This process takes approximately 5 to 20 minutes. The placenta is examined to verify whether it is complete and healthy.

The process of giving birth

Before a woman starts to go into labor, the baby's head positions itself at the exit to the maternal pelvis. For first-time mothers, this change of position can happen over a period of weeks, while for women who have given birth previously, it can take only a few hours.

The muscles of the uterus start to make irregular contractions and grow in intensity. These contractions are the ones that cause the rupture of the amniotic sac that envelops the baby (referred to as when a woman's "waters break").

The cervix starts to dilate until it reaches a diameter of some 4 inches, enabling the baby to pass through. The contractions become increasingly intense and intermittent.

During a normal labor, the first thing to exit the birth canal is the baby's head. If the mother is not sufficiently dilated, it is necessary to make a small incision in her perineum–i.e. the area extending from the vulva to the anus–to avoid complications.

After the head appears, the baby's body turns around and emerges from the birth canal.

Once the baby has been born it is still connected to the placenta by the umbilical cord, which has to be cut. The placenta remains inside the woman.

Roughly a quarter of an hour after delivery, the woman expels the placenta, the remainder of the umbilical cord, and all other residue.

Caesarian section

This procedure is performed if vaginal delivery is not an option or might be risky for either mother or baby. The operation is done either under general anesthesia or using an epidural anesthetic. In the first case, a woman is completely unconscious, while in the second she is awake but feels no pain.

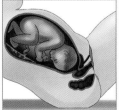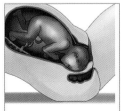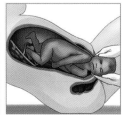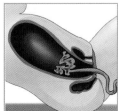

Men during pregnancy

When a man learns he is to be a father, the feelings and concerns that immediately race through his mind are easily imagined. On the one hand, he will feel overjoyed; on the other, he will feel worried. He will be assailed by thoughts about whether he will be able to look after his partner and his future child; he will wonder whether he will be a good father, what his new life will be like, whether he will be able to cope financially for a family... All of these doubts are normal, and the man should realize that every good father has asked himself the same questions at some point during pregnancy.

The baby is not just the mother's but the father's, too, and, he should therefore, also be involved throughout the whole process. A father-to-be has an important role to play during pregnancy: he is responsible for ensuring that his partner follows all the advice given to her by her doctor, while at the same time he needs to act as her rock throughout this period of major physical and psychological changes.

How can I help?

Check your partner's diet and weight. A man should take responsibility for his partner

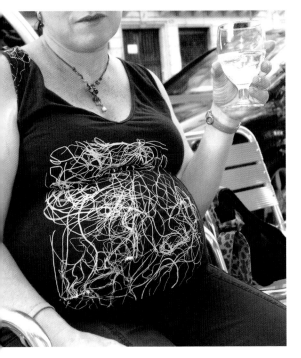

getting a proper, balanced diet: a lot of grains, meat, vegetables, milk, and fruit. It is important for him to assist in choosing the type of food that is healthiest and most appropriate. Weight gain throughout pregnancy should not exceed 35 lbs.

Avoid smoking. A pregnant woman who smokes risks giving birth prematurely or delivering an underweight baby, which can result in the baby suffering from complications. If the father smokes, he should avoid doing so when around his partner; passive smokers also suffer from the effects of tobacco smoke. If both parents-to-be smoke, this is an excellent time for them to quit.

Take some days off after the birth. After the birth and the arrival at home of the new member of the family, it is advisable for the father to take paternity leave from work so that he can get to know his child more quickly and experience everything possible together with his partner. After the birth, a woman needs a lot of emotional support and help to adjust to all the changes that she is undergoing.

No to drugs. Any drug carries with it risks to the pregnancy. It is vital that the man helps his partner to avoid taking any type of drug, illegal or otherwise, that has not been officially prescribed.

Avoid alcohol. Pregnant women who drink large amounts of alcohol may run the risk of giving birth to a baby with physical or mental defects. Alcohol is a powerful toxin that can seriously harm the baby. It is not known precisely what quantity of alcohol can be stated as "safe" for a baby; however, to avoid any risk, it is sensible for a woman to avoid any type of alcoholic beverage until she has given birth.

Share domestic chores and looking after pets. During pregnancy, a woman should avoid doing strenuous chores or making sudden movements, and she should avoid contact with toxic cleaning agents that might affect the baby's development. She should also avoid touching animals and their feces to prevent infections that, although harmless to the mother, might have a serious effect on the baby (such as from cats, for example). Cat feces can contain microbes that cause a disease called toxoplasmosis, which is harmful to the normal development of the baby.

Keep well informed, and accompany your partner throughout her pregnancy. It is essential to be up–to date on what is hap-

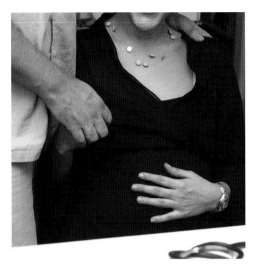

pening throughout the pregnancy. A man should attempt to keep abreast of everything that pregnancy involves, accompany his partner to her antenatal checkups, get to know the medical team monitoring the pregnancy and assisting at the birth, attend pre-birth parenting classes, and, if both parties wish, be present during labor. It has been shown that the presence of the father in the delivery room creates a sense of tranquility and security for the mother that is not achieved if he does not participate.

Communication between the parents. Both parents-to-be may feel apprehensive faced with the new situation and the responsibilities that it brings. This is a completely normal reaction, which it is always best for couples to share. Smooth communication helps them cope with the emotional roller coaster.

Advice on how to start being a doting father

- Your paternal instinct is real; let it take its own course. There is no need to be embarrassed if your attention is suddenly seized by baby clothing, if you start reading parenting magazines, if you feel emotional when you see the first ultrasound scan, or if you marvel at how your companion's body is changing. It is important not to be led by stereotypical expectations of masculinity that label these things "a woman's department." Men who do not take part in pregnancy lose out on one of the most intense experiences in their lives, and this makes it much more difficult for them to establish close bonds with their children afterward.

- Do not be afraid to caress your partner's belly and to speak to it and your child within. If you get into the habit of doing it at the same time every day, the little one inside will be expecting you and will recognize your voice and your caresses.

- Be present at medical checkups. Thanks to ultrasound scans, you will be able to see your child in the first few months of pregnancy, observe its movements, and listen to its heartbeat—experiences that create an inseparable bond between you and your child before it is even born.

- Be present in the delivery room if you can, assuming that this is what you and your partner both want. Being present at the birth of your child is an emotional experience and, without any doubt, will bring you even closer to both mother and child.

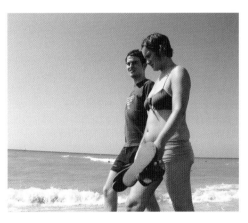

Do some kind of exercise together as a couple. Pregnancy is a good time for any type of joint exercise or physical activity, as long as the woman is capable of doing it. Walking outdoors, apart from being a healthy activity, also gives a couple opportunities to discuss the future.

This new situation represents a time of momentous change in your life. Show your partner your feelings, share the experience of pregnancy and birth with her, and help your new family and baby get off to a good start. Always remember that a baby is a project for two people and that, once it becomes a reality, it is a shared responsibility.

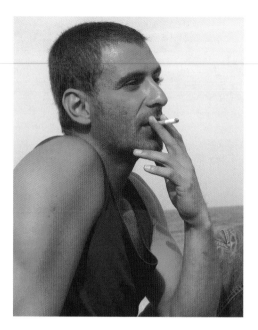

Tobacco is bad for the developing baby. Your partner's pregnancy is the perfect time to give up smoking.

He may also feel insecure about whether the baby will be born healthy or whether he will be able to handle properly his new responsibilities as a father. These are all temporary concerns that can be dealt with by talking them through as a couple or with other fathers, friends, or family members who are also parents.

During the first few months of a newborn baby's life, its pace of growth, learning, adaptation, mimicry, and understanding of language—not merely verbal—is swift and intense. It is important not to miss out on these precious moments.

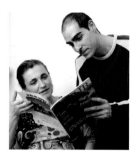

The future father should know that as the fetus starts to grow in its mother's belly, so too do its senses and that, from the fifth month onward, he can start to communicate with the baby. The baby senses everything that happens outside the womb.

By the fifth month, the baby is already moving and responding to its mother's movements and can hear and start to make tactile responses. Its first taste and smell sensations begin in the sixth month. The baby can hear everything that happens outside the mother's body through its tiny ears and with increasing clarity the more it develops. Brain activity takes off at full speed in the seventh month, as the baby is almost ready to be born. The baby becomes in full-time communication with its environment through its various senses.

A father goes through distinct emotional phases in parallel to those of the mother as the pregnancy progresses. Changeability of mood and temperament are not exclusive to women. At times, men may feel worried and anxious about the health of their partner. And a woman's physical changes cause a man to adopt a protective attitude toward the mother because of the feelings of tenderness they instill in him.

What happens afterward?

- The parents are then able to see their child, touch it, hear it cry, feed it, and start to communicate more directly with it.

- A newborn is quick to start using all its senses: the baby looks around, gazing at its mother, at its father, and everything else in its environment, especially if it moves. The baby also listens, touches, and feels cold, heat, pain, softness, and roughness; it can grip, suckle, and smile—all of this in the first seconds, minutes, hours and days.

- At first, babies spend many hours sleeping. This is because their high activity levels require them to take a great deal of physical rest, although their brain and biological activity continue to work unabated, organizing and classifying everything that their senses have picked up.

- While a father cannot nurse the baby, he can still perform all the other activities essential to its development and growth: he can give the baby its bottle, bathe it, change its diaper, put it to bed, etc.

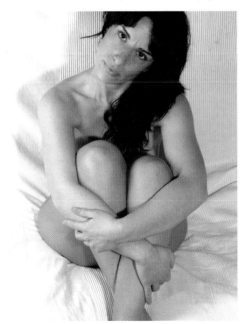

infertility and sterility

Fertility guarantees the future of humanity, and societies and cultures throughout the world have always placed a premium on it. Children play an important symbolic role in their parents' lives: they represent a link to the future, continuity, and the culmination of a union between two people. A couple's ability or inability to have children can have an effect on their emotional and physical health. Consequently, it is sensible to consult a specialist if your attempts to have children are unsuccessful. In most cases, couples can be helped to produce offspring of their own.

What is infertility and sterility?

Until relatively recently, infertility was considered to be an exclusively female problem. A man was considered fertile as long as he could manage an erection sufficient to penetrate a woman and then ejaculate.

Approximately 10—15 percent of couples with a normal sex life present infertility prob-

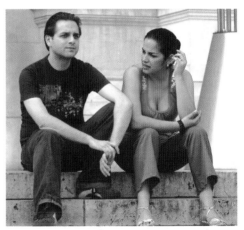

Nowadays, medical professionals prefer to analyze a man's semen as the first step when studying a couple's infertility before subjecting a woman to a whole range of gynecological examinations. The reason for this is that if the cause of infertility lies with the man there are always variations in both the concentration and quality of sperm.

According to the World Health Organization (WHO), a couple cannot be considered infertile until they have tried for a baby unsuccessfully over the course of one year without using any form of contraception.

lems. 40 percent of these cases relate specifically to the woman, another 40 percent specifically to the man, and 20 percent relate to conditions involving both partners. In other words, a man's fertility is at issue in half of all cases.

Infertility is defined as a couple's inability to conceive after a year of trying for a baby without using any contraception. Although the majority of couples manage to conceive within a year, some couples are unable to do so.

The term "sterility" is often used interchangeably with "infertility", but implies a more permanent situation, with no possibility of treatment.

Primary infertility: when a couple has failed to conceive after a year of trying for a baby without any protection.

Secondary infertility: when a couple that has already produced one child fails to conceive after two or more years of trying for another baby. Technically, secondary infertility cannot apply when there has been a change of partner.

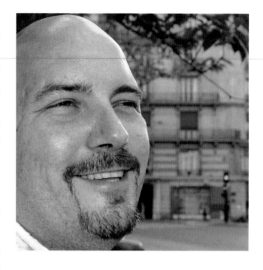

Men and women's period of greatest fertility is between the ages of 20 and 40. 75 percent of couples trying for a baby are found in this age group, and they are usually able to conceive after trying for a period of less than nine months.

A couple's sex life can become affected. In part, this is due to the difficulty they may have in accepting their inability to conceive; but, in addition, it shouldpointed out that frequent diagnostic and treatment-related procedures are bothersome and prevent sexual spontaneity, eventually turning sex into a duty and making it a stressful experience.

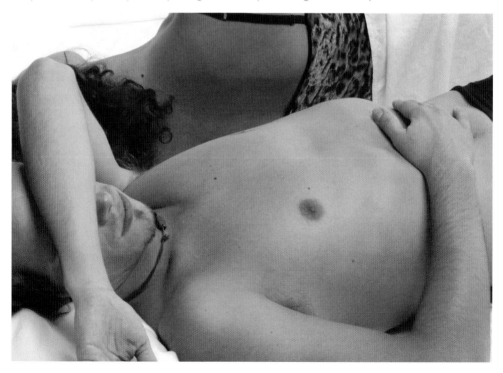

Causes of infertility or sterility

Infertility or sterility in men:

- General causes:
  Fatigue, stress, depression
  Excessive drinking, smoking, or drug abuse
  Sexual hyperactivity
  Erectile dysfunction and sexual impotence
- Developmental causes:
  Cryptorchidism
  Germinal cell aplasia
  Hypospadias
  Klinefelter's syndrome
- Endocrine causes:
  Hypopituitarism
  Acromegaly
  Thyroid conditions
  Adrenogenital syndrome
  Severe diabetes
- Genital-related causes:
  Varicocele
  Epididymitis
  Prostatitis
  Orchitis
  Traumatic injury, inflammation, surgery
  STDs
  Mumps during puberty

Infertility or sterility in women:

- General causes:
  Poor diet
  Severe anemia
  Emotional conditions (hormonal)
  Frigidity
- Developmental causes:
  Absence of uterus or uterine hypoplasia
  Uterine malformation
  Swyer syndrome (gonadal dysgenesis)
  Kallmann syndrome
- Endocrine causes:
  Hypopituitarism
  Hyperprolactinemia
  Thyroid conditions
  Adrenogenital conditions
  Polycystic ovarian syndrome
- Genital-related causes:
  Pelvic inflammation
  Tuberculosis
  Tubal obstruction
  Endometriosis
  Fibroids (leiomyomata)
  Endometrial polyposis
  Cervicitis; vaginitis
- Combined causes:
  Emotional imbalance
  Misunderstandings about sex
  Immunological incompatibility

Although not strictly speaking an illness, infertility can create significant emotional problems between two people. The inability to conceive can cause profound changes in a relationship. It can lead to a reduction in the frequency that a couple makes love, sexual dissatisfaction, stress and anxiety, and depression, and plunge them into a vicious circle that serves only to fuel their inability to conceive.

Fertility has repercussions on a person's mental and physical health. On the other hand, some situations connected with stress and emotional

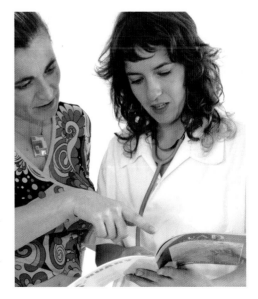

As in any crisis situation, the discovery of one's infertility usually leads to phases of shock, incredulity, and even denial. It is important to demystify the situation and, above all, to avoid feelings of guilt. Once insecurities have been dealt with and the news has been accepted, a couple can move on and try to find a solution.

problems may lead to a state of temporary infertility; and once these are resolved, a couple is able to conceive again. Infertility is not due solely to genetic or hereditary factors, or to unsatisfactory lovemaking techniques, as the feelings of frustration and guilt that accompany a couple's inability to procreate can also be contributing factors in themselves.

Investigating male infertility

When investigating male infertility, the first thing that the uroandrologist (specialist in the male urinary and reproductive system) will do is to compile a clinical history and general examination of the patient, as well as an assessment of his reproductive system.

Hypospadias

Hypospadias is a birth defect in which the opening of the urethra (the urethral meatus) is located at any point from near the anus to the end of the glans, which is where it is found normally. Treatment always requires surgery.

Semen analysis

Semen analysis (seminogram) is essential to the investigation of male infertility; it involves the study of a semen sample both biochemically and under the microscope.

Semen analysis should include the following areas of inquiry:
• **Volume.** If the quantity of semen is deficient, it indicates disease in the seminal vesicles: e.g. diabetes or tuberculosis.
• **Sperm count.** A normal sperm count measures between 20 million and 300 million spermatozoa per milliliter. Sperm counts lower than this are considered subfertile.
• **Motility.** Motility concerns the percentage of mobile spermatozoa, as well as the type of movement that they make. It is considered normal when 40–50 percent of them are mobile. Continual, forward motion is normal. Circular or static motion is considered abnormal motility and characteristic of subfertile sperm.
• **Morphology.** Approximately 20 percent of all spermatozoa are strangely shaped, double-headed, or have multiple flagella (tails). Sterility

Stress, emotional problems, depression, poor diet, drugs, and many other factors can have an effect on fertility.

arises when the proportion of aberrantly formed sperm is higher than normal.
• **pH.** The normal pH (acidity or alkalinity) of semen is between 7.2 and 7.6. Infections of the urinary tract can produce variations in the pH, which can cause sterility.
• **Liquefaction.** When a medical condition is present, the time it takes for semen to liquefy after ejaculation varies from the norm.
• **Agglutination.** When an inflammation is present, the spermatozoa agglutinate and lose their capacity for movement.

▪ Semen analysis

Semen analysis is a highly valuable diagnostic test, but it has its limitations: a semen analysis that comes back as normal is not a guarantee of fertility, and only a total absence of spermatozoa (azoospermia) or their total lack of motility makes conception unviable. As long as his semen contains some mobile spermatozoa, a man remains (theoretically) fertile and capable of fertilizing an ovum.

Clinical history and physical examination

- Your medical records will contain information on the amount of time you have been trying to conceive, any previous evidence of fertility, gynecological examinations performed on your partner, and some of the contraception methods used in the past.

- Every individual has his or her own fertility quotient. If both parties in a relationship, male and female, have a low fertility quotient, the likelihood of conception diminishes accordingly. On the other hand, a man with low fertility may be successful with a woman who has above-average fertility.

- Your clinical history may reveal factors that indicate possible infertility or sterility: urogenital system conditions (cryptorchidism, hypospadias, traumatic injury and inflammation, STDs, surgery, parotitis (mumps), prostatitis, etc.).

- Similarly, your clinical history will include any toxic habits, i.e. whether you smoke, drink alcohol, or take drugs; whether you have been exposed to radiation (x-rays), or high levels of heat in the area of the testicles; whether you are taking any medication, etc.

- In addition, your family history will also be examined: the fertility of your siblings, family birth defects, and hereditary illnesses.

- It is also necessary to examine your primary and secondary sexual characteristics: the shape, size, and position of the testicles, epididymis, vas deferens ducts, penis, and prostate gland, as well as your distribution of facial and body hair.

Every individual has his or her own fertility quotient. If both parties in a relationship, male and female, have a low fertility quotient, the likelihood of conception diminishes accordingly. On the other hand, a man with low fertility may be successful with a woman who has above-average fertility.

▪ WHO criteria

A normal ejaculation of semen according to the criteria of the WHO:
Volume > 2 ml
Concentration of spermatozoa > 20 million/ml
Motility > 50 percent advance or > 25 percent advance swiftly
Morphology (strict criterion) > 15 percent with normal morphology
Leucocytes < 1 million/ml
Immunoglobulin enveloped < 10 percent covered

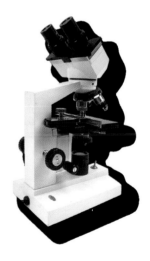

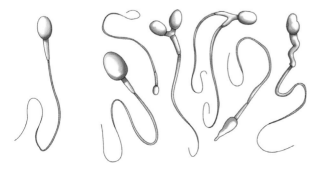

Despite the quality control carried out by the epididymis on the production of spermatozoa, approximately 20 percent of them present an abnormal type of morphology. If a high proportion of these have an abnormal form, it follows that this is the probable cause of infertility.

Diagnosis	Semen analysis
Normospermia	All the parameters are normal.
Oligozoospermia	Reduced concentration of spermatozoa. Slight–moderate: from 5 to 20 million/ml.
Astenozoospermia	Reduced motility (< 50 percent advance or < 25 percent advance swiftly).
Teratozoospermia	Increase in abnormal morphology (normal spermatozoa < 15 percent)
Oligoastenoteratozoospermia	Presents all of the abnormal variables.
Azoospermia	There are no spermatozoa in the semen.
Leucocytospermia	Increased number of leucocytes (> 1 million/ml).
Necrozoospermia	None of the sperm is viable or mobile.
Hyperspermia	An excessive volume of semen can lead to excessive dilution of the spermatozoa and make it difficult for them to concentrate in a woman's cervical mucus.
Polyzoospermia	An excessive concentration of spermatozoa can cause agglutination and reduce their motility, resulting in infertility.

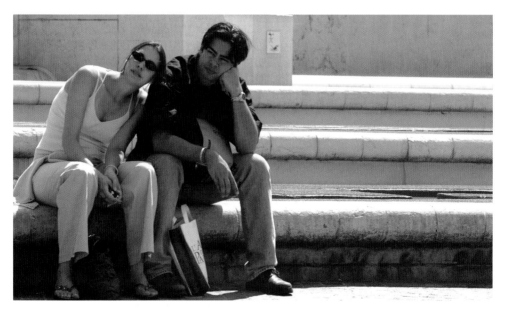

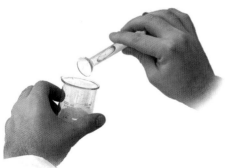

It is advisable to have at least two or three semen analyses performed at intervals of eight or ten days due to the great variation that occurs in all men, in terms of both the quantity and the quality of semen produced.

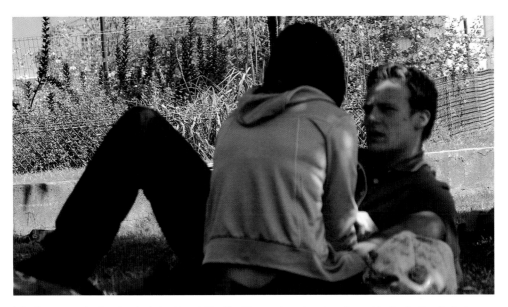

Infertility can greatly affect the physical and mental health of the couple, and can have far-reaching implications for their relationship. In most cases, treatment from an infertility specialist can help the couple to have children.

Points to remember when providing a semen sample

- Abstain from sex for at least two to three days before providing the sample.
- Do not apply any ointments or scrupulously wash your penis before providing the sample.
- Provide the sample by masturbating. To obtain a significant quantity of fluid, it is sensible to become highly aroused beforehand.
- The semen sample is collected in a sterile container. A sample provided in a condom or any other "homemade" receptacle is invalid. Ideally, the sterile container in which you collect the sample should be at body temperature, and it must be kept at the same temperature during its subsequent journey to the laboratory. The procedure should be completed quickly.

▪ Hormonal tests

- A hormonal analysis is usually performed together with the semen analysis.
- The hormones investigated are luteinizing hormone (LH), follicle-stimulating hormone (FSH), testosterone, and prolactin.
- Increased levels of FSH indicate damage to the testicles. When sperm production (spermatogenesis) is nonexistent, the pituitary gland increases its secretion of FSH in order to boost production. Therefore, men with azoospermia or low sperm counts usually have higher levels of FSH in their bloodstream.
- Reduced levels of LH and testosterone are responsible for changes to sperm; in these cases, treatments that complement such hormonal deficiencies are very effective at improving sperm production.
- A reduced level of spermatogenesis and erectile dysfunction are linked to increased levels of prolactin.

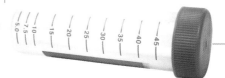

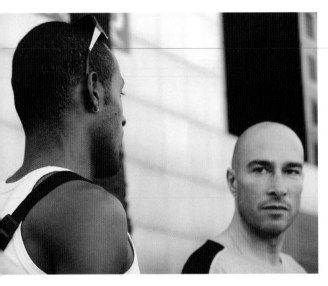

Sperm donors are usually young men—generally, college students—and are evaluated before being accepted as candidates. They undergo a medical examination and answer all types of personal questions about their medical history: the existence of any hereditary illnesses or conditions in the family, blood tests, HIV tests, etc. In addition, those selected will have semen that best fits the criteria for fertilization. Donated sperm is processed, frozen, and kept in storage until it is needed.

Treatment for male infertility

Once it has been confirmed that the infertility is male in origin, a range of medical and surgical treatments can be provided in an attempt to solve the problem.

The most serious conditions relating to semen have a poor prognosis, as treatment for them has not yet been developed. One of the possible future uses of embryo stem cells is to create a means of curing male sterility problems.

Some of the treatments currently available to achieve conception, and thus overcome male infertility, include:

- **Artificial insemination:** This involves placing a relatively high number of pre-selected, healthy spermatozoa either at the entrance to the cervix or in the woman's uterus to make their journey to the Fallopian tubes easier. This can be done either using a man's own semen (homologous artificial fertilization) or that of a donor.

- **Type 2 diabetes:** This is generally diagnosed in childhood. The body produces little or no insulin. In such cases, daily insulin injections are necessary for survival.

- *In vitro* **fertilization, or gamete intrafallopian transfers and other techniques.** *In vitro* fertilization is commonly used when the infertility male in origin. As with artificial insemination, in vitro fertilization and similar techniques allow sperm to be pre-selected and prepared in the test tube to facilitate the fertilization of an ovum (egg).

- **Microsurgical fertilization** (microinjection techniques, such as intracytoplasmic sperm injections or ICSI). This treatment is performed to ensure that sperm enter the ovum (egg), and is performed using an injection of a single sperm directly into the ovum. Fertilization is done in the laboratory under a microscope and, afterward, the fertilized ovum is implanted in the woman's uterus.

- **Pharmacological treatment:** Men who are infertile because of a hormonal condition can be given a drug-based hormonal therapy. Treatment with antibiotics is required if the reason for infertility is an infection.

- **Surgery:** Surgical intervention is the solution when the cause of infertility is an anatomical abnormality, as in the case of epididymis blockages, varioceles, or hypospadias.

How to improve semen quality

Independent of surgical procedures and medical advice for the treatment of male infertility, there are a few basic rules to follow for improving the quality of seminal fluid and successfully conceiving:

- **Reduce stress:** A stressful situation or prolonged anxiety can cause infertility.

- **Eliminate toxic substances:** Many studies show that tobacco immobilizes the spermatozoa and reduces semen quality. Some drugs, such as marijuana, affect both hormonal levels and spermatozoa quality. Heroin and other drugs reduce libido, make erection difficult, and reduce the quality and quantity of the spermatozoa.

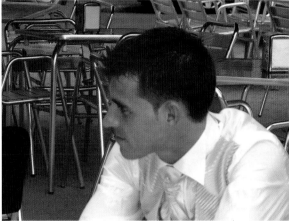

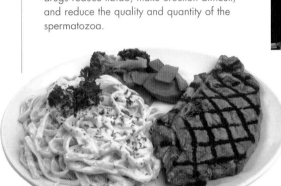

- **Temperature:** An increase in testicular temperature has a very adverse effect on sperm production. The testicles are about 5°F below body temperature, which is the ideal temperature for spermatogenesis. Sperm production is halted if the temperature rises and remains higher for long enough. Once the temperature stabilizes again, testicular sperm production reverts to normal.

- **Diet and weight:** A diet that is low in calories or lacking in protein causes male infertility. Obesity reduces the quality and quantity of the spermatozoa.

- **Prescription drugs:** A number of drugs affect male fertility: antidepressants, antipsychotics, antiepileptics, antibiotics, etc.

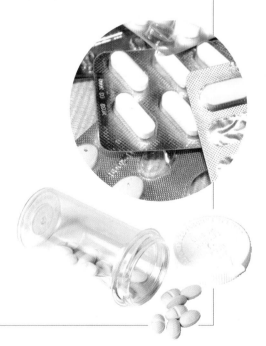

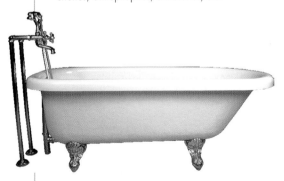

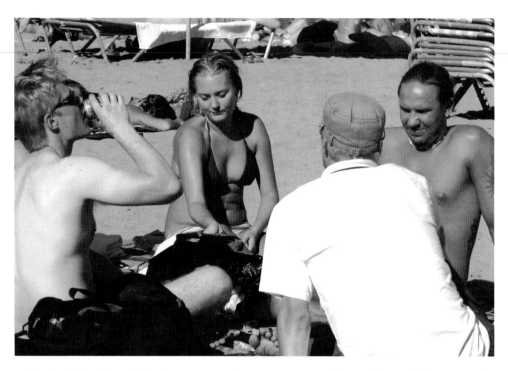

A microinjection of just one sperm into an egg can be performed in cases of severe male infertility (low sperm count, atypical morphology), failed cases of *in vitro* fertilization, or a high content of antispermatic antibodies. The process is similar to that performed in *in vitro* fertilization; it differs only in the way in which the egg is fertilized. In *in vitro* fertilization, eggs are left to incubate with the spermatozoa, whose task it is to penetrate them. In microinjection, a single sperm is selected and injected into an egg.

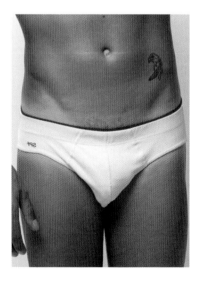

Saunas and long, hot soaks in the bathtub can cause infertility due to the increase in testicular temperature. Fevers have the same consequences. Tight-fitting underwear, particularly briefs, should be replaced with looser, cotton garments, such as boxer shorts. The testicles should be able to hang loose, free of the body, allowing them to keep at a lower temperature.

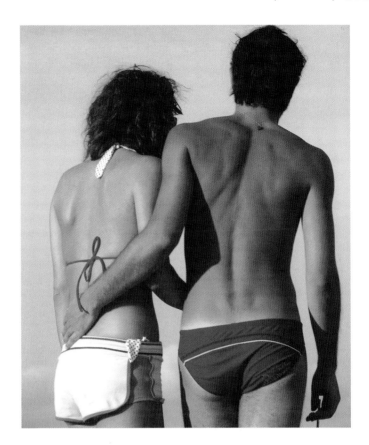

Sexually transmitted diseases can cause infertility.

◼ Investigating female fertility

- Analyzing basal temperature: this verifies whether menstruation is regular.

- Hormonal analysis: this consists of investigating the plasmatic level of progesterone during days 22 and 23 of the cycle; it is also detects any endocrine conditions.

- Endometrium biopsy: a tissue sample analysis to detect abnormalities or diseases that might prevent the implantation of the fertilized egg.

- Transvaginal ultrasound scan: this visualizes malformations or anatomical abnormalities (e.g. uterine fibroids (leiomyomata))

- Laparoscopy: examination of the abdomen and pelvis by inserting an optical device that allows an assessment of the internal reproductive organs and establishes whether adhesions are present and whether endometriosis can be diagnosed.

- Hysteroscopy: the optical inspection of the uterus using an instrument called a "hysterocope"; this is useful for the diagnosis of uterine polyps and Asherman's syndrome (scars in the uterus), the presence of adhesions, and whether endometriosis exists.

- Hysterosalpingography (HSG): x-ray of the uterus and the Fallopian tubes using the injection of a radio-opaque material into the cervical canal.

- Postcoital test (PCT) or Sims-Huhner test: this evaluates the interaction of spermatozoa with the female reproductive system. In the test, a sample of cervical mucus is taken during ovulation and 5 to 15 hours after sexual intercourse. This sample is then analyzed to determine its physical characteristics and the presence of spermatozoa.

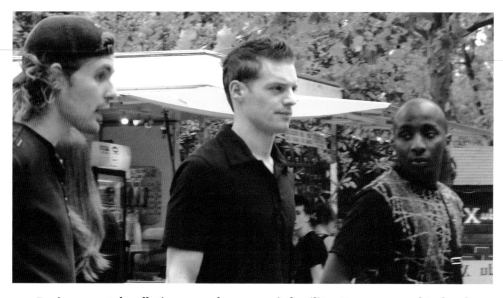

Environmental pollution can also cause infertility. Men exposed to lead pollution put their sperm quality at risk. There are many sources of lead pollution. The most common of these include drinking water (through contact with old plumbing), contact with some types of paint (until 1978, paints used for interior and exterior painting often contained lead), or breathing in the gases emitted by vehicles that use lead-based gasoline.

Some sexual positions make it more difficult for semen to remain in the vagina. After intercourse, it is important for the woman to remain lying down to prevent the ejaculated semen from being expelled. Full penetration is also important, as is withdrawing the penis only once it has become completely flaccid. Some sexual positions make fertilization easier by enabling semen to be deposited more deeply inside the woman.

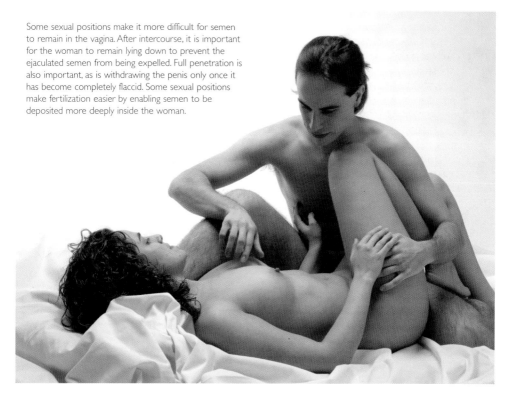

erectile dysfunction

Erectile dysfunction is a very common condition that affects about half of all men between the ages of 40 and 70. Erection problems can have a profound physical and mental impact on a man, causing loss of self-esteem, anxiety, and depression, as well as emotional isolation that can have a negative effect on the relationship with his partner. Male stereotypes and the mythology that surrounds male sexuality often prevent men from seeking help for a condition that can be remedied with medical treatment in the majority of cases.

What is erectile dysfunction?

Erectile dysfunction, also referred to as impotence, means the inability to achieve and/or maintain a sufficiently hard and sustained erection for sexual relations that require penetration.

Erectile dysfunction is usually associated with other health problems. In fact, erectile dysfunction is usually a symptom of some other underlying health issue.

Erectile dysfunction affects men to different degrees and can roughly be classified as follows:
- **Minor.** The ability to obtain and sustain an erection is slightly reduced. Men who suffer from minor erectile dysfunction feel a slight degree of dissatisfaction with their sex lives.
- **Moderate.** In this case, the ability to achieve and maintain an erection is moderately reduced. Most men who ask for advice present this type of dysfunction and usually show clear dissatisfaction with their sex lives.
- **Severe.** When the ability to obtain and sustain an erection is very low or nonexistent.

What are the causes?

Generally speaking, there are two major causes of erectile dysfunction: psychological and physical.

Erectile dysfunction that is psychological in origin is much more common in young men. Conversely, erectile dysfunction in older men usually has some physical cause.

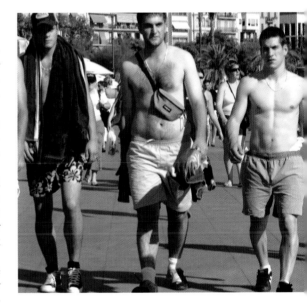

Erectile dysfunction is a common condition among the male population. It is estimated that, throughout the world, 152 million men over 40 suffer from it and, because of fear, taboos, or lack of information, only 10 percent of them ask for medical help. If you are suffering from erectile dysfunction or think you might be, it is important to realize that there are solutions to the disorder and that treatments for it are becoming ever simpler, safer, and more effective.

Erectile dysfunction affects a man's emotional well-being by preventing him from enjoying sexual activity pleasurably and naturally.

Chance or chronic dysfunction?

Many men suffer erection problems occa-

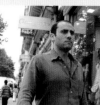

sionally or temporarily, but this does not necessarily mean that they have a chronic condition. Erection failure must recur regularly for the problem to be diagnosed as erectile dysfunction.

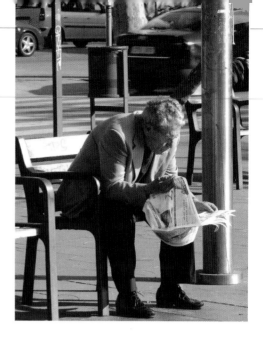

In fact, erectile dysfunction is usually the result of a combination of both factors: it affects emotional well-being to a some extent, and emotional well-being affects a man's sexual response.

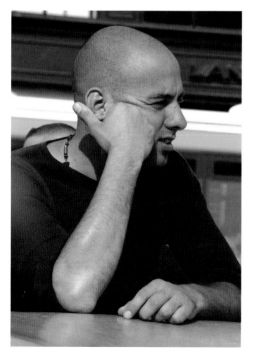

How is erectile dysfunction diagnosed?

Medical and psychosocial history. Before following any other lines of inquiry, physicians will first try to obtain a patient's medical history. They will discuss all current and past medical problems with the patient, any illnesses that he has suffered or is suffering from, the types of medication that he is taking, whether he is a smoker, etc. They will also discuss a patient's psychological history: whether he suffers from stress, anxiety, or depression. Physicians will inquire about a patient's sex life as well: the length of time that a patient has suffered from sexual dysfunction, the frequency, quality, and duration of his erections, the presence of erections on waking, etc. In addition, they will investigate the reasons for the patient seeking treatment and his expectations. Because erectile dysfunction tends to be a problem experienced by two people, and it may be appropriate for a couple to participate jointly in the process to resolve it.

As a man gets older, he notices that it takes him longer to become erect, or that his erections are not as hard as they used to be, or that it takes him longer to reach orgasm. These changes are normal and are inextricably linked to aging but should not be confused with erection disorders. Erectile dysfunction is not an inevitable part of aging and, if it happens, it can be treated.

An erection is a very physiologically complex phenomenon that depends on many factors, including among which the correct function of the nervous system, vascular system, endocrine system, and erectile tissue. Any change or condition affecting one of these mechanisms can lead to the an erection disorder.

Physical examination. This involves the man having a complete checkup to allow the doctor to diagnose any physical problems that might be a cause of dysfunction. Some of the basic tests include taking blood pressure, physically examining the reproductive organs, a rectal examination, and checking secondary sexual characteristics, such as the hairline, which may indicate a hormonal problem.

■ Physical causes of erectile dysfunction

- Alcoholism
- Fatigue
- High blood pressure and vascular diseases
- Atherosclerosis or hardening/furring of the arteries
- High cholesterol levels
- Diabetes
- Cerebral or spinal cord injuries
- Low levels of testosterone
- Liver or kidney conditions
- Prostate gland conditions
- Multiple sclerosis
- Parkinson's disease
- Radiation therapy on the testicles
- Drug abuse
- Some types of surgery on the prostate gland or bladder
- Some types of medication, such as for high blood pressure, antidepressants, and anxiolytics
- Penile malformations, such as Peyronie's disease
- Birth defects

■ Psychological causes of erectile dysfunction

- Feeling anxious about sex, probably due to a bad memory or experience or due to a previous episode of impotence.
- Stress, either relating to work or a family situation.
- Problems and lack of communication with your sexual partner.
- Depression and lack of self-esteem.
- Feeling so inhibited that you are unable to enjoy sex.
- Lack of information that results in fearfulness and false beliefs about sex.

Laboratory analysis. This involves techniques that can help to diagnose the causes of erectile dysfunction. Usually, they consist of analyses of blood and urine samples, which establish the profile of fats and glucose levels in the bloodstream, markers for prostate gland tumors, and the levels of creatinin and hepatic enzymes in a patient's blood.

Hormone levels. Hormonal disparities of testosterone, gonadotropins, and prolactin can also be a cause of impotence. If a patient complains of decreased interest in sex, the cause of his dysfunction may relate to changes in the levels of testosterone and endocrine system disorders.

Monitoring "nocturnal penile tumescence." This test detects the spontaneous erections that occur while a man is asleep. Its

Sometimes erectile dysfunction is simply a symptom of another medical condition. Moreover, the impotence may be caused by an undiagnosed illness. Therefore, it is important to have routine medical checkups and to visit your doctor if you are suffering from erection problems, thus possibly detecting underlying condition early.

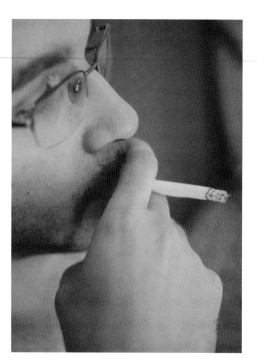

Smoking accentuates the effects of other risk factors, such as circulation problems, high blood pressure, or heart conditions. Smoking 20 cigarettes a day increases your likelihood of suffering from erectile dysfunction by 60 percent.

principal use is to distinguish between sexual dysfunction that is psychological in origin and dysfunction that has a physical basis.

The test can determine whether an individual is following a normal pattern of penile activity

This questionnaire has been designed to help determine whether you suffer from erectile dysfunction. There are various possible answers to each question. You should note down the answer number that most closely describes your situation, and try to select only one answer to each question.

Over the past six months	SCORING				
	1	2	3	4	5
How would you rate your confidence about being able to achieve and maintain an erection?	Very low	Low	Moderate	High	Very high
When you had erections through sexual stimulation, how often were your erections sufficiently hard to achieve penetration?	Never or almost never	Occasionally, but much less than half of the time	Sometimes, about half of the time	Often, more than half of the time	Always or almost always
During sexual intercourse, how often were you able to maintain your erection after penetrating your partner?	Never or almost never	Occasionally, but much less than half of the time	Sometimes, about half of the time	Often, more than half of the time	Always or almost always
During sexual intercourse, how difficult was it for you to maintain your erection all the way to orgasm?	Extremely difficult	Very difficult	Difficult	A little difficult	It wasn't difficult
When you attempted to sustain sexual intercourse, how often did you feel satisfied by it?	Never or almost never	Occasionally, but much less than half of the time	Sometimes, about half of the time	Often, more than half of the time	Always or almost always

Add together your scores for Questions 1–5. If your total score is 21 or less, you may show signs of erectile dysfunction and should consult your physician.

during his sleep, according to which a man has three to five erections a night, each lasting for 25 to 50 seconds. These erections do not occur if the cause is physical, but if they do occur, the cause is psychological.

Ultrasound scan diagnosis. Ultrasound makes it possible to obtain a clear anatomical image of all the component parts of the penis and, due to the technique's low invasiveness, it is very useful in studying normal and abnormal erectile function.

What therapeutic options are there?

First and foremost among these is a change of lifestyle. As with all illnesses, modifying the day-to-day habits that affect your health will ameliorate the problem and aid its treatment. The first steps toward overcoming erectile dysfunction are to quit smoking, not to take drugs, moderate your drinking, eat a balanced diet and reduce your consumption of fat, take exercise, and attempt to live a more relaxed life, avoiding anxiety and stress.

Switch or reduce the dosage of medications that cause impotence. Impotence can be a side effect of some pharmaceutical drugs. It is important to switch such medication or reduce its dosage.

Psychotherapy and behavioral therapy. Irrespective of the cause of erectile dysfunction, all patients are recommended to follow some type of psychological, behavioral, or sexual therapy, ideally accompanied by their partner.

These types of therapy try to reassert a man's self-esteem, strengthen communications with his partner, and eliminate fears, taboos, and obsessive thoughts.

Transurethral and injection therapy. This involves injecting the penis with a medical substance to dilate the blood vessels of the corpus cavernosum, relax the muscles, and allow erection. It is a safe, effective type of therapy and is suitable for many cases of erectile dysfunction. The results are immediate and cause a full erection that can last for between 30 and 60 minutes. Adverse reactions are usually minimal, although prolonged and painful erections can occur (priapism). An alternative to injection is to apply the same medication using a plastic device, a catheter, that is inserted into the urethra.

Hormonal treatments. Testosterone therapy is advised only for men with low levels of the male hormone (hypogonadism). It can be taken orally or absorbed through skin patches. Testosterone is never recommended to men with normal levels of the male hormone because, although it improves a man's sex drive, too high a level can cause irreversible damage to the prostate gland and liver.

Vacuum pump. This is a piece of equipment that aims to produce an artificial erection by means of creating a vacuum around the penis. The effect can be achieved with a manually or electrically powered pump that is connected to a tube that encases the penis. Once

Overwork, tension, family issues, and a lack of communication with his partner or other relationship difficulties increase a man's likelihood of suffering erection problems.

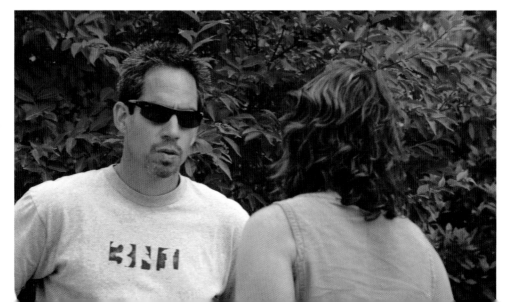

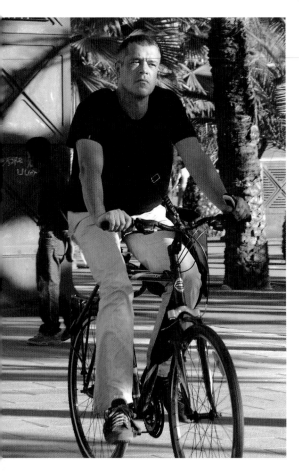

As with any medical condition, it is very important to avoid or reduce, any factor that causes erection problems as far as you can; in other words, quit smoking, avoid alcohol and drugs, take exercise, eat a balanced diet, avoid fats, keep your weight under control, and generally stick to a healthy lifestyle both mentally and physically.

▪ Transurethral and injection therapy

Although this procedure is very safe and much less expensive than surgical therapy, the treatments are often abandoned over time, as the loss of spontaneity during sex leads to a loss of interest in continuing with the procedure.

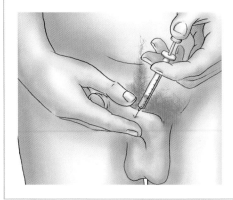

an erection or semi-erection has been achieved due to the engorgement of the penis with blood, a rubber ring previously attached around the tube is loosened and fitted around the base of the penis thus maintaining the erection by constricting the veins and so preventing the outflow of blood.

Penile implants. Penile prostheses, or implants, are devices inserted surgically into the corpora cavernosa of the penis, allowing a man suffering from impotence to become rigid enough to achieve penetration. These prosthe-ses are made in different sizes—both in terms of length and width—to adapt to the characteristics of each individual. This type of surgery is not the best solution for impotence, but in some cases it is the only means capable of providing a solution for erection problems.

Revascularization surgery. Revascularization may be performed if the source of the problem is the poor condition of the veins in the penis. It involves surgically connecting a leg artery to the arteries at the back of the penis thus increasing blood flow.

Fewer than 10 percent of men suffering erection problems seek medical help. Safe and effective treatments exist nowadays, although none of them provides miracles. The type of treatment used depends on the specific problem that is causing the impotence. The first step is to identify and define its source and then try to find the simplest solution to the problem.

pharmacological treatment of erectile dysfunction

In the 1990s, a chance finding made during medical research revolutionized the treatment of erectile dysfunction: the discovery of sildenafil citrate (Viagra®). This drug a potent selective inhibitor of phosphodiesterase type 5 (an enzyme that is present in relatively high concentrations in the corpora cavernosa of the penis) and is capable of improving a man's erectile function if it is deficient. The discovery of Viagra® provided impetus to other pharmaceutical laboratories, which have been launching drugs onto the market with a proven high degree of clinical effectiveness in the way that they improve the flow of blood to the penis for the treatment of this male disorder.

Sildenafil (Viagra®)

This was the first prescription drug to come onto the market for the treatment of erectile dysfunction that could be taken orally. Sildenafil works by inhibiting selectively activation of the enzyme phosphodiesterase type 5 (PDE5), thus increasing blood flow in the penis in a natural way so that sexual arousal causes a man to get an erection.

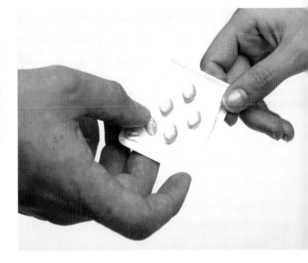

Viagra® is a prescription drug that has received a surge of interest, but there can be side effects and contraindications. It cannot be prescribed without a consultation. If you have erection difficulties, you should visit your doctor and explain your problem; but you should not take these pills without medical advice.

Viagra® is not an aphrodisiac, nor is it a hormone or a substance that causes an erection by itself. All it does is help achieve an erection when there is sexual stimulation.

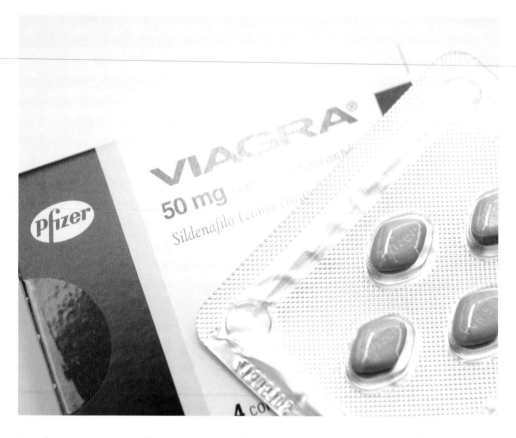

Viagra® is one of the pharmaceutical drugs most commonly prescribed for impotence; however, remedial action is sometimes simpler than just reaching for "the little blue pill." Smoking, high blood cholesterol, diabetes, and physical inactivity are some of the factors that can cause impotence, and for some men, simply a change of lifestyle and personal habits is all that is needed.

Viagra® can be taken when needed or wanted. It starts to work half an hour after being swallowed and can last for up to four hours.

It is not recommended to take more than one pill a day.

Among its side effects are stomach upsets, vomiting, diarrhea, headaches, blocked sinuses, facial flushing, muscular aches, and, in some cases, blurred vision.

As with other drugs that treat impotence, use of Viagra® is not recommended for men suffering from heart problems, particularly if they are taking medication to treat angina (e.g. glyceryl trinitrate). If both these drugs are taken together, they can cause a sudden and dangerous lowering of blood pressure.

N.B.

• To be fully effective, Viagra® should be taken at least four hours after your last meal. It is absorbed rapidly, its effects appear half an hour after swallowing, and it can remain effective for up to four hours if you are in good health. One of its limitations is that its effects can be delayed by up to an hour if it is taken immediately after a high-fat meal.

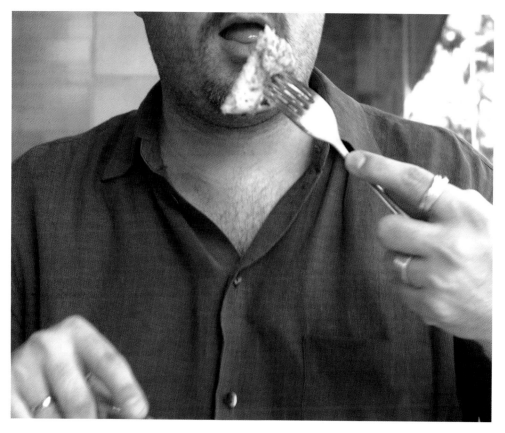

Apomorphine hydrochloride (Uprima®)

This is a pharmaceutical drug that acts on the central nervous system. It modifies the level of neurotransmitters, amplifies the nervous signal that causes an increase in blood flow to the penis, and thus facilitates an erection.

As with Viagra®, a sexual stimulus is necessary for the drug to be effective.

It is taken sublingually (under the tongue), approximately 20 minutes before sex.

Some of the side effects include nausea, headaches, dizziness, and fainting.

Uprima® has the advantage that it can be taken by patients who are prescribed nitrate drugs for heart problems; previously they had been unable to use this type of medication.

Vardenafil (Levitra®)

As with the prescription drugs discussed previously, Levitra® works by increasing blood flow to the penis and thus causes an erection, as long as there is some source of sexual stimulation.

The erection

As a result of sexual arousal, a nitric oxide (NO) is released from the neural system referred to as the "non-adrenergic/non-cholinergic system" (NANC). This substance sets in motion a series of changes—mediated by cyclic guanosine monophosphate (cGMP)—that cause a relaxation of the smooth muscle cells surrounding the blood vessels of the corpora cavernosa in the penis. This allows the blood vessels to dilate (vasodilation), resulting in an erection. However, cGMP is degraded by an enzyme—phosphodiesterase type 5 (PDE5)—and this is responsible for making an erection subside. Sildenafil is a potent, and highly selective, PDE5 inhibitor, which prevents the degradation of cGMP, thus stopping the penis from becoming flaccid and encouraging erection.

■ Percentage of patients with improved erections

This graph shows the percentage of patients with different types of dysfunction whose erections have improved thanks to sildenafil. An equal number of subjects were given a placebo. A placebo is a pharmacologically neutral substance which will have a positive effect on certain individuals if they believe or assume that the substance might be effective. All substances used for a curative or palliative ends have a double effect when administered: the true pharmacological effect and the effect caused by autosuggestion. In tests, patients are not told whether they have the actual drug or the placebo.

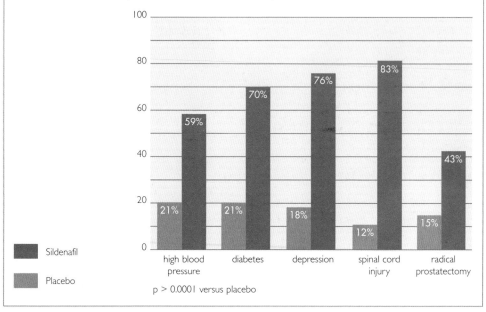

■ Sildenafil

▨ Placebo

p > 0.0001 versus placebo

Its principal agent is vardenafil, a PDE5 inhibitor.

If vardenafil is taken together with a high-fat meal, its absorption can be reduced, and it may take over an hour for its effects to be felt, which will then be less pronounced.

It should be taken between 25 and 60 minutes before sex, and its effects can last for up to 12 hours.

Its most common side effects are headaches, facial flushing, nausea, dizziness, rhinitis (runny or blocked nose), and dyspepsia (heartburn).

Tadalafil (Cialis®)

The principal agent of Cialis®, tadalafil, is a potent PDE5 inhibitor and, just like the other prescription drugs described above, it increases blood flow to the penis, in the context of sexual stimulation.

It needs to be taken approximately half an hour before having sex.

Tadalafil can remain effective for up to 24 hours. Moreover, food does not affect its absorption.

Its most common side effects are headaches, facial flushing, and aching (back) muscles.

ejaculation problems: premature ejaculation

"Premature ejaculation" refers to a situation when a man ejaculates too soon without being able to control it. In severe instances of this disorder, a man may ejaculate before his penis receives any, or hardly any, direct stimulation. This is a common problem, and there are solutions.

Premature ejaculation

Most men suffer, have suffered, or will suffer from this condition at some point in their lives without needing to worry about it.

Premature ejaculation becomes a problem only when it occurs during most experiences of sex.

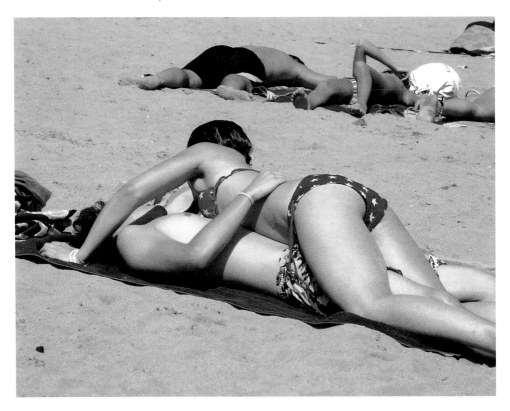

▟ How to tell whether you suffer from premature ejaculation

During sex, a man's excitement increases gradually until he reaches the "plateau phase," which can be sustained through self-control and thus allows more time for sexual enjoyment until the moment when climax is reached (orgasm).

A man who ejaculates prematurely is unable to linger in the plateau phase; instead, his arousal is rapid and beyond his control, which results in him experiencing swift, involuntary ejaculation.

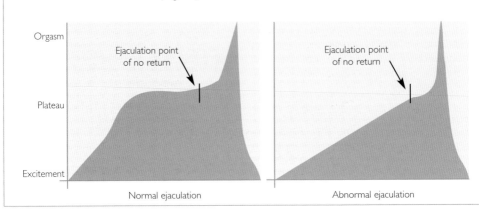

Orgasm

Ejaculation point
of no return

Plateau

Excitement

Normal ejaculation

Ejaculation point
of no return

Abnormal ejaculation

Persistent premature ejaculation can have a very negative effect on sex lives—for both men and women.

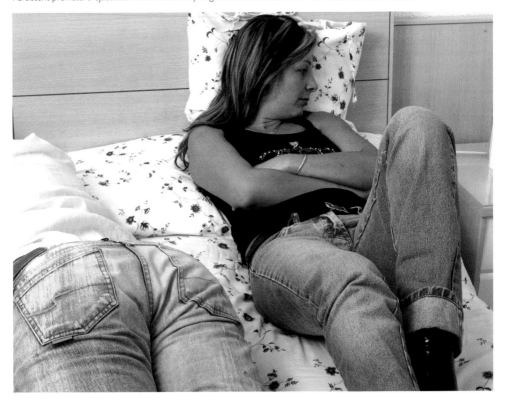

Premature ejaculation can arise at any age, but it is most common in young, inexperienced men. It is usually associated with first-time experiences, sexual impetuousness, and new situations (adolescence, a first sexual experience with a particular person, or special or unusual circumstances).

Often, a man suffering from premature ejaculation feels a loss of sexual desire or less sensitivity while ejaculating, which can lead to erectile dysfunction. This usually happens because a man is concentrating so hard on not reaching orgasm too soon that he cannot actually enjoy the act of sex itself.

A distinction can be made between primary premature ejaculation (in which a man has always had the problem and has never been able to control ejaculation) and secondary premature ejaculation (which might happen unexpectedly at some point in life).

Physical causes of premature ejaculation

Physical causes include: urogenital complaints of the posterior urethra and prostate gland, neurological disorders, degenerative conditions, vascular disorders, pharmaceutical drugs (antidepressants, drugs treating high blood pressure, stimulants), hypersensitivity of the glans, hormonal imbalances, and all illnesses that affect the reflex mechanisms for ejaculation.

Psychological causes of premature ejaculation

The immediate psychological causes of premature ejaculation include: a decline in the pleasure or sexual desire felt during sex; a repressed childhood and upbringing; lack of information about sex; pressure from a partner; underlying family issues; anxiety; stress; fear of failure; fear of not being able to control sexual stimuli; a partner who is inept, frigid, or indifferent; and lack of attraction to a partner (whether for physical reasons or because of hygiene, lack of communication or intimacy, the partner's gynecological problems, having suffered sexual abuse as a child, depression, problems at work or with friends, etc.).

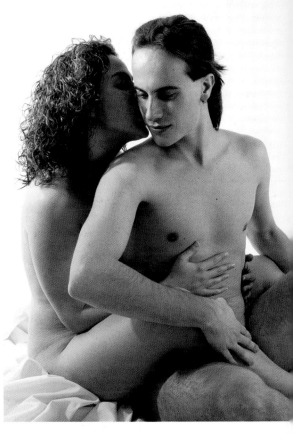

Very commonly, men who suffer from premature ejaculation reduce the time devoted to foreplay, which leaves a partner under-aroused and results in sexual activity that lacks much pleasure, and it may even be painful for a woman, due to lack of stimulation. When this happens, it only serves to increase tensions—and can even lead to a downward spiral of yet shorter periods before a man ejaculates, and thus even less satisfaction for his partner. Ultimately, this results in sexual activity diminishing.

Treatment

Firstly, a man should always talk this problem through with his sexual partner. Communication is very important in solving premature ejaculation.

Premature ejaculation is the sexual problem most commonly experienced by men, affecting some 40 percent.

Apart from removing the fear of things "going wrong," **solitary masturbation**, without the partner being present, helps a man to get to know his body better and identify the sensations that he feels during arousal and ejaculation, thus encouraging better self-control.

Stopping and starting exercises. A man can practice a variety of exercises to help him regain control. These involve stimulating the penis for a while (either yourself when masturbating or during sex with your partner) and then stopping the stimulation just before ejaculation. Revert to stimulation after a rest period of 30 to 60 seconds, and stop once again just before ejaculating. These stopping and starting exercises should be repeated five or six times before reaching orgasm (and thus ejaculating).

Compression method. A man is sexually stimulated until he alerts his partner that he is on the point of ejaculating. Then, either he or his partner should gently grip the end of the penis, at the point where the glans joins the shaft, for some 30 seconds. After this interruption, sexual stimulation can resume. The man or his partner can repeat the exercise until he wants to ejaculate.

Use of anesthetic creams, sprays, or gels with a localizing effect. These are able to numb the penis wherever they are applied and are partially effective, although they do present some difficulties: the anesthetic removes some of your pleasurable sensations; and the anesthetic can also take away some of your partner's sensitivity and pleasure.

■▪ Some recommendations for overcoming premature ejaculation:

- Spread excitement to all parts of the body, and do not concentrate only on the genitals and ejaculation.
- Play with your penis when erect, either alone or with your partner, so that you learn how to control your arousal and emotional tension.
- Recognize the ejaculation reflex and the sensations that occur before ejaculation so that you learn to control your arousal and do not go straight through to the point of no return.

Other types of therapy. These include the use of drugs such as some antidepressants that have a delaying effect on ejaculation as a side effect. These are not advised for the treatment of premature ejaculation, even if they are used with that aim: antidepressants can cause erectile dysfunction.

Another therapeutic option is the **use of vasodilatory drugs** in the corpora cavernosa of the penis. This involves injecting the medication into the penis yourself. It has a localized effect and maintains an erection for between 40 and 60 minutes. This totally natural erection does not subside after ejaculation, thus enabling you to carry on with sexual intercourse until your partner is satisfied.

male sexuality

It is important to understand that there are multiple and varied ways of interpreting and experiencing your sexuality: it is not a secondary part of your personality but is at the very heart of it, being vital to your happiness and development as a person. Human sexuality, unlike that of other animals, is infused with innumerable elements that go well beyond a mere genital focus. Understanding this is the basis for accepting the different ways in which we express our emotions and our sense of what is erotic or sexually arousing.

Male sexuality

Sex education should take into account all human beings' realities and forms of expression and should be capable of helping those who feel different from the majority so that they can live according to their personal reality and achieve happiness.

For centuries, sexual behavior that did not conform to the heterosexual model was considered to be a pathological aberration and deviant. However, homosexuality and bisexuality have ceased to be officially treated as illnesses for decades. The lack of empathy and understanding toward people with these sexual orientations has resulted not only in discrimination against them but often in them also suffering frequent persecution and even violence.

The phrase "alternative sexual orientation" is sometimes used as it not only emphasizes the way in which people identify their sexual desires, but jost as importantly includes the

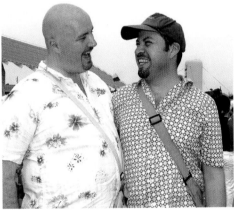

Leaving aside stereotypes and long-abandoned notions of conventionality, it is worth stating that sex and forming relationships as a "couple" are part of living and enjoying life. For these values to operate well depends to a large extent on how emotionally stable and generally well balanced a person is.

Both parents and teachers should ensure that children are given wide-ranging, quality information on the subject of sex and sexuality, without prejudice or subject to conditions, because, in the absence of this, children may get ill-informed answers from the wrong sources to their questions or concerns.

direction taken by their emotional and romantic feelings—a direction that differs from that of the heterosexual majority. People who follow the model that is considered "normal" see the opposite sex as the object of their desires. However, while the percentage of people in the population attracted physically and emotionally to the same sex, or to both sexes, is much lower than the percentage of those who fit into to the purely heterosexual model, it is not so low as to be considered abnormal.

Sexual orientation

Why do different types of sexual orientation exist? There are many different theories to explain the reason for this: psychological, endocrine, neuro-anatomical, genetic, etc. None of these has been scientifically proven in any conclusive way. What is certain is that an individual does not choose his or her sexual orientation; it cannot be modified and, of course, it is not contagious either. It is a personal orientation: a way of being. For gay men and lesbians, homosexuality that is natural, just as an orientation toward the opposite sex is natural for heterosexuals. Expecting people to behave in a way that goes against their nature and sexual orientation endangers their state of mental equilibrium and physical health.

Bisexual people can be aroused sexually by either men or women, and are able to satisfy their emotional needs with people of either sex.

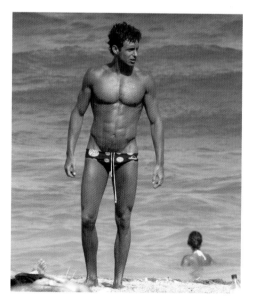

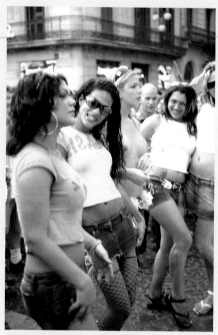

Transsexuality

A gay or lesbian orientation should not be confused with someone who is transsexual, transgender, or a transvestite.

- **Transsexual** describes people physically born as one sex but who feel strongly that they are a different sex mentally. They want to be rid of their primary and secondary sexual characteristics and to live as members of the opposite sex.

- **Transgender** describes people who are more androgynous, incorporating both masculine and feminine elements in their appearance. They may live partly as a man and partly as a woman, or wholly as a member of the opposite sex but without plans for genital surgery.

- **Transvestite** (crossdresser) describes people who enjoy dressing in the clothing of the opposite sex, but who have no desire to change sex.

Transsexuals, transgenderists, and transvestites may be male or female, heterosexual, homosexual, or bisexual. Distinctions need to be made at all times between a person's sex, sexual orientation, and sexual practice.

Generally speaking, male homosexuals see themselves as like any other men, regardless of sexual orientation. They do not usually have a gender-based identity problem, and many of them even emphasize their masculinity to the greatest possible extent. In most cases, the stereotype of the effeminate homosexual is a misleading one.

Of course, an individual can *choose* whether or not to act on his feelings, or modify the degree to which he does so. However, the case of sexuality, forcing your sexual and emotional feelings in a direction opposite to your natural inclination can be a source of frustration and dissatisfaction.

Homosexuality

Homosexuality describes the sexual orientation of people who feel emotionally and sexually attracted to people of their own sex. Men who feel attracted to other men are referred to as "gay," and women who feel attracted to other women are "lesbians." People who feel attracted to both sexes are bisexual. These categories, as with any classification of human beings, are not necessarily fixed or exclusive.

Sexual orientation is completely involuntary. Although some people discover their homosexuality later in life, most start to sense it in childhood and develop their feelings in adolescence.

Transsexuality

In general, a man or woman's primary and secondary sexual characteristics go toward solidifying that person's sense of self and identity. However, some people feel that their body and genitalia do not belong together with their gender identity.

For example, an individual whose genitalia make him a man may feel and identify as female; similarly, someone with all the normal sexual characteristics of a woman may feel inside that she is a "he."

People living with this condition adjust to it in differing ways. Some may devise their own cosmetic changes to their appearance, while others require intervention from medical professionals.

Some individuals who are genitally male adopt a female role in their social lives, often in a way that is both satisfactory to them and convincing to others. They alter their physical appearance to become more feminine and sometimes manage to acquire a social and work-related status that allows them to function as women in society.

Aberrant sexual behavior

This includes uncommon, unusual activity that certain people require to become sexually aroused. (This does not mean isolated inci-

Aberrant sexual behavior

- **Transvestitism** (crossdressing). This involves wearing the clothing of the opposite sex to obtain sexual excitement. It is different from transsexuality and homosexuality—the majority of transvestites are heterosexual, but they need the clothing of the opposite sex in order to feel aroused.

- **Voyeurism.** Secretly observing people as they undress or while they make love.

- **Fetishism.** Becoming sexually aroused through using a particular inanimate object, usually one that suggests or evokes another person or some part of them (often shoes or other items of clothing). Such objects are used during masturbation and during sexual activity with another person.

- **Exhibitionism.** An exhibitionist shows or exposes his genitalia to strangers unexpectedly in public places. He does not expect this to culminate in a sexual act; the reaction from others that he hopes to provoke through his behavior is all that he needs.

- **Frottage.** Taking part in activities or having sexual fantasies that are based on touching or rubbing unexpectedly against another person and without their consent, with this activity being practiced repeatedly or exclusively as a form of sexual arousal.

- **Sadism and masochism.** "Sadism" refers to inflicting pain on another person repeatedly in order to achieve personal sexual arousal. "Masochism" refers to sexual pleasure being obtained through the pain or humiliation received at the hand of someone else. Each of the partners involved in this type of behavior usually assumes a specific role, either the dominant aggressor or the submissive victim.

- **Pedophilia.** A pedophile is an adult who fantasizes about and having sexual relations with them children.

- **Bestiality.** This involves performing sexual intercourse with animals.

dences of sexual experimentation.) The essence of aberrant sexual behavior is that it is essential and integral to that person and constitutes virtually their only means of sexual excitement.

sex addiction and inhibited sexual desire

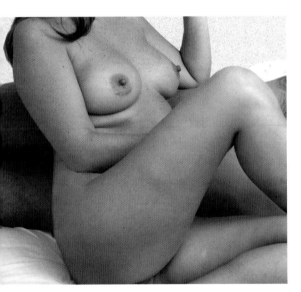

Addiction to sex is a form of compulsion that people admit to the least in our society. Often, compulsive sexual behavior is rationalized in some way, especially by men, who hope that by so doing they will minimize it or dilute the suffering that it causes to themselves or their families.

Mood swings are common for sex addicts, and this makes it more and more difficult for them to communicate with those around them.

It involves a type of dependency that cannot be described by means of a single type of behavior, as can be done for other addictions, since it can assume one or many different forms: compulsive masturbation, sexual relations

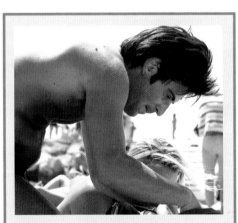

Sex addiction

Not all sexual deviancy can be termed an addiction, but the use of sex as a substitute for normal, healthy relationships within and with other members of society is a symptom of an addictive sexual disorder.

Sex addiction, as with any other type of compulsion, involves a pattern of behavior in which there is a loss of self-control concerning sexual behavior, alternating with periods of relative calm.

For sex addicts, sexually obsessive thoughts and sexual fantasies become increasingly necessary in order to cope with the problems of day-to-day life.

Sex addicts

Sex addicts experience sexual activity in the form of an uncontrollable urge and are more obsessed with desire than with the act of sex or reaching orgasm in itself. It is comparable to a physical addiction and abstinence is accompanied by agitation, irritability, trembling, and insomnia.

Sex online

Recently, a new means of becoming addicted to sex has arisen through the popularity of the Internet, because it is readily accessible, helps to preserve anonymity, and direct contact with a sexual partner is nonexistent, making it much easier to handle "contact," given the insecurities and fears that sex addicts typically feel. Nobody is there to judge them, and they do not have to reveal their identities—and as a result their problems (sexual problems, poor self-image, etc.) are reinforced and perpetuated. It has to be said that the principal characteristic that stands out about people who use this medium is the enormous loneliness that they feel. Without the existence of direct human contact, their feelings of loneliness only become more acute.

with multiple heterosexual or homosexual partners, encounters with strangers, use of pornography, prostitution, or telephone sex lines, etc.

Although at first, and from a frivolous perspective, it may appear that this addiction can only be a source of fun for the person involved, it should be remembered that, once out of control, sexual pleasure can be transformed into feelings of shame, self-loathing, pain, anguish, loneliness, etc.

These feelings, if sustained over a relatively long period of time, can result in the person succumbing to underlying depression, which serves only to worsen the initial symptoms.

Compulsive sexual behavior can lead to a range of outcomes on different levels. People can ruin themselves financially when they invest all their capital on satisfying their sexual needs—brothels, erotic massage parlors, telephone sex dating, etc. In cases where an addict is married or living with a partner, this behavior can lead to the breakdown of their relationship, especially when a man or woman learns of the continual deceit to which they have been subjected. It may also create problems relating to work, as a sex addict is unable to think of anything else other than his addictive behavior, putting everything else in second place.

Prognoses vary depending on the time that has passed since a person first started to

become addicted to sex. It should be borne in mind that many sex addicts will have had this problem from as far back as adolescence due to a lack of sex education and even, in many cases, due to sexual abuse or mistreatment.

The treatment for this addiction entails helping an individual to achieve control over his sexual response, while at the same time acquiring social skills that foster better communication and interaction in order to overcome feelings of isolation and loneliness.

Sex addiction usually operates on three levels:

Medical. A medical checkup is vital in most cases because antidepressants and anti-anxiety drugs can be prescribed to control sexual compulsions. This does not attempt to inhibit a person's sexual response completely or to enforce a life of celibacy, but to regulate a person's behavior until they return to a more acceptable level of conduct.

How does a sex addict behave?

Sex addicts are usually egocentric people interested only in their own satisfaction, be it through compulsive masturbation, use of pornography, prostitution, etc. Even when they have sexual encounters with others, these people are not treated like human beings—just as objects that satisfy their needs for the moment. On the other hand, addicts usually feel ashamed afterward. Their compulsive activity leaves them feeling blame, emptiness, and remorse about the experience. They suffer constant mood swings, making it difficult for other people to maintain any meaningful relationship with them. For addicts, sex is a way of dealing with their reality and everyday problems. They use it to ease tension, anxiety, and the inner malaise caused by these problems and others.

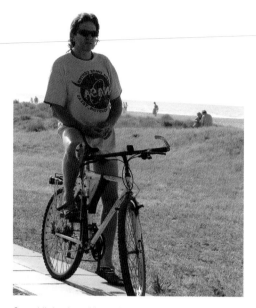

Sex addiction is a wide-ranging and complex condition, as it encompasses a variety of individual factors in terms of behavior and mentality. For that reason, recuperation is usually very gradual and involves many relapses until a balance is found.

Behavioral. The idea is to change a person's attitudes and help them regain self-control over matters such as buying pornography, calling telephone sex lines, and visiting prostitutes, by gradually reducing these activities and substituting alternative activities such as sport or leisure activities.

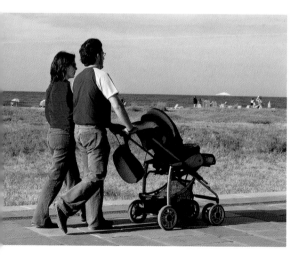

▪ Profile of a sex addict

- Experiences frequent mood swings
- Is egocentric and on a quest for self-satisfaction
- Thinks of people only as sex objects
- Has sexual relationships in which there is no tenderness or physical affection
- Thinks of sex as the only means of achieving personal satisfaction
- Feels ashamed and guilty about his sex life, keeping it secret
- Has low self-esteem
- Escapes reality by living in a world of sexual fantasy

Psychological. An addict has to change his negative mental attitude, raise his sense of self-esteem, and attempt to deal with any underlying reasons for his problem, such as depression or sexual abuse as a child.

What is inhibited sexual desire?

Inhibited sexual desire (ISD) refers to a low level of interest in sex that is expressed by a difficulty in initiating, or responding to a partner's desire for, sexual activity. This condition can be primary, in which a person has never felt much interest in sex or sexual desire, or secondary, in which a person used to have sexual feelings but no longer does. A person with ISD may feel this way only toward the partner with whom he or she currently has a relationship: he or she remains interested in other people, but not in the partner; or it may be general: he or she lacks sexual interest toward anyone.

In its most extreme form, sexual aversion, a person not only lacks sexual desire, but also finds sex repellent, disgusting, and unpleasant.

A sex addict's family suffers a great deal as a result of the problem, especially the spouse, and the addict's children may copy his addictive style of behavior in their adult lives.

epididymitis

Epididymitis is an inflammation of the tube (the epididymis) running from the rear of each testicle to its vas deferens, caused by a bacterial infection of the urinary tract.

Epididymitis

The epididymis is a tightly coiled tubular structure to the rear of each testicle that holds immature sperm generated by the testicles and stores them for several days. When a man ejaculates, the semen is propelled from one end of the epididymis toward the vas deferens. Subsequently, the semen is transported via the vas deferens toward the spermatic cord in the pelvic cavity beyond the ureter and behind the urinary bladder. At this point, the vas deferens joins the seminal vesicle forming the ejaculatory duct, which passes through the prostate gland and empties into the urethra.

The epididymis is located to the rear of each testicle and is a tightly coiled tube, which forms the first part of the duct that carries sperm away from the testicles.

Epididymitis is an inflammation of the epididymis.

Epididymitis usually affects only one testicle.

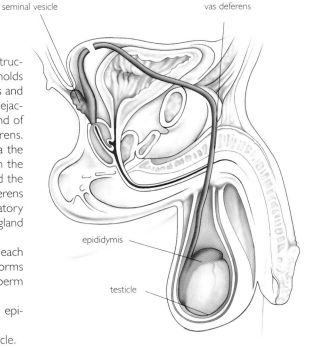

seminal vesicle

vas deferens

epididymis

testicle

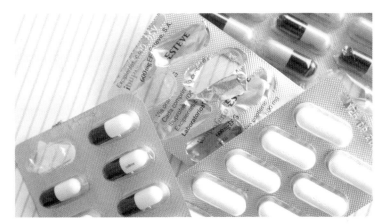

Sometimes, certain types of medication, such as drugs to treat cardiac arrhythmia, for example, can cause the epididymis to become inflamed. The inflammation does not respond to antibiotics in epididymitis of this type. The only treatment in these cases is to reduce the dose of the medication used or to change the medication.

237

Causes

- This is a common disease in young men between the ages of 19 and 35, although a man of any age can suffer from it.
- It is usually caused by the spread of a bladder or urethral infection.
- In young, straight men, the microorganisms that most commonly cause this type of inflammation are gonorrhea (*Neisseria gonorrhoeae*) and chlamydia (*Chlamydia trachomatis*).
- In children, young gay men, and older men, it is more commonly caused by bacterial organisms typical found in the urogenital organs, such as Escherichia coli, for example.
- Other bacteria that can cause epididymitis are *Microbacterium tuberculosis* and *Ureaplasma urealyticum*.

- Sometimes, certain types of medication can cause inflammation of the epididymis. This is true of some drugs used to treat cardiac arrhythmia. In epididymitis of this type, inflammation is restricted to the end of the tube and does not respond to antibiotics. The only treatment in these cases is to reduce the dose of the medication that is causing the swelling or even to change it.
- Sexually active men who are not monogamous and do not usually use condoms present the greatest risk of suffering from this type of infection.
- The risk of suffering from this type of infection is also increased following surgical procedures or when people with chronic conditions are using catheters.

Acute epididymitis causes inflammation of the scrotum, testicular pain, and is sometimes accompanied by fever, which can last for several weeks.

In rare cases, epididymitis can become a chronic condition if not treated early on or if treated inadequately. In such instances, there is only pain and no inflammation, and surgical intervention may become necessary.

■ Symptoms

- An increase in size of the testicle(s).
- The testicle is inflamed and more sensitive on the affected side.
- The area of the groin on the infected side is inflamed and painful.
- Testicular pain that worsens when passing feces.
- Fever.
- Discharge from the urethra.
- Pain during urination.
- Pain during sexual activity or when ejaculating.
- Blood in semen.
- Groin pain.

The first symptoms are a mild fever, shivering, a feeling of heaviness in one of the testicles, and increased sensitivity in the area if there is rubbing, pressure, or movement.

The scrotum around the testicle reddens and the testicle swells in size due to inflammation. Acute, intense pain is felt.

Discomfort may be felt in the lower part of the abdomen or in the pelvic region, and a feeling of heat and even pain may be felt when urinating.

There may also be a discharge from the urethra, blood in semen, or pain during ejaculation, but this is uncommon.

Included among the complications that can arise from epididymitis are testicular infarction, scrotal abscess, scrotal cutaneous fistula, chronic epididymitis, and infertility.

Treatment

Treatment usually relies on antibiotics to eliminate the infection. Normally, sexually transmitted infections require specific antibiotics and are usually prescribed as well to a patient's sexual partner to make sure the infection is completely eliminated.

In some cases, where there is inflammation and acute pain, the use of anti-inflammatory drugs and analgesics is also recommended.

Bed rest is advisable, as is ensuring that the testicles are supported close to the body, which prevents the inflammation from becoming exacerbated. To reduce swelling and heaviness, it can be a good idea to apply cold water or even ice-cube compresses to the affected area.

It is important for your physician to monitor the whole course of treatment and assess whether the infection has been completely eradicated. This is very important, because poorly treated epididymitis can cause severe testicular problems, scrotal abscesses, fistulas, chronic epididymitis, and infertility.

Preventive measures

Complications from epididymitis can be prevented if it is diagnosed early and if recommended treatment is closely followed.

Safe sex practices are the best way of preventing the cases of epididymitis linked to sexually transmitted diseases.

It is vital to treat both partners in a relationship to prevent possible reinfection.

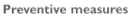

It is not a good idea to continue with sexual activity while the infection is present: there is a chance of passing on the infection or becoming reinfected, and also it is important to allow the testicle to rest while acute symptoms persist.

Diagnosis

- Diagnosis of epididymitis is done by a straightforward physical examination and some laboratory tests.

- Physical examinations sometimes reveal a reddish, hard lump that is very sensitive to the touch on the epididymis coming from the affected testicle.

- A man may present swollen lymph glands in the groin.

- The doctor may also want to investigate whether there is any discharge from the penis.

- In addition to a physical examination, the doctor may want to carry out other tests, such as a full urine analysis, a culture, or a urethral smear to detect which microorganisms are causing the infection.

- In order to discount other possible medical conditions, it may be necessary to undergo a testicular ultrasound scan.

hydroceles

A hydrocele is a buildup of liquid within the scrotum, surrounding the testicles. Hydroceles are common in newborn boys and usually disappear during the first months of life. The main symptom of a hydrocele is the painless swelling of a testicle, with the testicle feeling like a small, water-filled balloon. Generally speaking, hydroceles are not dangerous and are usually treated only if they become uncomfortable or bothersome, or if they are impeding the flow of blood to and from the testicle.

Causes

Hydroceles are common in newborn babies, and a buildup of fluid may be seen on one or both sides of the scrotum.

During normal development, the testicles descend from the abdomen toward the scrotum via a tube. Hydroceles form when this tube fails to close and the peritoneal liquid passes from the abdomen through the open tube. The liquid accumulates in the scrotum and remains trapped there, which is what makes it swell up.

Hydroceles normally disappear a few months after birth, but their appearance can cause parental alarm.

In some cases, a hydrocele may be linked to an inguinal hernia.

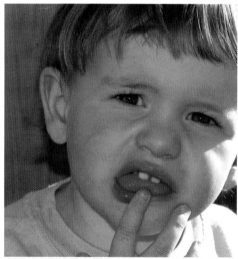

A hydrocele is a buildup of fluid within the scrotum, surrounding the testicles. This buildup of fluid is very common among newborns and generally disappears by itself during the first months of life.

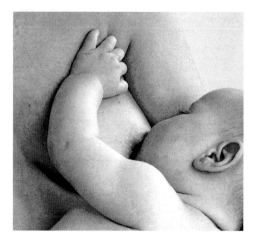

Hydroceles may also be due to an inflammation of or injury to the testicle or epididymis, or even the obstruction of the spermatic cord by fluid or even blood. This type of hydrocele is more common among older men.

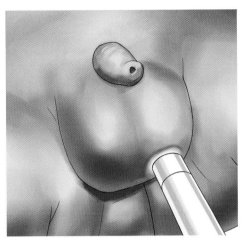

A hydrocele is easily identified: placing a flashlight against the inflamed part of the scrotum, the scrotum becomes illuminated if filled with fluid.

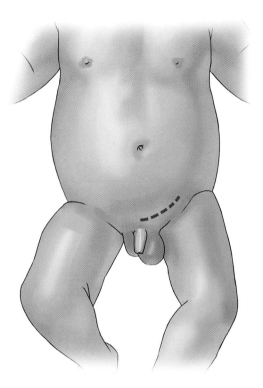

Preventive measures:
Surgery should be sought as soon
as possible for hydroceles linked to
an inguinal hernia, and hydroceles
that do not get better by
themselves within a few months
should be evaluated to decide
whether surgery is necessary.

An incision is made just above the groin while the baby is under general anesthesia. Repair work is done on the open conduit (inguinal canal) between the abdominal cavity and the scrotum, fluid is extracted from the scrotum, and the incision is closed.

A hydrocele forms toward the eighth month of fetal development. During this period, the testicles descend from the abdomen and locate within the scrotum. At this time, fluid that is normally present in the abdomen may accompany the testicle and follow it into the scrotum. Usually, the conduit between the abdomen and the scrotum closes up, and the fluid is reabsorbed (a noncommunicating hydrocele). In some cases, it does not close up, consequently allowing fluid to flow between the abdominal cavity and the scrotum (a communicating hydrocele).

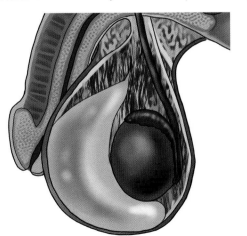

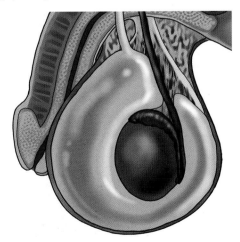

Signs, symptoms, and examinations

- The first symptom is a painless testicular edema (swelling) on one or both sides of the scrotum, feeling like a small, water-filled balloon. The scrotum swells in size and does not cause any pain.

- A hydrocele is referred to as a "closed hydrocele" if its volume is constant—i.e. it never changes size. The membrane containing the fluid (the tunica vaginalis) is filled at some point, then closes, and remains closed. The natural progression of this condition is its spontaneous disappearance—the fluid is gradually reabsorbed over a period of months. It almost never requires treatment.

- If the hydrocele changes in volume, it means that the membrane remains open and is allowing fluid to flow in and out. This is referred to

as an "open hydrocele." Very often, this sorts itself out. In other cases, it is usually linked to a hernia and may persist. If so, its treatment and that of the hernia will require surgery.

- Hydroceles can be detected through a simple physical examination. This is very easy, because it causes no pain. The scrotum appears enlarged and, very often, the testicle cannot be seen because of the amount of fluid surrounding it.

- The fluid in a hydrocele is usually clear; as a result, it is possible to shine a light through it via the skin of the scrotum, outlining the testicle, and indicating the presence of any fluid.

- An ultrasound scan may be performed to confirm the diagnosis.

■ Treatment

- Generally speaking, hydroceles are not dangerous, and they are normally treated only when they are causing the patient genuine discomfort.

- One option is to drain the fluid in the scrotum using a hypodermic syringe ("needle aspiration"). This method can cause infections, fibrosis, slight or moderate pain in the region of the scrotum and, furthermore, it is highly unlikely to resolve the problem—the fluid simply builds up again afterward. However, after needle aspiration, drugs can be injected to help close the opening present in the scrotal sac and thus help prevent a renewed accumulation of fluid. It is not the method most commonly used, but it is an alternative for patients for whom surgery might present a risk.

- The best option for treating a hydrocele that fails to disappear of its own accord is a hydrocelectomy. This is a minor surgical procedure for the correction of a hydrocele, often available as ambulatory surgery under general or local anesthesia. Postoperative patients are advised to apply ice to the area to reduce swelling and also to use an athletic supporter (jockstrap) for some time afterward. Blood clots

or bruising may appear after the operation and, occasionally, the scrotum may also become infected or damaged.

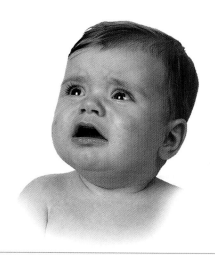

scrotal swellings

A spermatocele is a lump similar to a cyst that grows within the epididymis. It is usually filled with fluid and dead sperm cells. As with hydroceles, a spermatocele does not usually require treatment, unless it keeps growing or feels uncomfortable.

Causes

Depending on the reasons for them, scrotal swellings may be cancerous in origin or benign and harmless. Benign scrotal swellings include:

Varicoceles. These are networks of distended, thickened, and widened veins located in the scrotum, very similar to varicose veins (dilated veins). Varicoceles usually appear on the left side of the scrotum and feel to the touch like a bag of worms. A varicocele can be observed when a man stands up but usually disappears again when he lies down or reclines, because that posture reduces blood flow to the dilated veins. A varicocele can be corrected surgically if it is bothersome or if it might affect a man's fertility.

Hydroceles. This is an accumulation of fluid in the membrane that surrounds the testicles, causing a painless swelling to form around one of them. This condition can occur at the time of birth or else develop as a man ages. Hydroceles are generally painless, but they can grow so large that they require surgical removal to eliminate the problem.

Hematoceles. A hematocele is a collection of blood inside the scrotum.

Spermatocele. These are lumps inside the scrotum similar to cysts and contain fluid and dead sperm cells.

Scrotal swellings can also be caused by a variety of inflammatory illnesses or infections, such as, for example, epididymitis; a scro-

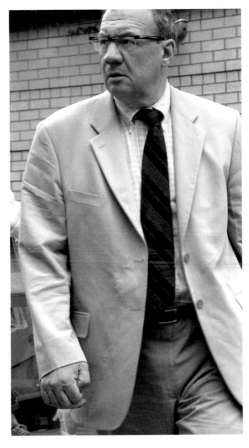

tal injury or physiological condition; inguinal hernia; or a tumor.

Treatment

Any lump, cyst, or scrotal swelling that you find should be checked out by a doctor.

Hematoceles, hydroceles, and spermatoceles are usually benign and if so do not require treatment.

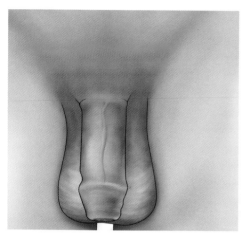

There can be various reasons for scrotal swellings, ranging from tumors, cysts, and inflammations to physical injuries or inguinal hernias.

If a scrotal condition appears suddenly or temporarily, it can help to apply ice to the area, or some other medium to relieve the swelling. In other cases, it may be necessary to take antibiotics or painkillers and anti-inflammatory drugs.

Using an athletic supporter (jockstrap) can provide some relief from the pain and discomfort associated with a scrotal swelling. In some cases, a hematocele, hydrocele, or spermatocele may need surgical intervention to remove the accumulation of blood, fluid, or dead cells.

Symptoms

- The first symptom of a problem may be a protuberance or lump inside the scrotum, which is frequently painless, or else an enlargement of the scrotum.
- Another symptom may be infertility.

Varicoceles are networks of dilated veins, similar to varicose veins but located in the scrotum. Varicoceles can be felt by gently pressing the scrotum, and they are sometimes even visible below the surface of the skin.

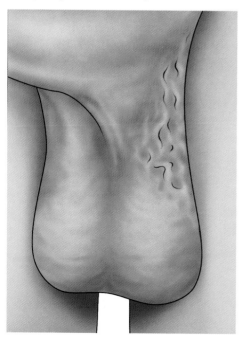

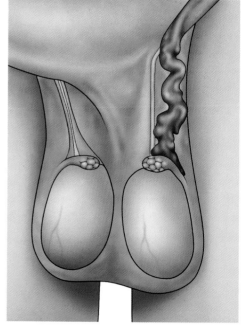

▪ Signs and physical examinations

- When performing a physical examination, lumps or masses may be found inside the scrotum that present a wide range of characteristics:

- Although a swelling typically appears on one side of the scrotum, it may be present on both sides.

- It may be sensitive or insensitive: i.e. it may or may not be painful.

- To the touch it may feel rounded, smooth, lumpy, or granular.

- It may feel firm, fluid, or solid.

- The groin's lymph glands on the affected side may be inflamed and feel sensitive.

- If a physical examination is insufficient for the diagnosis of a scrotal swelling, it may be practical to perform an ultrasound scan or a biopsy.

- It is important for all men to perform regular self-examinations of the scrotum and testicles and thus detect any lumps, swellings, or abnormalities early on.

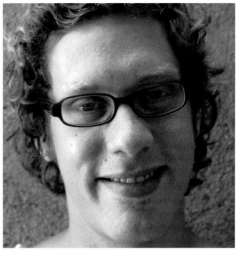

Most scrotal swellings are benign and do not involve long-term consequences or complications as they can be treated easily. Even a testicular tumor can be cured if it is diagnosed and treated early and effectively. It is very important to consult a specialist at the first sign of any symptoms, as early diagnosis is the key to curing cancer.

Preventive measures

- Scrotal swellings linked to sexually transmitted diseases, such as epididymitis caused by gonorrhea, for example, can be prevented by a responsible attitude toward sex and the use of condoms.

- Wearing sensible clothing when playing sports or working out can prevent injuries from occurring, which in the long term can result in the appearance of scrotal swellings.

- It is very important to examine your testicles every month for the early detection of any tumors, thus increasing your chances of recovery in the event of testicular cancer.

It is very important to examine your testicles each month and thus be able to detect any lumps or abnormalities early.

orchitis

Orchitis is an inflammation of the testicle. It is most commonly caused by mumps, especially when the illness occurs in adulthood. Orchitis can also appear after a prostate gland infection or epididymitis. Many less common illnesses can also produce orchitis.

Causes

- Many bacteria and viruses can cause orchitis, but it usually appears as a result of epididymitis (inflammation of the epididymis—the tube that connects the testicle to the vas deferens).

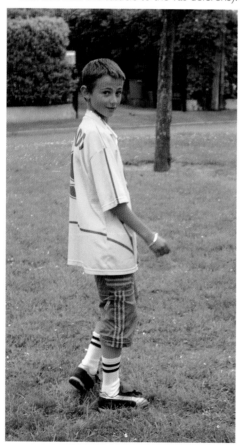

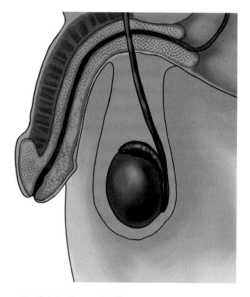

Orchitis is an inflammation of the testicle. It is usually caused by the pathogenic microorganisms typically present in the urinary tract, although many men who contract mumps may also develop orchitis.

- The most common viral cause of orchitis is mumps. Approximately 30 percent of patients who contract mumps after puberty go on to develop orchitis during the course of the illness. It is very common among adolescent boys (ten years old and above), generally appearing four to six days after the onset of mumps. One-third of boys who develop orchitis during mumps also present testicular atrophy. Orchitis as the result of mumps can cause men to be sterile.

- The most common bacterial causes among young, heterosexual men are gonorrhea (*Neisseria gonorrhoeae*) and chlamydia (*Chlamydia trachomatis*). Among children and the elderly, it is more usual for orchitis to be caused by the pathogens typically present in the urinary tract.

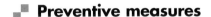

■ Preventive measures

- Mumps can cause orchitis. Vaccination against mumps prevents this.
- Safe and responsible sex prevents sexually transmitted diseases.
- Proper hygiene and a healthy lifestyle prevent infections and health-related conditions.

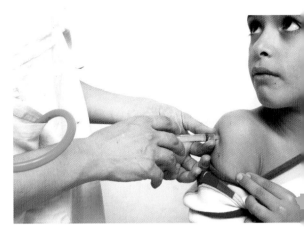

Mumps can cause orchitis. Vaccination against mumps prevents this.

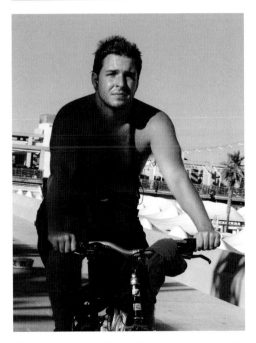

Orchitis can cause infertility and the atrophy of one or both testicles. Other potential complications include scrotal swellings, testicular infarction, chronic epididymitis, and scrotal cutaneous fistulas.

Symptoms
- Inflammation of the scrotum.
- A testicle that is sensitive, inflamed, and feels heavier than normal.
- Swollen lymph glands in the groin area, feeling more sensitive on the affected side.
- Fever.
- There may be discharge from the penis.
- Pain when urinating.
- Pain during sex or ejaculation.
- Groin pain.
- Testicular pain that may intensify when passing feces or feeling bloated.
- Blood in semen.

Treatment
If orchitis is bacterial in origin, antibiotics need to be taken to treat the infection. Anti-inflammatory and painkilling drugs are advised in cases of significant pain and swelling.

In the event of gonorrhea or chlamydia—sexually transmitted diseases—sexual partners need to be treated jointly to avoid reinfection.

Only painkillers are prescribed if a virus is responsible for causing orchitis, because viruses cannot be killed by antibiotics. Plenty of rest lying down is advised, thus reducing swelling and pain by preventing the scrotum from pulling downward. Applications of ice compresses to the affected area will reduce inflammation.

ORCHITIS RISK FACTORS (NOT SEXUALLY TRANSMITTED)	ORCHITIS RISK FACTORS (SEXUALLY TRANSMITTED)
Inadequate vaccination against mumps.	Unprotected (high-risk) sexual activity.
Age (older than 45)	Not using condoms.
Recurrent urinary tract infections.	If a partner has been suffering from an STD.
Birth abnormalities of the urinary tract.	Personal history of gonorrhea or other STDs.
Surgery or investigation of the urinary tract using medical equipment.	
Chronic catheterization.	

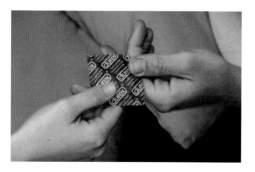

Unsafe sex can increase the risk of testicular infections.

Acute scrotal or testicular pain can mean an emergency situation. Therefore, you should see a doctor immediately if you experience pain in the testicles or scrotum.

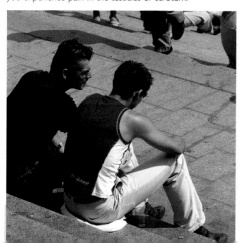

■ Signs and physical examinations

A simple physical examination can reveal whether you are suffering from orchitis. Swollen lymph glands in the groin, or a swollen or enlarged testicle, are all signs of possible orchitis.

A rectal probe may be necessary to assess whether the prostate gland has also become inflamed.

- As with other infections, it may be practical to carry out other tests to verify the cause of the condition, such as:
- Culture and analysis of a urine sample from the patient;
- Selective tests for chlamydia and gonorrhea.
- Full blood analysis.
- If the diagnosis is unclear, it may be necessary to perform other types of test, such as a Doppler ultrasound scan, in order to rule out any other medical causes.
- Testicular gammagraphy can also obtain images to discount the possibility of testicular torsion and confirm a diagnosis of orchitis by verifying an increase in blood flow.

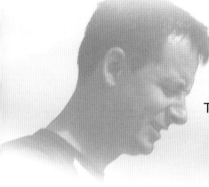

priapism

This is a male condition involving a prolonged erection that is not brought on by sexual stimulation and does not result in ejaculation. It can be painful and, in the long term, can result in impotence.

Priapism can be classified according to two types: primary or idiopathic priapism (without any apparent cause or reason) and secondary priapism.

45 to 60 percent of all cases are primary priapism, sometimes occurring when an erection fails to subside, persisting over time despite the end of any sexual stimulus.

The causes of secondary priapism are usually physical or neurological conditions. Among its neurological causes are abnormalities in the nerve mechanisms involved during erection, psychiatric conditions, diseases of the nervous system, trauma, high levels of alcohol in the bloodstream, particular types of medication, etc.

Prominent among its mechanical and physical causes are penile or pelvic injuries, infections, prostatitis, tumors affecting the urinary bladder, prostate gland, or rectum, and cardiovascular system problems.

Priapism can occur at any age, from infancy to old age, with the secondary form predominating among boys, and primary among adults.

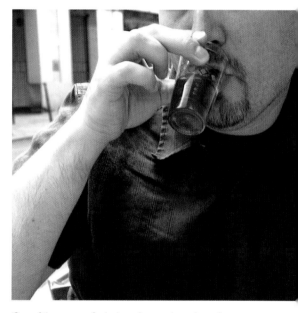

One of the causes of priapism—i.e. a prolonged erection not brought on by feelings of arousal and without ejaculation—can be the excessive consumption of certain drugs, such as alcohol.

Symptoms

- An erection creates a significant increase in blood flow. The process of a penis becoming erect, and then flaccid after ejaculation, occurs through the retention and subsequent release of blood flowing to and from the structures within the penis. Any factor that adversely affects the normal mechanics of this system can cause priapism.

- Engorgement of the penis is at its maximum extent in cases of priapism and can be identified from the flaccid state of the glans, which is not involved in the process.

- Acute priapism is painful and causes extreme exhaustion, usually accompanied by urine retention and fever.

- Some men may react violently to the condition, only making the pain worse.

- In some cases of priapism the penis is less rigid and, consequently, less painful.

- The penis may spontaneously return to normal, but this is impossible to predict.

Treatment

Treatment is wholly variable according to the type of priapism involved.

If priapism is venous in origin (failure of blood to drain from the penis via its veins)— "low-flow priapism"—some possible treatments include:

- Doing some kind of moderate physical activity, after which many cases normalize by themselves;
- Draining blood from the penis and repeated cleansing of the corpora cavernosa using saline solution;
- The most severe cases require pharmacological injections into the penis to encourage a return to the flaccid state, such as epinephrine, methoxamine, or phenylephrine. In such instances, it is advisable to check a patient's heart rate and blood pressure, as this can vary when these substances are introduced.
- If the priapism still persists, doctors proceed with a surgical procedure to prevent permanent damage to the erectile tissue of the penis.

When priapism is linked to injections to treat impotence, alternative types of therapy have to be used instead or the dosage has to be carefully readjusted. Cases of priapism due to drug treatments to relieve impotence are increasingly uncommon thanks to the development of effective, orally administered forms of medication.

If priapism is arterial in origin (high-flow priapism), there is no danger of it causing damage to erectile tissue, and its treatment is less urgent. Although some cases are resolved simply with medication, most require occlusion of the damaged blood vessel.

A range of nonspecific measures can be of practical use in reducing an erection, such as performing a firm prostate massage, or applying an ice pack or cold compress.

Priapism is linked to certain lifestyles. Men susceptible to this condition often have hectic sex lives, drink heavily, or take drugs that stimulate the nervous system. Some undergo prolonged erections when sleeping, with this situation lasting for months at a time. Sometimes the penis fails to return to its flaccid state after sexual intercourse, and this can make sex a traumatic experience.

A painful erection that has lasted for more than four hours justifies urgent medical attention.

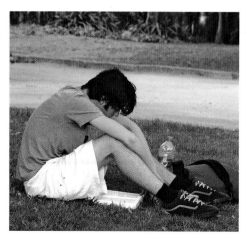

Medical examination and diagnosis

- Thorough discussions with a patient are vital to a physician's diagnosis of the likely cause of that patient's priapism. Understanding the cause is invaluable if a patient is to receive the correct treatment.

- In order to assess whether the cause of priapism is low flow (venous) or high flow (arterial), a blood sample is taken from the corpus cavernosum. If, despite all efforts, the cause cannot be discovered, it may be necessary to perform a Doppler ultrasound scan.

testicular torsion

As is well understood, the testicles are located in the scrotum, free of the abdominal cavity. This position outside of the body allows the temperature of the testicles to be lower than body temperature, which is vital if they are to function properly. Each of the testicles is attached to a structure—the spermatic cord—that feeds its blood supply. Occasionally, a testicle will twist around and become entangled with the spermatic cord, unable to return to its original position. This entanglement stops blood from flowing to the testicle and can cause irreparable damage as a result.

Causes of testicular torsion

Testicular torsion (strangulation) can sometimes occur for no apparent reason, even during the night. At other times, the cause may be more obvious, such as after an intensely physical workout, for example.

Some men are more predisposed to testicular torsion than others as a result of malformation or hereditary abnormalities in the connective tissue inside the scrotum. However, an injury or blow can also cause it.

Testicular torsion is a medical emergency—albeit rare— and can occur at any age, although it is more likely to happen during puberty and infancy.

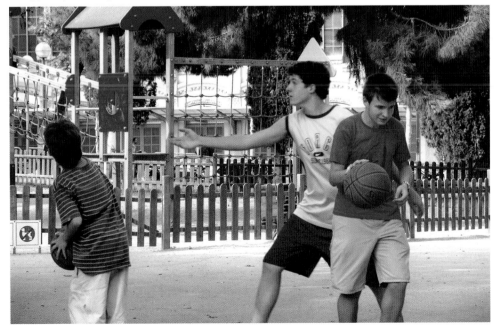

◾ Signs and symptoms

- Acute, intense pain begins suddenly in one testicle with or without any prior warning or apparent reason.
- Inflammation on one side of the scrotum.
- Swelling.
- The affected testicle is higher than normal.
- Nausea and vomiting.
- Giddiness.
- Blood in semen.
- Lump in the testicle.

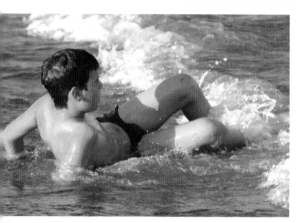

Testicular torsion is a rare medical emergency that occurs in approximately 1 in every 4,000 men.

It can happen at any age but is most common during puberty between the ages of 12 and 18 and among babies less than one month old.

Symptoms include major pain in the testicular area, feeling very intense and acute, radiating toward the groin, and changing position fails to reduce it. It may be accompanied by fever and vomiting.

Treatment

Testicular torsion generally requires immediate intervention. The seriousness of the torsion depends on whether the testicle or testicles have been completely strangulated or only partially. The more twisted the testicle, the more urgent it is to proceed with surgery, which involves opening the scrotum, untwisting the testicle, and holding it in place with stitches to prevent it from strangulating again.

If there is the slightest doubt, urologists usually decide to operate on patients, particularly children and adolescents, with a view to saving the testicle. If the operation is performed within the first six hours of the complaint, there is a much greater chance of the testicle's survival even though it is somewhat purplish in color. After six hours, the testicle usually blackens and it is impossible to resuscitate it, leaving its removal as the only option.

Diagnosis

- Testicular torsion is usually diagnosed through a physical examination and by considering a patient's complete medical history. An immediate diagnosis is vital, because prolonged testicular torsion can cause irreversible damage to the testicles leaving it impossible to repair them and forcing the surgeon to remove them and replace them with silicon testicle prostheses.

- The medical practitioner's examination of the scrotum is very painful and, at times, impossible, as the testicle is higher than normal and the scrotum will be swollen with fluid.

- It may be necessary to perform an ultrasound scan or other types of examination that allow the degree of testicular torsion to be diagnosed with greater accuracy.

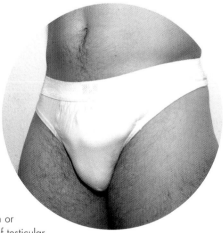

twisted spermatic cord

untwisted spermatic cord

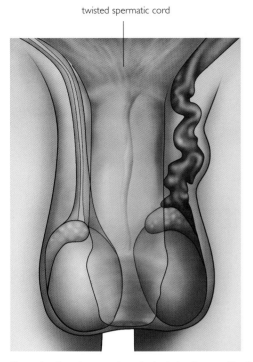
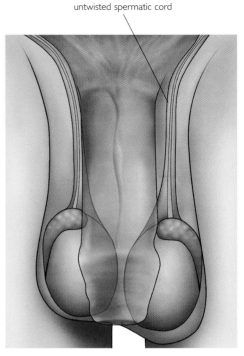

The patient is under general anesthesia during the operation, leaving him deeply unconscious and feeling no pain. An incision is made into the scrotum, the testicle is untwisted, and dissolving stitches are put in place to prevent the testicle from turning around again. The unaffected testicle is also fixed in place with stitches, as the problem tends to occur on both sides, and the healthy testicle is at high risk of suffering similar torsion subsequently.

To minimize any long-term problems, it is advisable to perform the operation within six hours of the first symptoms occurring.

The other testicle is also operated on, even if unaffected, to prevent any future torsion.

Even when the operation is successful, and recovery apparently complete, 50 percent of strangulated testicles go on to produce abnormal semen.

The testicle can atrophy (die) days or months after the operation to correct torsion. Another potential complication is a severe testicular and scrotal infection due to the restriction of normal blood flow during torsion.

Torsion of the testicular appendix

At each upper pole of the testicle and epididymis is a small appendix that can become twisted on the pedicle that links it to the testicle. The torsion of these appendices is one of the most frequent causes of acute testicular pain—it is officially known as torsion of the hydatid of Morgagni—and is responsible for 90 percent of all cases. Its cause is unknown, although it is thought to be the result of accidents involving injury or perhaps sporting activities. Other hydatids (vesicles) can become twisted as well and have similar clinical symptoms. These symptoms include reddening and swelling of the scrotum, which varies greatly in intensity from case to case. This can range from significant symptoms to symptoms that are barely noticeable but which recur frequently.

In the case of mild symptoms, patients follow a conservative course of treatment involving anti-inflammatory drugs and bed rest; however, if the symptoms are serious, surgical removal of the hydatid is advised in order to eliminate the pain and any complications, such as testicular atrophy.

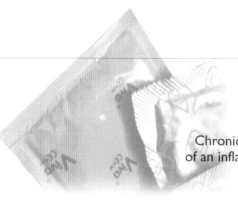

chronic urethritis

Chronic urethritis, or urethral syndrome, consists of an inflammation and irritation of the urethra and can last for weeks or even months.

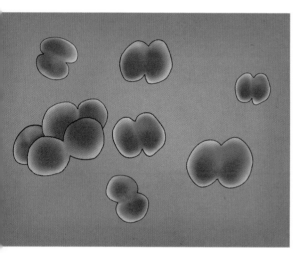

Bacteria that cause chronic urethritis.

Causes, effects, and risk factors

Chronic urethritis is normally caused by a bacterial infection or an anatomical problem, in which the duct that carries urine away from the bladder, the urethra, has become distended, although it can also be the result of a wide variety of systemic illnesses and can even be linked to emotional problems and stress levels.

Urethritis is a condition that affects men and women equally.

Its main symptoms are: pain when urinating and an increased need to urinate.

Between 50 and 70 percent of all people presenting symptoms of urethritis have a bacterial infection of the urethra or of the bladder (cystitis). This type of infection can be recurrent.

In the case of urethral syndrome, the symptoms of chronic urethritis are present, but there is no evidence of bacterial infection.

The possible causative agents of chronic urethritis include all the organisms that start infections in the urinary tract, whether bacterial, viral, or fungal in origin.

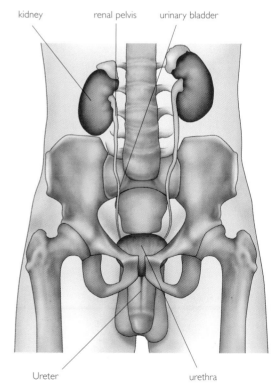

kidney   renal pelvis   urinary bladder

Ureter   urethra

The symptoms of urethritis appear very often and account for five to ten percent of all consultations with physicians.

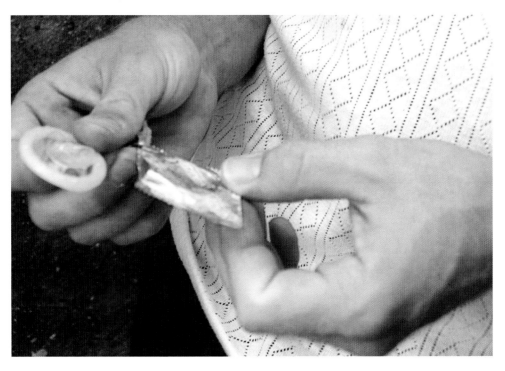

Signs and symptoms

- Increase in the urgency and frequency of a person's need to urinate.
- Discomfort when urinating, which includes a burning or itching sensation in the urethra and lower part of the abdomen.
- Sensitivity or inflammation of the groin area and/or the penis.
- Appearance of a discharge of pus from the urethra that may be bloody.
- Pain during sex or when ejaculating.
- Blood in semen.
- The symptoms can become chronic.
- If left untreated, or treated ineffectively, an infection of the urethra by gonococcus can cause the urethra to narrow (stenosis). This stricture increases the risk of a more acute form of urethritis arising and, sometimes, the formation of an abscess surrounding the urethra. The abscess can cause a deterioration of the urethral wall (urethral diverticula: pouch-like enlargements of the urethra) which can also become infected.
- A prolonged infection, left untreated, can progress and eventually infect the kidney, the epididymis (epididymitis), or cause damage to the tissues of the urinary tract.

Diagnosis

A complete physical examination of the urinary tract is necessary, including an examination of the abdomen, the region containing the kidneys and bladder, the penis, and the scrotum, and a digital exploration of the rectum. These examinations may reveal an enlargement or sensitivity of the inguinal (groin) lymph nodes, as well as any discharge from or sensitivity and swelling of the penis.

Having a urine analysis done is also advisable, as it will reveal whether or not there is any infection.

A culture is grown from the urine sample to confirm an infection, discover the organism responsible, and determine the best course of treatment.

If a patient has a urethral discharge, it may be practical to analyze this as well and to grow a culture in order to rule out any sexually transmitted diseases as the cause.

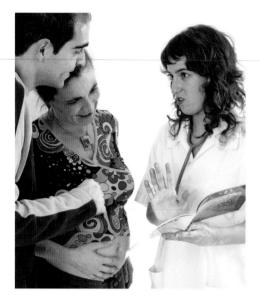

Behaving in a responsible way about sex and using condoms reduces the risk of contracting sexually transmitted diseases and, therefore, suffering from urethritis.

In certain cases, a cystoscopy (an endoscope examination of the bladder via the urethra) may be performed to examine the urethra directly. This is not always necessary; however, it may be carried out on a patient if the urethritis fails to clear up or its cause cannot be determined.

Treatment

Depending on the source of the problem, antibiotics or anti-viral drugs will be prescribed if the evidence points to an infection. It is very important for the patient to have routine check-ups to ascertain whether his treatment is working and to prevent any relapses.

People suffering from urethral syndrome—in other words, people who present symptoms but who do not otherwise show any evidence of infection—are prescribed medication to help reduce their discomfort.

Drinking large quantities of liquid often gets rid of a minor infection of the urinary tract. The stream of urine flushes the bacteria out of the body, while the body's natural defenses eliminate the remainder.

If the patient is in a stable sexual relationship, it is important for both partners to receive treatment simultaneously to avoid reinfection.

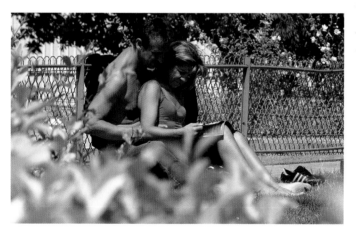

Preventive measures

- Drinking a lot of water helps prevent urinary infections.
- Urinating after sexual intercourse, particularly for women, can also prevent infections from arising.
- Maintaining a good state of personal hygiene is very important, both for the person affected as well as for his or her sexual partner. Good hygiene does not have to be excessive and can be accomplished using mild soap suitable for the genital area.
- It is important to consult a specialist as soon as symptoms appear to prevent any significant harm from arising, such as structural tissue damage.

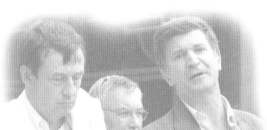

Peyronie's disease

This disorder involves the formation of hardened fibrous tissue in the structures that make up the penis. This hardening causes curvature of the penis, making erections difficult, painful, and crooked.

What is Peyronie's disease?

Peyronie's disease was mentioned for the first time by Gabriello Fallopio in 1561, although was first described by the French surgeon François de la Peyronie in 1743. Peyronie defined it as a hardening of the penis and classified it as a form of impotence. Nowadays, impotence is recognized as a factor associated with Peyronie's disease, but it is not always present.

Peyronie's disease involves the development of plaques or hard lumps in the erectile tissue of the penis. This fibrous growth causes curvature during an erection, and this is usually painful, making sexual intercourse difficult or even impossible.

Peyronie's disease develops as an exaggerated response to a local inflammation. The protein

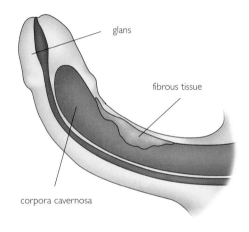

glans

fibrous tissue

corpora cavernosa

fibrin is deposited initially, and ends up like real scar tissue; but, unlike scars visible on the skin, this does not disappear over time.

Most patients with Peyronie's disease undergo two phases: in the first, or active, phase, erections are painful and the penis starts to become deformed; the later, less aggressive, phase is typified by stabilization of the curvature, erections that are not as painful as they once were, and stabilization of the whole process.

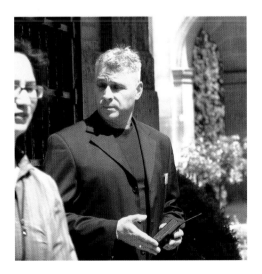

Around 38 in every 1,000 men develop Peyronie's disease. This condition is rare and usually occurs in men over the age of 40, although the average age at which it appears is 53.

257

Causes

- No definitive cause exists for Peyronie's disease, but all studies point to its initiation being mainly conditional on the multiple micro-traumas produced during intercourse. Certain positions and movements during sexual intercourse are more likely to lead to these micro-injuries—in which the woman is positioned on top of the man or the man repeatedly fails to penetrate correctly. This theory may explain the more acute cases of this condition, but it does not explain why there are cases in which it develops gradually or why the disease can exist without apparent trauma.

- If a patient recovers from the disease within a year, his fibrous tissue will not grow back and the condition will not develop any further than the initial inflammatory phase. However, if the disease persists for years, the hard fibrous tissue which often appears will calcify, causing curvature of the penis.

- It has been observed that there is a greater incidence of Peyronie's disease in men with diabetes, Dupuytren's disease or contracture (involving the appearance of fibrous nodules on the palm of the hand), Paget's disease (a bone disorder that causes deformities), gout, high blood pressure brought on by medication, and men who use or have used some type of urethral instrument (e.g. a catheter).

- There is evidence to indicate a possible genetic link to Peyronie's disease. In other words, this condition may be genetic in origin and thus a man may have a genetic predisposition to suffer from the disease.

Diagnosis

A physical examination is enough to diagnose curvature of the penis. The hard plaques or lumps can be felt with or without an erection. To evaluate the curvature, it is necessary for the penis to be erect; to facilitate this, it may be necessary to induce an erection by injecting the penis with a drug.

Otherwise, the patient can validate his curvature by taking a series of photographs of his penis when erect in the privacy of his home.

Although not essential, a medical practitioner may ask for a (Doppler) ultrasound scan to be performed to identify any damage that is causing the curvature.

Treatment

For men affected by Peyronie's disease, the general objective of treatment is to keep them sexually active. An important part of treatment is to explain the nature of the condition and how it develops.

Treatment is unnecessary in some cases, given that the problem often occurs as a mild condition and improves without intervention within the space of 6 to 15 months.

Symptoms

- Painful erection

- During erection, the penis is curved in one direction or another depending on where the fibrous tissue is located. In cases where fibrous tissue is located in both the upper and lower part of the penis, fissuring and shortening of the penis may occur.

- The diameter of the penis becomes narrower during erection.

- It is possible to discern a thick, cord-like line of hard tissue within the penis, like a scar, including when the penis is erect.

- The pain, curvature, and emotional upset can be an impediment to sexual intercourse and cause impotence.

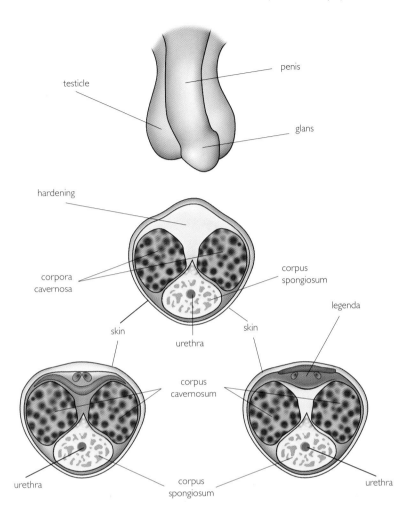

If necessary, treatment may include:

- Palliative treatment, if pain and discomfort is involved;
- Surgery. Experts recommend surgery only in those cases where the condition has stabilized completely and the presence of the deformity is making sexual intercourse difficult. Surgical corrections can lead to impotence;
- Surgery that attempts to eliminate curvature using a prosthetic penile implant. The prosthesis straightens out the penis and allows erections to be sustained and prolonged. It is recommended for men who experience severe pain during erection or to those suffering erectile dysfunction as a result of the disease;
- Vitamin E. In some cases, it has been observed that taking vitamin E has alleviated some of the suffering associated with the disease; however, control studies to establish the effectiveness of this treatment are not yet available;
- Injections of medication into the fibrous plaques. Trials have been done injecting therapeutic medicines directly into the damaged area. The greatest area of study has been done on therapies using corticosteroids, verapamil, interferons, collagenase, and orgotein. However, none of these treatments has produced any statistically significant improvement and, in some cases, they can complicate subsequent surgery;
- Radiation therapy. This involves applying radiation to the part of the penis containing the fibrous tissue in an attempt to reduce pain. This technique only reduces the symptoms, not the fibrous tissue itself.

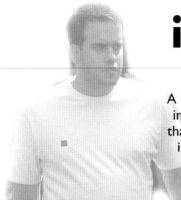

inguinal hernia

A hernia occurs when part of an organ—generally the intestines—protrudes through the thin muscular wall that keeps the body's organs in position. In the case of inguinal hernias, the intestine pushes through a weak point or a tear in the abdominal wall.

Causes

Usually, there is no obvious cause for the development of a hernia, although the appearance of a hernia is very often linked to the lifting of heavy objects.

People with any of the following symptoms are more likely to develop a hernia:

- If there is a history of hernias in the family.
- Cystic fibrosis.

Hernias are common occurrences for babies and children. With children, hernias usually appear because the muscular wall containing the abdominal organs did not close completely before they were born, resulting in inguinal or umbilical hernias. Inguinal hernias are more frequent among boys than girls.

- Testicles that have not descended.
- Being overweight.
- Chronic coughing.
- Enlarged prostate gland as a result of efforts made to urinate.

There are several types of hernia:

- **Inguinal hernia:** This appears as a bulge in the groin or within the scrotum. This type of hernia is more common among men than women.
- **Femoral hernia:** Similarly to inguinal hernias, this appears as a bulge in the upper part of the thigh. This type is more common among women than men.
- **Incisional hernia:** A hernia can protrude through the scar tissue of people who have undergone abdominal surgery.
- **Umbilical hernia:** Causes a bulge around the navel, which occurs when there is a weakness or opening in the surrounding muscle tissue.

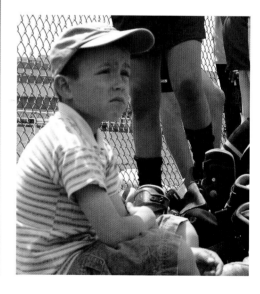

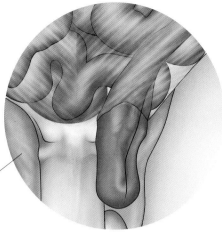

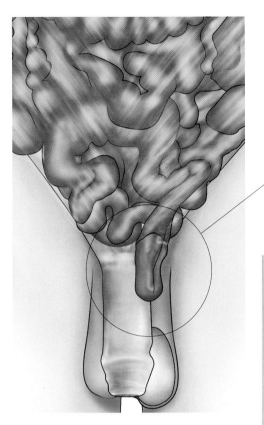

An inguinal hernia is a common condition among men (2 percent) and can appear as an indirect hernia (when a portion of the intestine protrudes into the scrotum) or as a direct hernia (when the intestine protrudes into the groin).

Symptoms
- Discomfort or pain in the groin that worsens when bending down or lifting weights.
- Appearance of a protuberance in the groin or scrotum, which may or may not be painful.
- In boys, the appearance of a protuberance or lump in the groin or scrotum without any associated pain.
- A person should see a medical practitioner immediately if nausea, vomiting, and fever occur, or if the skin changes color around the area of the hernia.

Sometimes, the appearance of a hernia may be to the result of lifting heavy objects.

Examination and treatment

- A physician can confirm the presence of a hernia through a simple physical examination. The protuberance is seen to enlarge when the patient coughs, bends down, picks up an object, or strains in some way. In the case of babies and children, a hernia may not be visible unless they cry or cough.

- Most hernias can be pushed back into the abdominal cavity. However, if they are not repositioned, this portion of the intestine can become strangulated and die because it has no blood supply. Immediate surgery is required if this happens; otherwise, gangrene can take hold, killing the patient.

- Almost all hernias require surgery, preferably before complications appear—such as the loss of part of the strangulated intestine or weakening of the abdominal muscles.

- Hernia repair involves ambulatory surgery under either local or general anesthesia. Firstly, after making an incision, the herniated part of the intestine is relocated within the abdominal cavity and, subsequently, the muscle and skin is sutured to repair the hernia. A synthetic mesh prosthesis is commonly incorporated to reinforce the defective abdominal wall.

Preventive measures

- Lift weights using a sensible lifting technique.

- Avoid becoming overweight.
- If you suffer from constipation, eat more fiber, drink more liquid, and go to the bathroom as soon as you feel the need, to avoid straining.
- Take regular physical exercise.
- Avoid chores that require excessive effort.

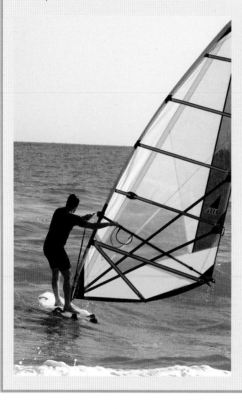
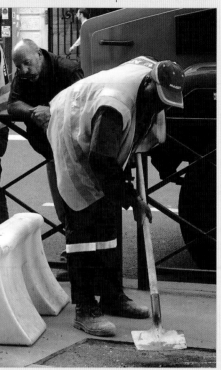

Surgery involves making an incision above the hernia and replacing the protrusion inside the muscle wall, afterward repairing the muscle tissue and inserting stitches.

Surgery

Surgery is recommended in cases where:

- A large bulge is protruding through a small hole, because of the increased risk of strangulation and hospitalization;

- The hernia is very painful or the protuberance in the groin is very large.

- Both adults and children are recommended to move and walk about immediately after hernia

surgery. However, in the weeks after the operation, it is important to avoid knocking the area of the incision, straining, or lifting heavy objects because this could reopen the wound, although the hernia repair is not at risk. Recovery is complete after four weeks.

HIV/AIDS

It is estimated that 40 million people worldwide are affected by HIV/AIDS. The cause of this epidemic is a virus that attacks the immune system. It is transmitted through contact with blood, semen, or vaginal secretions from people infected with the virus. To halt this global epidemic, it is important to understand the nature of the disease and how to prevent its transmission, and to eliminate the myths and taboos that surround it.

HIV/AIDS

Acquired immunodeficiency syndrome (AIDS) describes the long-term progression of a disease caused by a retrovirus: the human immunodeficiency virus (HIV). This virus attacks the immune system by installing itself in the body's T4 lymphocyte cells; thse are the cells responsible for protecting the body against external attack. As the body's defenses are progressively destroyed, people infected with HIV go on to

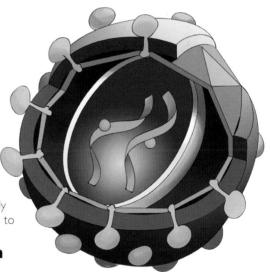

▪ Can HIV be passed on in other ways?

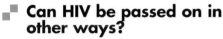

HIV has been detected in various bodily fluids (saliva, tears, urine) but, due to the low level of HIV found in them, there has been no confirmed transmission of HIV by these routes. Therefore, saliva, sweat, and tears do not transmit the virus. Similarly, it is not transmitted by insect bites, or through contact with household pets, as these are not carriers of the virus. HIV cannot be transmitted by acupuncture needles, tattoo equipment, medical instruments, etc. if basic hygiene precautions are observed (they should be sterile or for single use).

Retroviruses are viruses that have genetic information in the form of RNA (ribonucleic acid). These viruses need the DNA (deoxyribonucleic acid) from the cells that they invade in order to replicate their RNA and the proteins that surround them.

suffer serious infections and cancers unless provided with antiretroviral medication.

There are three ways in which HIV is typically contracted:

- Through sexual contact via semen and vaginal secretions.
- Through contact with blood: i.e. sharing needles or syringes, contaminated medical instruments, or the transfusion of infected blood.

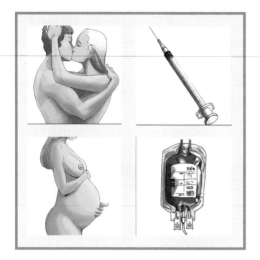

The most common means of transmission are: unprotected sex with an infected partner; sharing needles with an infected person; transmission to the fetus from an infected mother; blood transfusions using infected blood products.

During pregnancy:
• Treatments exist to reduce the risk of viral transmission from mother to baby during pregnancy and birth.
• An infected mother can also opt for a lawful termination of the pregnancy.

How to reduce the risk of developing AIDS
• Avoid reinfection with HIV (use condoms, avoid sharing syringes, etc.).
• Prevent "opportunistic infections" (an infection that normally does not cause disease but becomes a problem only when the body's immune system is impaired and unable to fight off infection, as in HIV).
• Do not take drugs (they can be a source of reinfection and are immunodepressants: i.e. they diminish the body's natural defense mechanisms).

• By a baby during pregnancy or birth (if the mother is an HIV carrier).

Transmission of the virus is limited by the following factors:
• HIV is weak and poorly equipped to survive outside of the body, which is why it needs to penetrate an organism's interior.
• Transmission requires a minimum amount of virus to enter the body. Below that level, the body is able to eliminate HIV, which explains why some bodily fluids found to contain low levels of the virus do not transmit it.

Preventive measures
Prevention is very important in restricting the spread of the disease and requires changes in sexual behavior and avoidance of high-risk situations.
In relation to sexual activity:
• Have a responsible attitude toward sex.
• Always use condoms correctly (whether for men or women).
• Avoid oral, vaginal, or anal contact with semen.
• Other situations:
• Do not inject drugs.
• If you cannot give up injecting drugs, always use sterile equipment and avoid sharing syringes, needles, and the equipment used to prepare the dose (spoons, filters, etc.).
• Always use disposable or sterile equipment for acupuncture, tattoos, or piercings.
• Do not share toothbrushes or razor blades for shaving.

Progression of HIV infection

From the time of infection until the appearance of the first symptoms, a person passes through different stages of disease progression:

• **Initial phase or acute phase of primary infection.** For some people, the symptoms are similar to those for infectious mononucleosis ("mono" or the "kissing disease") or influenza. The person feels feverish, suffers aching muscles, and has swollen lymph glands. These symptoms can occur within three months following infection.

• **Intermediate or seropositive phase.** This is the phase in which the infection is chronic and an infected individual shows no symptoms.

• **Final phase or AIDS.** Immunodeficiency worsens, the number of lymphocytes diminishes, and opportunistic infections take hold, which are usually both extremely debilitating and responsible for a person's subsequent death.

- Live a healthy lifestyle, including a balanced diet and good personal hygiene and avoiding stress, smoking, and alcohol.
- Visit your physician regularly, and take your medication as prescribed.

Diagnosis

Diagnosis involves detecting the antibodies that the body produces in response to HIV. If the result is positive, it means that a person has been infected. If the result is negative, it means either that a person is healthy or that their body has not yet produced the antibodies. Tests are available at Planned Parenthood health centers and from most physicians, hospitals, and health clinics free of charge.

What does being HIV+ mean?

A person is described as HIV+ (seropositive) when they produce antibodies against the HIV virus. HIV+ status means that:

- A person has been in contact with and become infected by HIV.
- A person can transmit the virus to others because he is a carrier of the virus.

However, being HIV+ does not mean that a person has AIDS, nor does it predict that he or she will go on to develop the disease. All HIV+ individuals have to take precautions to reduce the risk of the infection developing into AIDS and, above all, to avoid passing the virus on to somebody else.

Treatment

Treatment using combinations of antiretroviral drugs and prophylactic therapy against opportunistic infections have changed HIV's ability to develop into AIDS, transforming it into a chronic disease. Vaccination would be the ideal way to combat HIV, but the invention of a vaccine is presenting technical difficulties. Therefore, prevention remains the best way to avoid the spread of this disease.

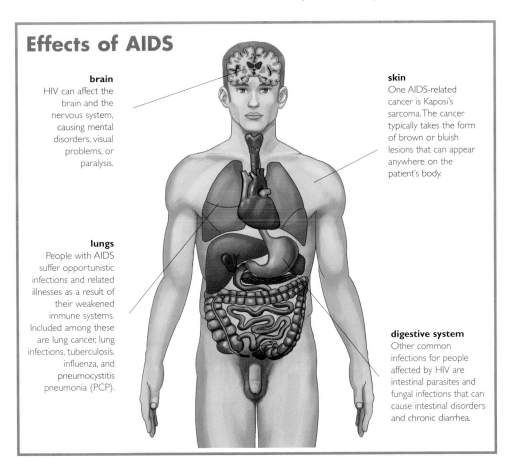

Effects of AIDS

brain
HIV can affect the brain and the nervous system, causing mental disorders, visual problems, or paralysis.

skin
One AIDS-related cancer is Kaposi's sarcoma. The cancer typically takes the form of brown or bluish lesions that can appear anywhere on the patient's body.

lungs
People with AIDS suffer opportunistic infections and related illnesses as a result of their weakened immune systems. Included among these are lung cancer, lung infections, tuberculosis, influenza, and pneumocystitis pneumonia (PCP).

digestive system
Other common infections for people affected by HIV are intestinal parasites and fungal infections that can cause intestinal disorders and chronic diarrhea.

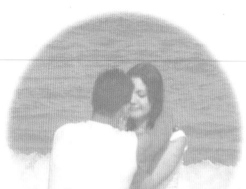

sexually transmitted diseases

Sexually transmitted diseases (STDs) cover everything from viruses, such as the human immunodeficiency virus (HIV), for example, to visible insects, such as crab lice. Although these diseases are commonly the result of vaginal, oral, or anal sex with an infected person, transmission does not always require penetrative sex and, occasionally, some are passed on through kissing or close body contact. Some of these microorganisms can be transmitted by food and water, from blood transfusions, contaminated medical instruments, or between drug addicts who share needles.

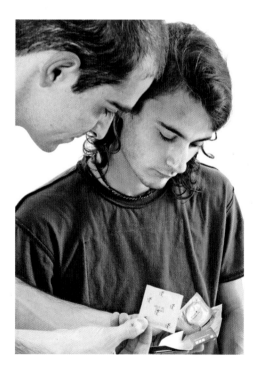

Look after your health by talking openly and frankly with your physician about your sex life and your concerns regarding your sexual health. Remember that tests, examinations, and treatment for sexually transmitted diseases are always handled in strict confidence.

Incidence and classification

Venereal diseases are among the most common infections in the world. Each year, more than 250 million people worldwide become infected with gonorrhea and another 50 million with syphilis. Other sexually transmitted diseases (STDs), such as trichomoniasis and genital herpes, are probably even more commonplace, but statistics for them are unreliable because physicians are not obliged to report instances to public bodies in such cases. Nowadays, the treatments for most STDs are fast and effective, which helps to prevent them spreading. The control of venereal diseases depends in large measure on encouraging safe sex practices and explaining how to avoid the spread of these diseases, in particular promoting the use of condoms.

Traditionally, five diseases were classified as venereal: syphilis, gonorrhea, chancroid, *Lymphogranuloma venereum* (LGV), and granuloma inguinale.

However, many others can be sexually transmitted: genital herpes, hepatitis, *Molluscum contagiosum*, crab lice, scabies, or HIV infection (the virus that can lead to AIDS). Sometimes, other infections are passed on during sexual activity, such as salmonella or giardiasis; however, these are not generally considered sexually transmitted diseases.

Venereal diseases are generally grouped according to the symptoms and signs that they produce: infections, sores or ulcers, or other symptoms.

Syphilis

Syphilis is caused by the bacterium *Treponema pallidum*. Treponema begins to multiply rapidly at its point of entry as soon as a person becomes infected. Subsequently, it spreads through the bloodstream to the rest of the body.

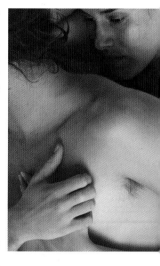

If left untreated, these bacteria can remain in a person's body for life and cause deformities, neurological disorders, and even death. The number of registered cases of syphilis has fallen in recent years thanks to the use of condoms and treatment with effective antibiotics.

Syphilis is passed on by vaginal, anal, or oral sex, through saliva, and from mother to baby during pregnancy. Syphilis is particularly contagious when there are open sores (chancres), and the pus is very infectious.

The effect of syphilis on a fetus is very serious. Left untreated, there is a high risk that the child will be stillborn or born malformed. Diagnosing syphilis is simple, and the treatment for it is effective: penicillin. Early diagnosis is important, as is thorough treatment.

The disease can progress through various stages and does not always follow the same pattern. Symptoms vary at each stage but, in general, the disease does not present obvious symptoms.

- **Primary stage:** The first sign of syphilis is the appearance of a chancre—a painless, open sore or ulcer. These appear three weeks to three months after infection and last for three to six weeks. They are mainly found on the genitals, vagina, on the cervix, labia, mouth, breasts, or anus.
- **Secondary stage:** After the appearance of the chancre, other symptoms appear and disappear spontaneously over a number of years, such as a non-itchy rash on the palms of the hands and soles of the feet, fever, fatigue, sore throats, hair loss, weight loss, headaches, and muscular aching.
- **Latent stage:** A person shows no symptoms. A latent stage can occur during any of the other stages.

◾ Diseases that can be transmitted sexually

The diseases first recognized as being sexually transmitted:

- Syphilis
- Gonorrhea
- Chancroid
- Granuloma inguinale
- Lymphogranuloma venereum (LGV)

Sexually transmitted diseases recognized more recently:

- Chlamydia infections
- Crab lice
- Candidiasis (thrush)
- Genital herpes
- Genital warts
- HIV infection
- Molluscum contagiosum
- Urethritis (non-gonococcal)
- Scabies
- Trichomoniasis

Diseases occasionally transmitted by sexual means:

- Amoebiasis
- Campylobacter infections
- Cytomegalovirus infections
- Giardiasis
- Hepatitis A and B
- Salmonellosis
- Shigellosis

- **Tertiary stage:** One-third of people with syphilis who have not received treatment go on to suffer serious damage to the nervous system, heart, brain, and other organs. It can be fatal.

Chancroid

The symptoms of chancroid are painful, inflamed ulcers or sores found on the genitals. It is caused by the bacterium *Haemophilus ducreyi* and it has an incubation period of two to five days. It is easily diagnosed because of its obvious symptoms:

- Among men, the first ulcer usually occurs on the foreskin, under the ridge of the glans, on the glans itself, or at the opening of the urethra. Among women, it may appear on the labia majora, on the clitoris, and adjacent areas, as well as in the vagina and on the cervix.
- The chancroid ulcer starts out as a small blister that soon breaks open and turns into a painful sore with irregular borders and a whitish area in the center. It can leave scars.

Gonorrhea

Gonorrhea, also referred to by its slang term as "the clap," is caused by the bacterium *Neisseria gonorrhoeae*. The sites that it infects mostly are the external genitalia or the anus, but it can also appear in the mouth, throat, and joints.

Its incubation period is about six days. In men, it produces a discharge of pus from the penis, sometimes referred to as "gleet."

If left undiagnosed and untreated during this initial stage, the infection can spread through the internal urogenital system, causing infections of the prostate and urethra.

In most cases, gonorrhea shows no symptoms in women, but they remain capable of infecting their sexual partners. Diagnosis is very simple, relying on samples of urethral discharge or urine, and effective treatment is available using penicillin or related antibiotics.

Practicing safe sex reduces the risk of sexually transmitted infections. "Safe sex" refers to all the methods used to minimize the risk of catching or passing on sexual infections.

Genital herpes

This is caused by a virus called herpes simplex virus type 2, which is different from herpes simplex virus type 1 (the virus responsible for cold sores).

In women, multiple ulcerations and lesions appear on the vulva, causing a stinging sensation, pain, and discomfort during sex. In men, lesions appear on the glans and foreskin. Genital herpes usually produces a burning sensation when urinating and symptoms very similar to influenza.

There is no specific treatment, and with painkillers and good personal hygiene it goes into remission of its own accord. There is no cure, and lesions often reappear in certain circumstances, such as when under stress or when suffering from other diseases.

Because of its continual reappearance and the ineffectiveness of treatments for it, this viral infection can also have a psychological effect. It seems to have some effect on the development of genital tumors. It increases the risk of miscarriage among women, and babies born to carrier mothers may present serious medical conditions.

Granuloma inguinale

This condition develops over time and is not as contagious as the infections described above. Typically, ulcerous lesions appear in the genital, groin, and perianal regions. In rare cases, it can affect other areas of the skin, mucous membranes, or even internal organs.

For men, lesions appear mostly on the penis (foreskin, glans, or where both meet), the opening of the urethra, and the scrotum. For women, lesions most commonly affect the labia, the vagina, the cervix, and the pubis.

Hepatitis

This is an infection caused by a specific virus that is transmitted through blood (blood trans-

Candidiasis (thrush) is an infection caused by the fungus *Candida albicans*. This organism lives in moist areas around the genitalia in small quantities without causing problems; but if the body's defenses weaken—whether as a result of stress, fatigue, an illness, or lengthy medical treatment—these organisms start to reproduce rapidly and present physical symptoms. Men experience irritation and a burning sensation around the glans of the penis accompanied by a whitish secretion in the same area. Women experience burning, swelling, and increased discharge, with these symptoms becoming even worse in the days immediately before menstruation.

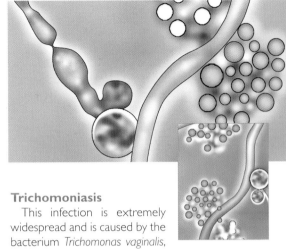

fusions, sharing needles), body fluids during sexual intercourse, or during pregnancy or birth from mother to child.

Hepatitis affects the liver, causing an infection that either clears itself or becomes a chronic condition depending on the person and the type of hepatitis concerned. Its most typical symptoms are fatigue, headaches, fever, rashes, loss of appetite, vomiting, dark-colored urine, and jaundice (yellowing of the skin).

Once the disease has been diagnosed, patients are advised to follow a healthy lifestyle, eat a balanced diet, and avoid reinfection, using condoms during penetrative sex.

Chlamydia infections

These are among the world's most widespread infections and are caused by the bacterium *Chlamydia trachomatis*. Unlike women, who commonly experience no symptoms, signs of this among men include penile discharges and pain or irritation when urinating.

If not treated in time, it can cause epididymitis in men and pelvic inflammatory disease in women, and for both sexes it can lead to infertility. The disease can be cured easily using antibiotics, if it is diagnosed in time.

If an expectant mother has chlamydia, it is possible for her to infect the baby when giving birth, leading to aggressive conjunctivitis – which if untreated can leave the baby blind – as well as chronic pneumonia. A variant of chlamydia, *Lymphogranuloma venereum* (LGV) is rare in developed countries like the United States. Unlike an ordinary chlamydia infection, LGV is a systemic disease that may cause painful swelling of the lymph nodes (glands) in the groin area.

Trichomoniasis

This infection is extremely widespread and is caused by the bacterium *Trichomonas vaginalis*, affecting men and women equally.

Among women, it causes an infection of the urethra and vagina. It can also affect the urethra among men. It causes discomfort, but it is not dangerous.

Men usually have no obvious symptoms, although it can irritate the glans and make urination uncomfortable. Any urethral discharge is analyzed when diagnosing the condition, and treatment is effective.

Fungal or yeast infections

Fungal infections mostly come from food or water, but if someone is infected—male or female—these infections can be transmitted via intercourse.

Genital warts

Genital warts, also known as condyloma acuminata, are caused by the human papilloma virus (HPV), which can be transmitted during either vaginal or anal intercourse, or even through the hands coming into contact with the genitals. The first wart usually appears on or around the genitalia one to three months after infection. The warts are small and pinkish and do not cause pain. They may typically appear on the glans and foreskin. They are easily diagnosed as they can be identified by sight or from analysis of a tissue sample.

Treatment takes a long time and is not very successful because of the tendency of the warts to reappear and because of their long incubation period, which can be as much as nine months. If creams or solutions to treat the warts have no effect, the warts have to be removed surgically by burning (using a cauterizing scalpel), laser, or cryosurgery.

Crab lice (pubic lice)

Crab lice (*Pthirus pubis*) are different from the lice found on the head in hair (*Pediculus humanus capitis*). Their bites produce irritations that, when scratched, produce scabs that can become infected and make the symptoms worse. Crab lice can be caught easily through close physical contact with a person carrying the lice, whether this is from sharing a bed, towels, bathroom, or from sexual activity.

It is treated using an antiparasitic lotion specifically against crab lice. The parasites usually disappear after one week of treatment. In addition to applying the lotion, it is important to pay close attention to personal hygiene, which includes washing all clothing and material that has been in contact with the skin.

Sexually transmitted diseases that infect the intestinal tract

There are a number of sexually transmitted intestinal infections. Various bacteria (*Shigella, Campylobacter,* and *Salmonella*), viruses (hepatitis A), and parasites (*Giardia* and other amoebas) that cause bowel infections can be transmitted sexually, particularly through activities that involve oral contact with the genitals or anus. The symptoms are those typical of the specific organism transmitted, and many can cause a combination of diarrhea, fever, nausea and vomiting, abdominal pain, and jaundice. These infections are frequently recurrent, particularly among gay men with multiple sexual partners. Some infections are asymptomatic.

Urinary infections

These are caused by bacteria that have spread from the rectum to the vagina or penis and then on to the urethra and the bladder. They can be sexually transmitted. Symptoms include burning and pain when urinating, the need to urinate when the bladder is almost empty and at night, incontinence, abdominal pain, and even fever. They affect women more than men, because a woman's urethra is shorter and closer to the anus than a man's, and bacteria can reach the bladder more easily.

These infections are easily diagnosed from urine or discharge samples, and effective treatment is available using erythromycin or other antibiotics. If untreated, these infections can cause fertility problems for both men and women, although particularly in the case of women, who can develop pelvic inflammatory disease.

THE SYMPTOMS OF SOME SEXUALLY TRANSMITTED DISEASES	
CHLAMYDIA	• 75 percent of the women and 50 percent of the men who are infected do not show any obvious symptoms. • Discharge of pus from the genitals. • Burning sensation when urinating. • Women may feel abdominal pain and/or back pain and pain during sexual intercourse.
GONORRHEA	• Discharge of pus from the genitals. • Burning sensation when urinating. • Pain in the pelvic region. • Women do not usually show symptoms.
SYPHILIS	• Painless ulcers in the genital region (appearing between ten days and three months after infection).
HUMAN PAPILLOMAVIRUS (HPV)	• Genital warts (sometimes internal and thus not visible).
GENITAL HERPES	• Sores and blisters (these go away but can reappear at a later stage).

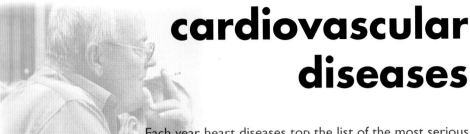

cardiovascular diseases

Each year, heart diseases top the list of the most serious health problems in the developed world. The main causes of heart deterioration are unhealthy lifestyles, ignorance about cardiac disorders, bad diets, high blood pressure, lack of exercise, stress, smoking, alcohol abuse, high cholesterol levels, and diabetes.

The cardiovascular system

The cardiovascular system, comprising the heart and blood vessels, is responsible for circulating blood around the body to supply it with oxygen and nutrients, simultaneously carrying away the body's waste products.

Although being male is an automatic risk factor in relation to cardiovascular diseases (due to the hormone testosterone), evidence over the past few decades shows that women run the same risk after the menopause.

Atherosclerosis

- This is caused by a buildup of plaques on the internal walls of the artery. Plaques are formed by deposits of fatty substances, cholesterol, the cells' waste products, calcium, and the protein fibrin, and they can develop in larger or medium-sized arteries.
- Atherosclerosis is a slow, progressive disease that could even have its beginnings in childhood. However, the disease can also progress rapidly.
- It is not understood precisely how atherosclerosis starts, nor what its cause is, but it is thought that certain risk factors can be linked to its development, including:
  - High levels of cholesterol and triglycerides
  - High blood pressure
  - Smoking
  - Diabetes mellitus (diabetes type 1)
  - Obesity
  - Physical inactivity

The heart is composed of:

- Four chambers (two atria and two ventricles) that receive blood returning from the body and pump it back again.
  - The atria receive the blood that returns to the heart.
  - The ventricles pump the blood away from the heart.
- The blood vessels are composed of a network of arteries and veins that transport blood throughout the body.
  - The arteries carry blood from the heart to the various parts of the body.
  - The veins carry blood back to the heart.

- The signs and symptoms of atherosclerosis appear gradually and, in its initial stages, may not even seem to exist. Moreover, symptoms vary depending on the artery that is affected.
- If it is blocking an important artery, an atheroma may cause a heart attack, a stroke (cerebral hemorrhage), an aneurysm, or a blood clot.
- Treatment includes:
  - Lifestyle changes to reduce risk factors: regular exercise, a balanced diet, and not smoking.

▮▪ How does the heart work?

With each beat that the heart makes, the chambers of the heart relax and fill with blood (diastole) and then contract and expel it again (systole). The two atria relax and contract together, as do the two ventricles. Deoxygenated blood saturated in carbon dioxide returning from all over the body enters the right atrium through the two largest veins: the superior vena cava and the inferior vena cava.

When the right atrium is full, it passes the blood through to the right ventricle, which pumps that blood to the pulmonary arteries, sending it to the lungs. Within the lungs, the blood flows through tiny capillaries, where it absorbs oxygen and releases its carbon dioxide. The oxygenated blood circulates through the pulmonary veins to the left atrium. This circuit from the right side of the heart to the lungs and back to the left atrium is referred to as pulmonary circulation.

Once the left atrium is full, it expels the oxygenated blood toward the interior of the left ventricle, which, in turn, pushes the blood to the aorta—the largest artery in the body and responsible for supplying blood to all of it.

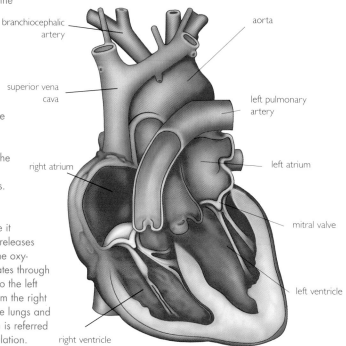

branchiocephalic artery

aorta

superior vena cava

left pulmonary artery

right atrium

left atrium

mitral valve

left ventricle

right ventricle

ATHEROSCLEROSIS

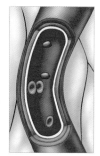

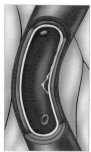

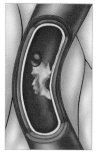

There is a gradual buildup of plaques, and the arterial walls become increasingly thick and inelastic, reducing blood flow and thus reducing the supply of oxygen to the body's organs.

Normal artery

Tear in the lining of the arterial wall

Accumulation of fat and cholesterol

ANEURYSM

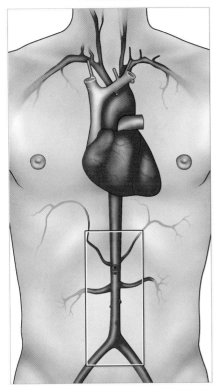

An aneurysm is dangerous because it can continue to grow until the blood vessel ruptures. An aneurysm that ruptures in a major blood vessel or the heart results in a fatal hemorrhage. If an aneurysm bursts in one of the brain's blood vessels, it can cause an embolism or a stroke.

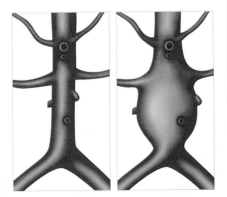

normal aorta   aorta with a large abdominal aneurysm

ANEURYSM

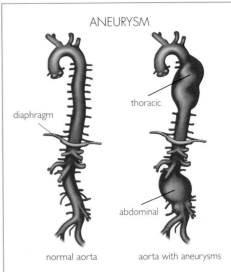

diaphragm

thoracic

abdominal

normal aorta   aorta with aneurysms

Aneurysms of the thoracic aorta are caused by hardening of the arteries (atherosclerosis), high blood pressure (hypertension), congenital conditions such as Marfan syndrome, injuries (frequently due to falls or road accidents), or, less commonly, syphilis. For these types of aneurysm, surgery is advised to replace the weakened section of the aorta or to implant a stent (a tube).

– Coronary angioplasty. This involves attempting to create a larger opening in the obstructed blood vessel.

Aneurysm

• This is the ballooning or formation of a bulge in a weak part of the wall of a vein, an artery, or the heart.

• Its cause may be an illness, such as atherosclerosis or high blood pressure, an injury, or a birth defect.

There are several types of cerebral vascular disease (diseases affecting the brain's blood vessels). A cerebral embolism is the sudden interruption of blood to the brain, usually caused by a blockage in the cerebral arteries (causing a thrombotic or ischemic stroke).

Another type of cerebral vascular disease is a cerebral hemorrhage (hemorrhagic stroke), which occurs as a result of ruptured blood vessels in the brain. The effects of a cerebral

ARRHYTHMIAS

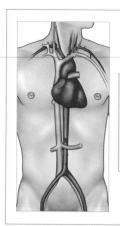

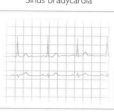

| Normal heart rate | Sinus bradycardia | Ventricular tachycardia |

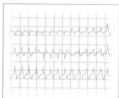

Bradycardia refers to a slower than normal heart rate.

Tachycardia means a faster than normal heart rate when at rest.

embolism depend on the part of the brain that is affected and the seriousness of the damage that it causes. Cerebral embolisms can cause debilitation, numbness, speech problems, loss of vision, or paralysis.

Angina pectoris

- This describes recurrent chest pain or discomfort, which occurs when some part of the heart is not supplied with enough blood and is thus deprived of oxygen.
- Angina is a symptom of coronary heart disease.
- The most common symptoms of angina are:
  - An oppressive pain that produces pressure or tightening in the chest just below the sternum.
  - A pain that radiates to the arms, shoulders, jaw, neck, and/or the back.
- The chest pain caused by angina generally starts after physical exercise. Other causal factors include emotional stress, intense heat or cold, heavy meals, excessive consumption of alcohol, and smoking. The pain usually disappears after a few minutes of rest or after taking medication prescribed for this condition.
- Angina can be diagnosed using an electrocardiogram (ECG), an exercise test, or a coronary angiogram (a medical imaging technique using x-rays).
- Treatment for angina usually concerns changing a person's lifestyle: not smoking, losing weight, and lowering cholesterol and blood pressure. Some medications alleviate the pain by dilating the blood vessels. The most common of these is nitroglycerin.

Cardiac arrhythmia

- Cardiac arrhythmia, also called cardiac dysrhythmia, is an abnormal heartbeat that can cause the heart to pump blood less efficiently.
- Cardiac arrhythmia can cause the heart to beat too rapidly, leaving the heart with an inadequate supply of blood; or it can cause the heart to beat too slowly or irregularly, preventing it from pumping enough blood to the body.
- In these situations, the body does not get the amount of blood it needs.
- The effects are very often the same, whether the heartbeat is too fast, too slow, or too irregular:
  - Weakness;
  - Fatigue;
  - Palpitations;
  - High or low blood pressure;
  - Dizziness and fainting.

Cardiomyopathy

- Cardiomyopathy is a disease of the cardiac muscle of the heart, making it lose its ability to pump blood. In some cases, it produces a change of cardiac rhythm, causing irregular heartbeats or arrhythmias.
- The causes of cardiomyopathy are sometimes unclear, although one of them may be a viral infection.
- There are three types of nonischemic cardiomyopathy:
  - **Hypertrophic cardiomyopathy.** The muscle mass of the heart's left ventricle is thicker than normal, or the partition between the two ventricles (the septum)

enlarges and obstructs the flow of blood from the left ventricle, preventing the heart from relaxing correctly between heartbeats, and filling with blood, which ultimately restricts the pumping of blood.

- **Dilated cardiomyopathy.** This is the most common type of nonischemic cardiomyopathy. The chambers of the heart are enlarged and stretched, resulting in them weakening and failing to pump normally.
- **Restrictive cardiomyopathy.** The myocardium of the left and right ventricles becomes excessively stiff, affecting the process that fills the ventricles with blood between heartbeats.

Congestive heart failure

- Congestive heart failure is a medical condition in which the heart is unable to pump enough oxygenated blood to satisfy the needs of the body's other organs. The heart still pumps, but not as efficiently as a healthy heart. In general, this reduction of pumped blood is symptomatic of an underlying heart condition.

- Congestive heart failure can be the result of:
  - Diseased heart valves due to rheumatic fever or other infections;
  - High blood pressure;
  - Infections of the heart valves and/or of the cardiac muscle, i.e. endocarditis;
  - A previous heart attack or attacks (the scar tissue from previous heart attacks interferes with the cardiac muscle's capacity to function normally);
  - Coronary heart disease;
  - Cardiomyopathy;
  - Congenital heart diseases or defects;
  - Arrhythmias;
  - Chronic lung disease and pulmonary embolism;
  - Heart failure induced by drugs;
  - Hemorrhages and anemia.
- Congestive heart failure interferes with kidney function, causing the body to retain fluid, which leads to swollen ankles and legs or a sensation of breathlessness in the lungs.
- The most common symptoms of congestive heart failure are:
  - Weight gain;
  - Visible swelling of the ankles, legs, and, sometimes, the abdomen;

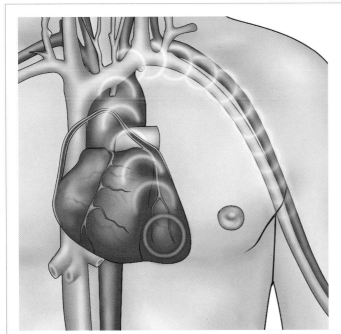

HEART ATTACK
(myocardial infarction)

The emergency medical services need to be called as soon as possible if a person suffers a heart attack. One of the signs indicating a possible heart attack is pain spreading from the chest to the arm.

- Breathlessness when at rest or exercising;
- Fatigue;
- Loss of appetite and nausea;
- Persistent coughing.

- Congestive heart failure can be diagnosed by taking a chest x-ray, using an electrocardiogram, or an echocardiogram.
- Treatment depends on the cause of heart failure. Surgery is usually carried out if it is due to a heart valve disorder. If the heart failure is caused by an illness, such as anemia, treatment is given for the medical condition responsible.
- The objective of treatment is to improve a person's quality of life. This means lifestyle changes and pharmacological therapy. It is important for the patient to avoid becoming overweight, to restrict his dietary intake of salt and fat, and not to smoke or drink alcohol.
- There are many medications for treating this condition: drugs that increase the strength of the heart's palpitations, drugs that reduce blood pressure, diuretics, and vasodilatory drugs. In very extreme cases, it is necessary to perform a heart transplant.

Heart attacks or myocardial infarction

- A heart attack, or myocardial infarction, occurs when one or more parts of the cardiac muscle experience an acute or prolonged restriction in their supply of oxygenated blood.
- An obstruction to blood flow is often the result of furring of the arteries (atherosclerosis). The atheroma or plaque that forms in an artery impedes and obstructs the circulation of blood and thus the flow of oxygen to the heart, simultaneously resulting in reduced blood flow to the rest of the body.
- If blood flow becomes reduced either suddenly or over a long period of time, the heart's muscle cells undergo serious and irreversible damage and die. The result is a lesion or death of part of the heart.
- The risk factors linked to heart attacks are either hereditary or acquired. Hereditary or genetic risk factors are those that a person is born with. Acquired risk factors are caused by a person's activities or lifestyle.
- People are at a greater risk of suffering a heart attack if:
  - They suffer from hereditary high blood pressure, hereditary high cholesterol or hyperlipidemia, and have a family history of heart disease;
  - They are elderly;
  - They have diabetes;
  - They are post-menopausal women;
  - They smoke;
  - They are under significant stress;
  - They take little or no exercise and are overweight.
- The most common symptoms of a heart attack are:
  - Severe pressure, feeling of an upset stomach, tightness of the chest, pain and/or discomfort in the center of the chest that lasts for more than a minute or two;
  - Pain or discomfort that extends to the shoulders, neck, arms, or jaw;
  - Chest pain that increases in intensity;
  - Chest pain that does not decrease when resting or taking medication for the heart;
  - A cold sweat breaking out over the skin, which feels clammy and/or turns pallid;
  - Lack of air;
  - Nausea, vomiting, dizziness, or fainting;
  - Inexplicable fatigue or weakness;
  - Rapid or irregular pulse.
- The objectives of treatment consist of alleviating pain, keeping the cardiac muscle functioning, and thereby avoiding death.
- Once a patient has been diagnosed and is stable, it may be necessary to perform a coronary angioplasty or bypass to re-establish normal blood flow to and from the heart.

A heart bypass involves an operation that uses a section of a vein from one part of the body to bypass the damaged or obstructed part of a vein or artery. The procedure creates a new route through which blood can flow, enabling the heart to receive the oxygenated blood it needs to function properly.

penile cancer and testicular cancer

Medical conditions affecting the penis and testicles can be alarming and detrimental to both mental and physical health. The penis and testicles can be affected by injury, inflammation, or infection, including sexually transmitted diseases and cancer.

Penile cancer

- This is a malignant type of cancer that affects the penis. This means that it grows aggressively and has a tendency to spread throughout the body.
- Penile tumors frequently develop in the skin that sheathes it and the semi-mucous membranes covering the glans.

Cancer is not a single disease one of many separate conditions in which cells grow abnormally until they produce masses of tissue or tumors. Essentially, there are two types of tumor: benign (non-cancerous) and malignant (cancerous).

Benign tumors have six main features:
- They only grow to a certain size;
- They do not normally grow very fast;
- They do not destroy normal cells;
- They do not spread to the tissue surrounding them;
- They do not normally cause serious side effects;
- In general, they show a regular pattern of growth.

Malignant tumors can be identified by their ability to invade and destroy tissue and organs, both those in the vicinity of the original tumor as well as those far from it. Death occurs when the spread of the cancer causes so much damage to body tissue and vital organs that they are no longer able to function.

- Benign-type tumors exist, such as those produced by the human papilloma virus (HPV). These lesions look similar to warts and can be

◼ Stages of penile cancer

1st. Cancer is restricted to the glans and foreskin; it does not affect the shaft of the penis nor the corpora cavernosa.

2nd. Cancer has invaded the corpora cavernosa of the penis, but it has not spread to the lymph glands in the groin.

3rd. Cancer has spread to the lymph glands in the groin. At this stage, any cure depends on the number and extent of invaded lymph glands.

4th. The cancer is extensive; it has affected the lymph glands in the groin and may show signs of having spread much further (metastasis).

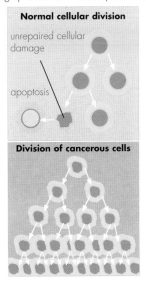

Normal cellular division

unrepaired cellular damage

apoptosis

Division of cancerous cells

easily confused with cancerous growths. It is estimated that around 25 percent of these benign types of growth may turn into malignant tumors if left untreated to develop of their own accord.

- Penile cancer is uncommon, representing approximately 1 percent of the tumors that affect men. However, its incidence may be greater in rural areas and regions where socio-economic status and personal hygiene are poor.
- The typical age at which penile cancer appears is between 50 and 60, although it can develop at any age.
- In most cases, the men who go for a medical consultation do so too late, often once the tumor is in a state of advanced development. This usually happens because of ignorance about the condition and its seriousness.
- Commonly, this type of tumor appears at the end of the penis at the juncture between the foreskin and the membrane of skin that covers the glans. It usually starts out as a hard, reddish blotch that, otherwise, causes no discomfort. Later, it tends to grow into a solid mass, similar to a wart. A common complication is the appearance of ulcers that can become infected and emit an unpleasant odor.
- This type of tumor can grow and spread, invading neighboring areas and affecting both surface and deeper body tissue, even making it difficult to urinate if it invades the urethra.
- If the tumor is located in the foreskin, treatment involves the local removal of the lesion. If it is located on the glans, a local amputation of the area affected by the tumor may be necessary. In cases where there is extensive cancerous growth throughout the penis, it may be necessary to amputate the entire organ. Radiotherapy is an option in the initial stages, although it is not very effective, because the tumor typically reappears once treatment has been completed.
- The survival rate is higher if this type of tumor is detected in the early stages. The rate of survival after five years is approximately 65 percent.

Testicular cancer

- Testicular cancer involves a cancer that develops in one or both testicles. It is a very treatable form of cancer and, usually, curable.
- Most testicular tumors develop between the ages of 15 and 40, although they can affect men at any age, including children and the elderly.
- The testicles contain several different types of cell, and one or more types of cancer can appear in any of them. It is important to distinguish between these types of cancer, because the prognosis and type of treatment available for each one is different.
- **Germ-cell tumors.** More than 90 percent of cancerous testicular tumors appear in the cells that produce spermatozoa (the germ cells). These cells suffer from two main types of tumor: seminoma and nonseminoma tumors.

The majority of the invasive cancerous tumors of testicular germ cells start out in a noninvasive phase of the disease called "carcinoma in situ" or "intratubular germ-cell neopla-

Klinefelter's syndrome

This is a chromosomal abnormality that affects only men, causing hypogonadism and sterility. A person's sex is determined by their X and Y chromosomes. Normally, the XY combination determines males, while the XX combination determines females. In Klinefelter's syndrome, the chromosomes have an additional X: in other words, men with this syndrome are XXY. This condition is common, affecting 1 in every 500 men. At birth, an XXY boy appears normal; however, the characteristics of the syndrome may develop during puberty: hypogonadism (reduced or absent secretion of hormones from the sex glands), lack of body hair, sexual dysfunction, growth of breast tissue, greater than normal height, learning difficulties, etc.

In the absence of obvious abnormalities, some mild cases may pass unnoticed, although most men with the syndrome will be infertile.

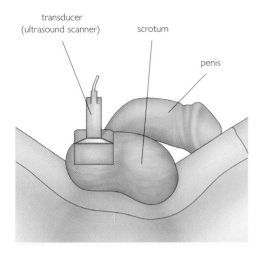

transducer
(ultrasound scanner)

scrotum

penis

sia." These tumors take about five years to progress and transform into invasive germ-cell cancer. When a cancer expands, its cells penetrate neighboring tissue and it may spread elsewhere in the body, either via the blood stream or lymph.

- **Seminomas.** About half of all testicular germ-cell cancers are seminoma tumors. They originate in the testicular cells that produce sperm. Two subtypes can be seen under the microscope: classical seminoma tumors and spermatocytic seminoma tumors. 95 percent are classical. Spermatocytic tumors grow very slowly and do not usually spread to other parts of the body. The average age for men diagnosed with spermatocytic seminoma is 55—about 10 to 15 years later than the average age at which classical seminoma appears.

- **Nonseminomas.** These usually appear at a much younger age than seminomas—generally among young men between the ages of 20 and 30. The main types of nonseminoma germ-cell cancer are embryonal carcinoma, yolk sac tumor, choriocarcinoma, and teratoma. Most tumors are a mixture of at least two different types, but this does not affect their treatment. All nonseminoma germ-cell cancers are treated in the same way.

- **Embryonal carcinoma.** This is a nonseminoma cancer in which the cells that are most abundant are of the embryonal type. This cancer causes 40 percent of testicular tumors. When viewed under the microscope, these tumors look like embryonic stem cell tissue during the first stage of life.

- **Yolk sac carcinoma.** The name refers to the similarity of these cells to those of the embryonic yolk sac during the first stage of life. This cancer is also known as "infantile embryonal carcinoma" or "orchidoblastoma." It is the most common type of testicular cancer among boys and adolescents. Treatment of these tumors is generally successful in childhood, but the tumors are more dangerous when they appear in adults.

- **Choriocarcinoma.** This is a very rare and aggressive type of testicular cancer. The tumors spread at great speed to various organs in the body.

- **Teratoma.** This is a germ-cell tumor with features similar to each of the three germ (cell) layers of a developing embryo. There are three main types: mature (benign) teratoma, immature (malignant) teratoma, and monodermal (highly specialized) teratoma, which may undergo malignant change.

Anything that increases the likelihood of developing a medical condition is referred to as a "risk factor." The risk factors for testicular cancer are:

- When one or both testicles have failed to descend into the scrotum (cryptorchidism);
- Abnormal development of the testicles;
- A personal or family history of testicular cancer;
- Having Klinefelter's syndrome;
- Being racially Caucasian;
- Infection with the HIV virus.

Stromal tumors

These can appear in supporting testicular tissue, in the cells producing hormones, or in the testicles' stromal (connective tissue) cells. The full name for these tumors is "testicular stromal cell tumors" and they account for 4 percent of testicular tumors in adults and 20 percent of testicular tumors in children. The two main types are Leydig cell tumors and Sertoli cell tumors.

- **Leydig cell tumors.** These originate in the Leydig or interstitial cells, which synthesize the male hormone testosterone. Although such tumors normally appear in adults, they can arise in childhood as well. While most of these tumors do not spread any further than the testicle and can be eliminated by surgical removal, a low percentage of them spread

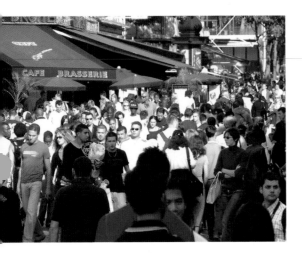

acute leukemia sometimes develop a testicular tumor. Secondary tumors can also spread to the testicles as a result of cancer of the prostate, lungs, skin, kidneys, and other organs. The prognosis for these types of cancer is usually poor because, by then, cancer is spreading throughout the body. Treatment depends on the specific type of cancer involved.

Testicular cancer is one of the most easily cured types of cancer. Studies show a successful rate of cure exceeding 90 percent.

Diagnosis of testicular cancer

Diagnosing testicular cancer may require a series of tests to be carried out, such as:

- A physical examination to identify any testicular lumps, abnormalities, inflammation, or pain;
- An ultrasound scan or diagnostic imaging techniques to confirm the presence of any solid masses;
- A blood sample to identify any tumor markers. Tumor markers are particular substances that, when cancer is present, are found in higher than normal concentrations in the blood. Some of the tumor markers used to determine testicular cancer include: alpha-fetoprotein (AFP), beta human chorionic gonadotropin (beta-HCG), and lactate dehydrogenase (LDH).

A testicular ultrasound scan is a technique that can produce images to examine the testicles and other tissue in the scrotum. This procedure is performed by moving the ultrasound transducer over the scrotum and observing the images generated. A testicular ultrasound scan allows a diagnosis to be made of any anomaly that might affect the scrotum and its contents. Therefore, it is useful when evaluating injuries, bruising, and

(metastasize). If so, the prognosis is poor, as it means that they have not responded well to either chemotherapy or radiotherapy.

- **Sertoli cell tumors.** These originate in the cells that nourish and support the sperm-producing germ cells. Like Leydig cell tumors, these are generally benign; however, if they do spread, they tend to be resistant to chemotherapy and radiotherapy.

Secondary testicular tumors

These tumors originate from another organ and spread to the testicle. Lymphoma is the commonest form of secondary testicular cancer. Among men aged 50 and above, testicular lymphoma is more usual than primary testicular tumors. A patient's prognosis depends on the type of lymphoma and the stage it has reached. The most typical course of treatment is surgical removal together with radiotherapy, chemotherapy, or both. Boys suffering from

---

Some of the possible symptoms of testicular cancer are:

- Painless lump or swelling on one of the testicles.
- Changes to the way a testicle feels.
- Dull pain in the lower part of the abdomen or in the groin.
- Sudden buildup of fluid in the scrotum.
- Pain or discomfort in a testicle or in the scrotum.

Testicular checkups

The testicles should feel firm but not hard. One of the testicles may hang lower or be slightly larger than the other, but this is not an abnormality. The testicles contain blood vessels and other structures that may lead a man to think that he has found a lump, but it is completely normal for these structures to be present.

If you perform your own checkups regularly, you will become familiar with your own anatomy and notice the appearance of any changes from the norm.

If you find any small, hard lumps, if one of your testicles starts to grow in size, or if any unusual symptoms appear that were not present when you last checked yourself, you must see your doctor immediately.

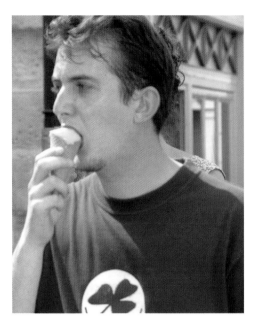

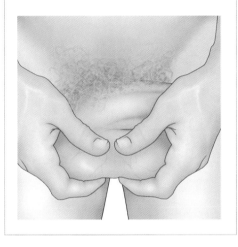

Testicular cancer has a good prognosis. In fact, it is one of the types of cancer to show the greatest rate of survival and cure. Statistics point to a near 100 percent probability of eradicating the condition. However, many taboos and fears continue to exist about cancer, despite the preventive strategies and types of treatment available having increased and improved enormously. These fears have more to do with the anxiety that a diagnosis of cancer causes than with what medical practitioners can do about it afterward.

inflammatory conditions, and when there is a suspicion of a tumor or inguinal hernia, etc.

Treatment of testicular cancer

• Once cancer has been detected, the first step is to determine the type of cancerous cells responsible by looking at them under the microscope. The next step is to determine the stage that the tumor has reached: in other words, if it has spread and the extent to which it has spread to other parts of the body:
– In stage I, the cancer has spread no further than the testicle;
– In stage II, it has spread to the lymph glands and the abdomen;

– In stage III, it has spread much further than the lymph glands, possibly reaching the liver or the lungs.
• Treatment depends on the type of tumor, its clinical stage, and the extent of the cancer. Three types of treatment can be employed:
– Surgical treatment, which includes removal of the testicle (orchidectomy) and the removal of any implicated lymph nodes (lymphadenectomy). This is normally performed in the cases of both seminoma and nonseminoma testicular cancer;
– For patients with seminoma-type cancer, radiotherapy may be employed after surgery to prevent reappearance of the tumor;

Chemotherapy is a treatment that uses medication to interrupt the growth of cancerous cells by eliminating the cells or preventing them from dividing and, as with radiotherapy, it may be used on postoperative patients as a complementary therapy. When chemotherapy is administered orally or injected into a vein or muscle tissue, the medication enters into the bloodstream and is able to reach cancerous cells throughout the body (systemic chemotherapy). When chemotherapy is put directly into the spinal column, an organ, or a bodily cavity, such as the abdomen, the medication mainly affects the cancerous cells in those specific areas (regional chemotherapy).

- At present, there is no way of entirely preventing testicular cancer. Many of its risk factors are genetic or unknown, making its appearance in some men inevitable. However, the early detection of any abnormality is of vital importance to the success of any treatment and to overcoming this type of cancer. Shortly after puberty, it is important for all men to be informed about this, to understand how to perform a testicular self-examination every month, and to have routine medical checkups.

The best time to carry out a testicular checkup on your own is after taking a bath or shower when the scrotum is looser. When doing a testicular checkup, if you are about to check your right testicle, you should position your right leg on some slightly raised surface, such as a stool or chair, for example. Do the opposite when checking the left testicle. Next, you should gently squeeze the scrotum until you find the testicle. Once found, you should move the testicle about gently but firmly between your thumb and the fingers of both hands in order to perform a thorough examination.

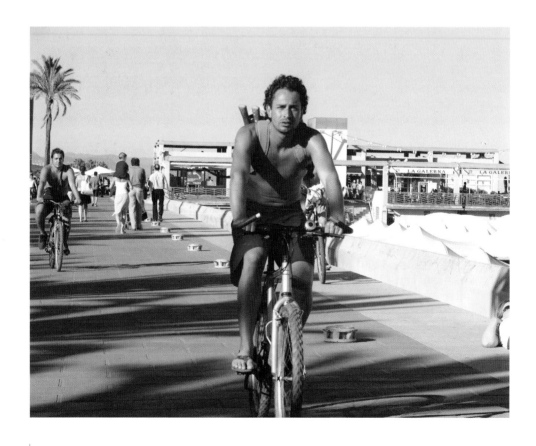

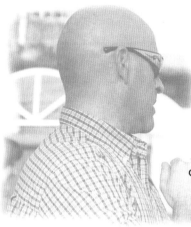

male baldness (alopecia)

"Alopecia" is the medical term that describes the partial or complete loss of hair, although it is known colloquially as "baldness." Hair loss, mainly experienced by men, tends to be inherited, but it is influenced by many more factors than simply genetic ones.

As people get older—men and women—their hair becomes weaker and loses its thickness. Normally, hair loss is gradual and limited to the hair on the head.

Men usually develop a typical pattern of baldness linked to the male hormone testosterone. It is called "alopecia androgenetica" or "male pattern baldness."

Male pattern baldness is a physiological condition that occurs among men who are genetically predisposed to it. During adolescence, these men produce greater amounts of the enzyme 5-alpha reductase, which is responsible for converting testosterone into dihydrotestosterone. This hormone inhibits hair growth, progressively reducing the number of hair follicles on a man's head.

As a result of the hair becoming weakened and the gradual decline of hair follicles, the hairline starts to recede from the temples and crown of the head. Ultimately, these bald patches meet, leaving a man completely bald apart from the sides and back of the head.

Typically, genetic baldness affects 25 percent of men before the age of 30 and another 50 percent before the age of 60.

Hair loss in patches, diffuse hair loss, brittle hair, or hair loss linked to psoriasis, flaking skin, and with pain, or rapid hair loss could have other causes or be related to other medical conditions.

A hair is a living structure in a constant state of development. Each hair follicle goes through various phases that allow hair to regenerate. The first stage is called the anagen phase, which is when hair grows. This phase

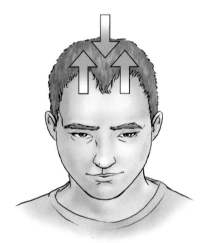

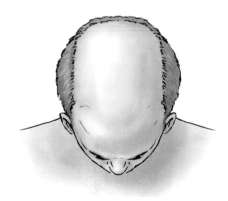

Alopecia areata is the partial loss of hair on the head (spot baldness), and alopecia totalis refers to a total loss of hair. Hair loss from everywhere on the body, including the eyebrows and eyelashes, is called alopecia universalis.

The average person has over 100,000 head hairs, and 100 hairs can be lost a day during the process of alopecia.

The life cycle of hair

Each individual hair lives for an average of four to five years, and during that time it grows at a rate of approximately 1/2 inch a month. In general, a hair will fall out in its fifth year and will be replaced by a new one within six months. Hereditary baldness is caused by the inability of hairs to regenerate and not by excessive hair loss.

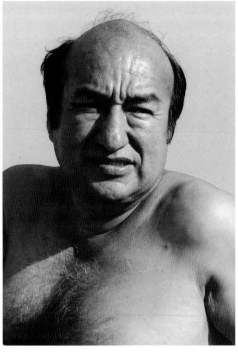

Male pattern baldness is a genetically linked trait handed down from mother to son. Therefore, men can predict their likelihood of suffering from baldness by considering their maternal grandfathers rather than concentrating on their fathers.

lasts for three to five years, and this includes 80—90 percent of all hair follicles.

The second stage—the catagen phase—describes a transitional or regressive period. It lasts for just seven to fifteen days and affects about 1 percent of all hair.

Finally, 15 percent of hair follicles are in the telogen phase, which lasts for two to four months. At the end of this process, the hair falls out with the follicle then returning to the anagen phase to reinitiate growth.

Many men accept the fact that their receding hairlines will become increasingly pronounced as they grow older; however, this fact remains a problem that affects sufferers to different degrees. Studies show that alopecia can affect sufferers' mental health and emotional well-being, denting their self-esteem in particular. Many men see alopecia as something that makes them less attractive and less virile, particularly when the process starts in their youth. Men who are losing their hair usually react in similar ways: at first, they ignore it, later they start to panic about the negative implications associated with baldness (a loss of sex appeal and masculinity, and a feeling of growing old), and afterward they feel a sense of powerlessness about being able to halt the process. Some become depressed, lose their self-esteem, and even avoid situations where they are obliged to put their incipient baldness on view. Many men who consult a psychologist have psychological

Trichotillomania

This is an impulse control disorder. It involves compulsive repetitive behavior in which hair is continually twisted and pulled. As a result, there are hair breakages and hair loss, usually in a specific area (although it can also be in irregular patches), with hair in some places appearing short and brittle or barely growing. Usually, the area most affected is the scalp, although the disorder can also affect the eyebrows and eyelashes.

conditions that can be linked back to hair loss.

A poor diet can contribute to hair loss and weaken its structure, causing breakages and slow regeneration. Hair problems caused by nutritional deficiencies can be corrected by following a more balanced, sensible diet. The main nutrients involved in this are vitamins A, B, and C, biotin, copper, iron, zinc, protein, and water.

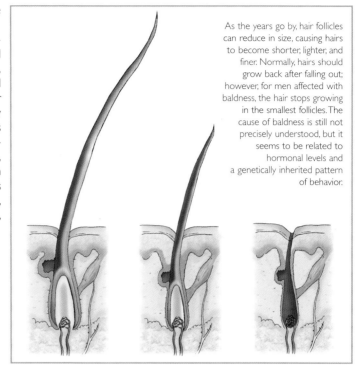

As the years go by, hair follicles can reduce in size, causing hairs to become shorter, lighter, and finer. Normally, hairs should grow back after falling out; however, for men affected with baldness, the hair stops growing in the smallest follicles. The cause of baldness is still not precisely understood, but it seems to be related to hormonal levels and a genetically inherited pattern of behavior.

Factors that can cause hair loss or alopecia

- Alopecia areata: alopecia of unknown origin that is characterized by patches of complete baldness.
- Hormonal conditions.
- Fever.
- Old age.
- Serious illnesses.
- Stress.
- An excess of vitamin A.
- Genetic factors.
- Cancer treatments.
- Agitation.
- Burns.
- Radiotherapy.
- Trichotillomania.
- If alopecia is a side effect of something else (stress, medications, fever, illness, etc.), the hair will recover and return to its normal condition once the primary cause has been eliminated or ended.
- Minoxidil or finasteride is used to treat hereditary alopecia. These are medications that are used for other disorders and illnesses, but which have been observed to produce hair growth as a side effect. They are usually used to reduce or halt the process of alopecia, although not all men benefit equally from such treatment.
- Hair transplants involve grafting small plugs of hair from areas where hair continues to grow and locating them in areas that are becoming bald. This procedure is slow and costly, but its results are effective and permanent.
- If hair starts to fall out rapidly without any apparent cause, it is necessary to consult a specialist, as it could be a sign of an underlying disorder or illness.

prostate conditions

The prostate gland is an organ that causes frequent problems. It is very common for men between the ages of 20 and 50 to consult their physician about a prostate gland inflammation or infection. For men above 50, the prostate can present a variety of medical conditions, including cancer. To prevent these problems, it is advisable for a urologist carry out regular checkups.

The prostate gland

The prostate is a gland forming part of the male reproductive system that is located in front of the rectum and below the bladder. It is the size of a walnut and surrounds the urethra (the duct that carries urine out of the body). The prostate is partly muscular and partly glandular with ducts that open into the prostatic section of the urethra. It is made up of three lobes: a central lobe and one on either side.

The prostate's main function is to secrete a viscous fluid that, together with seminal fluid and spermatozoa, forms a component part of semen. The muscular contractions produced during orgasm squeeze the fluid out of the

prostate and into the urethra, through which it leaves the body.

Normally, this gland increases in size with age, but it can become afflicted by infections or more complex medical disorders, such as tumors.

Prostate problems are commonplace, particularly among older men. It is estimated that 20 percent of the male population will develop some type of problem with this gland at some point in life.

Prostatitis

Prostatitis can be defined as an inflammation of the prostate. Its cause may be bacterial, non-bacterial, or it may involve congestion of the gland (prostatodynia).

In prostatodynia, the prostate becomes inflamed but without any evidence of infection. It is believed that stress, anxiety, and depression play an important role in causing the clinical symptoms shown by patients with prostatodynia.

Acute bacterial prostatitis

This is the least common form of prostatitis. Only five to ten percent of prostatitis cases are bacterial. Acute bacterial prostatitis can occur in men of any age, and its appearance is usually sudden. It is generally the result of bacteria entering the prostate via the urethra or bloodstream. The pathogen that is the usual culprit for acute prostatitis is the enterobacterium *E. coli*, although it can also be the side effect of a sexually transmitted disease (such as trichomoniasis, syphilis, or gonorrhea), or it may appear after

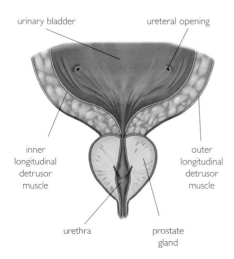

urinary bladder

ureteral opening

inner longitudinal detrusor muscle

outer longitudinal detrusor muscle

urethra

prostate gland

**Reproductive organs
of a young man**

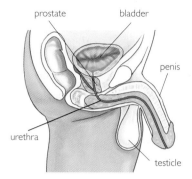

**Reproductive organs
of an older man**

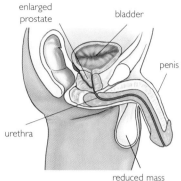

reduced mass
of testicular tissue

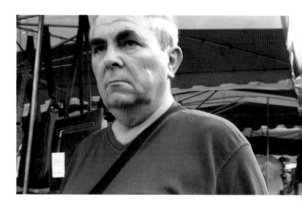

a surgical operation (a cytoscopy or catheterization).

Men with acute prostatitis have difficulty urinating and usually feel intense pain when doing so. Other symptoms can include fever, shivering, lower back pain, pain in the groin, needing to urinate more frequently, a burning sensation when urinating, as well as pain and discomfort throughout the body.

Chronic bacterial prostatitis

Although bacterial prostatitis is a relatively rare disorder, it can be recurrent and thus become a chronic condition. This turns it into a long-term infection that is difficult to treat. The symptoms of the infection are usually similar to the symptoms for acute bacterial prostatitis, but less intense and generally longer lasting.

Chronic non-bacterial prostatitis

Also referred to as "chronic pelvic pain syndrome" or "prostatodynia," this is probably the least well-defined type of prostatitis; however, it is the commonest form of the condition, as 90 percent of prostatitis cases fall into this category.

In chronic pelvic pain syndrome, symptoms may come and go without giving any sign or reason. The infection may be treated as an inflammatory condition, because no evidence of any infectious microorganisms is identified when samples of urine, semen, or other secretions are analyzed, and yet immune system cells are detected. It may be treated as a noninflammatory condition if immune system cells and any signs of inflammation are absent.

Benign prostatic hyperplasia (BPH)

This is a medical condition in which the prostate gland grows in size and interferes with urination.

BPH can raise the levels of the prostate specific antigen, or PSA, two or three times above normal. A high PSA level does not indicate cancer in itself; however, it should be borne in mind that the higher the antigen level, the greater the possibility that a patient will suffer prostate cancer at some point.

• Some of the signs of BPH and prostate cancer are the same. Even so, simply having an enlarged prostate does not increase the likelihood of a man going on to develop prostate cancer. Equally, a man with prostatic hyperplasia could also be suffering from prostate cancer at the same time or could go on to develop it in the future.

• The prostate goes through two stages of growth: during puberty and around the age of

Symptoms linked to prostate conditions include:

- Frequent desire or urgent need to urinate, especially at night.
- Pain when urinating.
- Difficulty and/or burning or stinging sensation when urinating.
- Difficulty in achieving an erection or loss of sexual desire.
- Painful ejaculation.
- Frequent pain or stiffness in the lower back, the hips, or the upper thighs.
- Total inability to urinate.
- Urine retention.
- Painful bowel movements.
- Unable to produce more than a trickle when urinating.
- Blood in urine or semen.
- Pain and/or pressure in the rectum.
- Fever and shivering (usually occurs when there is an acute infection).
- Inability to urinate simultaneously with bowel movements.

causes the prostate, because of its location, to press on the bladder and urethra, making the normal passage of urine more difficult.

- Most cancerous tumors of the prostate grow very slowly, although some can do so rapidly and even spread.
- Prostate cancer rarely occurs before the age of 55. Most men diagnosed with it are 65 or older.
- Early detection and treatment increase the likelihood of a cure. Moreover, prostate cancer is a very slow-growing type of cancer. When it develops toward the end of life, as frequently happens, the repercussions of this cancer are minimal, and even those men who have prostate cancer will often die of unrelated causes.

Preventive measures and risk factors

The reasons for cancerous growth processes are not yet understood, and very often it is unclear why malignant cells will sometimes appear in one patient but not in another. At present, many studies are investigating what these reasons might be and the risk factors that might increase a person's likelihood of suffering this disease. These factors include:

- **Age.** The probability of developing this type of cancer increases significantly after the age of 50. More than 80 percent of prostate cancer cases are diagnosed in men over the age of 65.
- **Diet.** Fatty foods seem to encourage the appearance of prostate cancer. Some studies have noted that men who have high-fat diets and who eat little fruit and green vegetables are at a higher risk of developing this cancer. The risk does not lie in fatty foods, as such, but in a diet that combines fatty foods with a low intake of fruit and vegetables.

25. At the start of puberty, the prostate doubles in size, and afterward, from the age of 25, it starts to grow again and continues growing in size for the rest of a man's life. This continual enlargement of the prostate does not usually cause problems, although it can lead to benign hyperplasia from middle age onward.

- Benign prostatic hyperplasia does not usually present symptoms before the age of 40. However, over half of men around the age of 60 show some symptoms, while 90 percent of men between 75 and 90 suffer from benign prostatic hyperplasia.

Prostate cancer

- This involves an uncontrolled growth of prostate gland cells that produces a malignant tumor in the gland. Among other things, this

Asymptomatic inflammatory prostatitis

This condition is notable for not producing the symptoms typical of other types of prostatitis and yet it does generate immune system cells to fight infection. Normally, this type of prostatitis is diagnosed during examinations for infertility or if prostate cancer is suspected, as well as in the course of tests for other conditions.

- **Physical exercise.** Regular exercise and keeping your weight down helps to reduce the risk of prostate cancer.
- **Genetic factors.** The risk of prostate cancer increases if a member of your family, such as your father or a brother, has suffered or is suffering from prostate cancer. It seems that the genes HPC1, HPC2, HPCX, and CAPB increase the likelihood of the disease.
- **Hormonal activity.** At first, testosterone initiates the growth of prostate cancer, but testosterone also manages to halt its growth when a tumor is at an advanced stage. The reasons for this dual effect are not understood at present, but numerous studies are investigating the role that testosterone plays in order to use it in the fight against this form of cancer.

Diagnosing prostate conditions

Following a general physical checkup, and after asking a series of questions about symptoms and medical history, an urologist will proceed with carrying out various examinations to determine whether a patient has a prostate condition and, if so, to identify its cause.

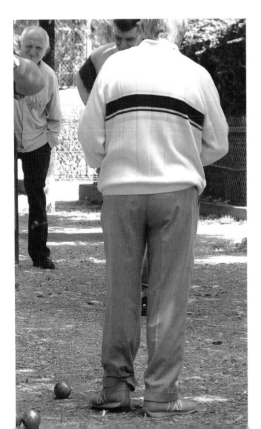

- **Digital rectal examination.** In this examination, the medical practitioner inserts a gloved, lubricated finger into the patient's rectum via the anus to detect any areas that feel irregular, hard, swollen, or lumpy, which might indicate a medical condition. Although slightly uncomfortable, the examination is quick and painless. It may also be necessary to examine the testicles to gauge their sensitivity and see whether any buildup of fluid is present (edema), as well as to check for any urethral discharge.
- **Blood sample or test to evaluate the presence of the prostate specific antigen.** This test is helpful for patients who are asymptomatic (show no symptoms) and involves taking a blood sample to detect the presence of a substance produced by the prostate: prostate specific antigen (PSA).
- **Urine sample.** A urine sample can reveal whether there are any abnormalities, such as prostatitis, prostatic hyperplasia, or tumor markers.
- **Transrectal ultrasound scan (TRUS).** This is a diagnostic imaging technique that uses sound waves to create an image of the prostate on a video screen, thus enabling the detection of abnormalities and small tumors. Placing the transducer in the rectum may be uncomfortable, but it is not painful.
- **Abdominal ultrasound scan.** This type of ultrasound scan is noninvasive. The instrument is passed over the abdomen to obtain an image of the interior on a video screen. It allows the medical practitioner to view any urinary tract or prostate conditions.
- **Prostate biopsy.** A diagnosis of prostate cancer can only be confirmed by taking a tissue sample (biopsy). The biopsy involves inserting a needle into the prostate in order to extract a sample of cellular tissue for subsequent analysis.
- **Intravenous pyelogram.** This involves using x-ray equipment after injecting a contrast agent into a patient's vein. This makes it possible to identify tumors, abnormalities, solid accretions (e.g. kidney stones), or any other type of obstruction in the urogenital organs, and also permits an examination of blood flow to and from the kidneys.
- **Cystoscopy or cystourethroscopy.** In this examination, a flexible tube with a small cam-

Prostate specific antigen (PSA)

- This is a protein produced by the prostate gland's cells. A PSA analysis measures the level of this protein in the blood. PSA is a biological or tumor marker, as it is a substance that the body produces that can be used to detect an illness.

- The amount of PSA in the blood is expressed in nanograms per milliliter. As a rule, a result below 4 ng/ml is considered normal. Results between 4 and 10 ng/ml are considered inconclusive. Those above 10 ng/ml are considered high and thus indicate a high probability that a patient has prostate cancer.

- These results provide an idea about how likely a patient is to have prostate cancer, but they do not confirm its existence.

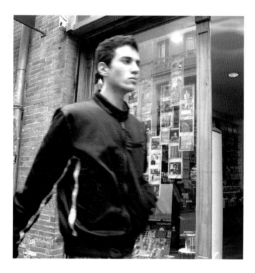

era is introduced through the urethra. It examines the bladder and the urinary tract, detecting any physical abnormalities or obstructions, such as tumors or solid accretions (stones).

- **Urinary flow analysis.** This involves an examination in which the patient urinates into a special container that measures the speed at which the urine flows. A reduction in flow speed may imply benign prostatic hyperplasia (BPH).

Treatment of prostate conditions

- Treatment for acute bacterial prostatitis usually consists of administering antibiotics and painkillers for several weeks. It is also highly advisable to drink a lot of fluids with this sort of infection.

- If prostatitis is chronic, antibiotics are usually administered for one or two months. This type of prostatitis is difficult to treat and erad-

icate, as it tends to recur very frequently. If the infection fails to respond to medication, low doses of antibiotics are often prescribed over long periods of time. If the infection still fails to clear up, surgery may be the only option.

- Drug therapies exist to help fight the symptoms of prostatitis:

- **Hormonal treatment.** Hormones such as 5-alpha reductase may be used over a long period of time and can reduce the size of the prostate by up to 30%.

- **Selective drug therapy** may be used, such as alpha-blockers, which work by relaxing the muscles of the bladder, urethra, and prostate, thus improving the ability to urinate and removing some of the discomfort that prostatic hyperplasia causes.

- The partial or total removal of the prostate gland can be performed in different ways:

- **Transurethral surgery.** This is performed via the urethra and does not require external incisions.

- The main knock-on effects of the partial or total removal of the prostate are impotence and incontinence. These effects are usually temporary but can be permanent in some cases.

- Removal of the testicles may be advised in some cases of advanced prostate cancer. These two organs are the body's principal manufacturers of the male hormone testosterone, which stimulates the growth of prostate cancer.

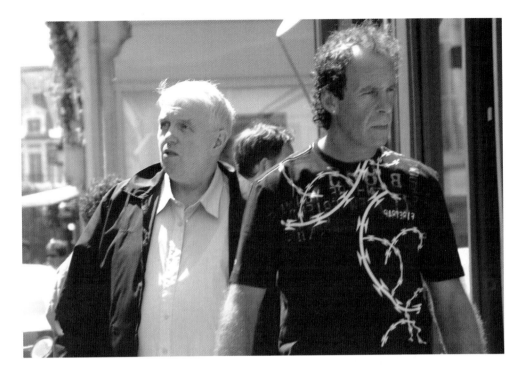

Apart from surgery...

- Apart from surgery, one or more of the following techniques may be advised for the treatment of prostate cancer:
- – Radiotherapy.
- – Chemotherapy.
- – Hormonal therapy.

- Male hormones (especially testosterone) can encourage the growth of prostate cancer. To halt this, female hormones or therapeutic drugs called agonists may be administered to reduce the amount of male hormones.

- **Transurethral resection of the prostate.** A medical instrument called a resectoscope is introduced through the urethra. It contains valves that eject an irrigating fluid, and at the end includes a tiny light and looped wire heated with an electrical current that is used to cut away tissue and seal (cauterize) the blood vessels. The surgeon uses this tool to remove the part of the prostate that is causing the obstruction.
- **Transurethral incision of the prostate.** This procedure is very similar to the previous one; in general, however, it only requires ambulatory surgery, being used for patients who have a relatively small prostate condition. It involves making a small incision in the tissue of the prostate to make more space for the urethra and the neck of the bladder, thus improving a patient's symptoms.

- **Laser surgery.** The laser vaporizes tissue obstructing the urinary tract.
- **Open surgery or prostatic adenomectomy.** This requires an external incision and is usually performed when the prostate is very enlarged, involves a tumor, or when the bladder has been damaged and needs to be repaired. This technique is complicated, but its success rate is high, and it does not usually require subsequent medical intervention. Surgery may be performed either by making an incision in the area between the scrotum and the anus (perineal prostatectomy) or by making an incision in the lower abdomen (retropubic prostatectomy).
- **Cryosurgery.** This type of surgery destroys the tumor by freezing.

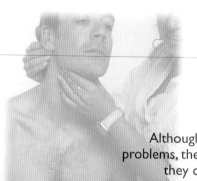

thyroid conditions

Although women are at greater risk of developing thyroid problems, these conditions are also important to men because they can be a cause of erectile dysfunction and sterility.

The thyroid gland

- The thyroid gland is located in the neck, just below the Adam's apple. It is butterfly-shaped with two lateral lobes joined at the center by the isthmus of the thyroid. It weighs approximately ¾ ounce and is responsible for producing the thyroid hormones T3 and T4.
- Thyroid hormones are vital to the function of every part of the body as they regulate its cellular metabolism.
- The thyroid gland itself is regulated by another gland called the "pituitary gland", which, in turn, is controlled by the brain. The pituitary gland keeps the thyroid stimulated by releasing thyroid-stimulating hormone (TSH).
- If thyroid function is sluggish, the pituitary gland increases its stimulus by sending out greater amounts of TSH. Conversely, if the thyroid is overactive, the pituitary gland reduces the level of TSH that it secretes.
- The thyroid hormones regulate the body's metabolism: i.e. the rate at which the body's various processes take place.

Two types of metabolic disorder are related to the production of these hormones:

1. Hyperthyroidism (overactive thyroid)
- This situation exists when there is an excess of thyroid hormone in the bloodstream.
- It occurs either because of an overproduction or disproportionate release of thyroid hormone, or because of too high a dose of thyroid hormone being administered to some people who need to take it.

- Hyperthyroidism can be caused for many reasons. The most common are Graves' disease (an immune-system disorder) and the appearance of a nodule (or benign tumor) in

▪ The thyroid gland

- The thyroid gland is situated in the middle of the throat, supported by the windpipe between the larynx and the trachea.
- Its size varies greatly from person to person and also depends on age and sex.
- The thyroid gland releases hormones that control growth and the body's metabolism, but it is the brain that dictates this release by means of the pituitary gland and the hypothalamus, thus affecting the balance of thyroid hormones circulating in the bloodstream.

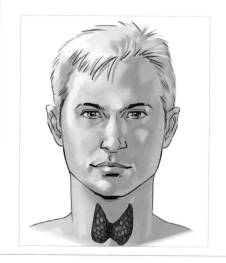

the gland. It can also arise temporarily in sub-acute thyroiditis—a condition caused by a viral infection or an inflammation of the thyroid gland.

- In rare instances, it is caused by overproduction of the hormone TSH by the pituitary gland or by a testicular tumor.
- Other symptoms can appear in Graves' disease (hyperactive diffuse goiter), such as swollen ankles (edema) and bulging eyeballs.
- Among older people, hyperthyroidism can produce less common symptoms, such as congestive cardiac failure, weight loss for no apparent reason, cardiac arrhythmia, psychiatric disorders, etc.
- It is relatively common for people receiving treatment with thyroid hormone for hypothyroidism to be affected by hyperthyroidism because of taking too high a dose. The dose of thyroid hormone has to be calculated and regulated very precisely for each individual. For that reason, regular medical evaluations and routine checkups are very important.
- The diagnosis of hyperthyroidism is very straightforward but the symptoms have to be clear to confirm suspicions that it is indeed

the medical cause. In the initial stage, it can be confused with anxiety or stress. Nevertheless, a patient's medical history and a physical examination may reveal some of the signs and symptoms of the disease that can be confirmed later in the laboratory.

- In cases of hyperthyroidism, TSH levels are lower than normal (or even undetectable) and, as time goes on, the levels of hormones T3 and T4 increase. In addition to taking blood samples to measure the levels of TSH, T3, and T4 in the blood, it may be necessary to perform an ultrasound scan or gamma camera imaging of the thyroid gland.

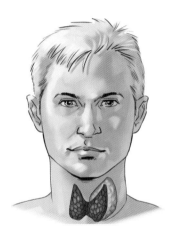

▪ Symptoms of hyperthyroidism

- Agitation and hyperactivity.
- Palpitations and trembling.
- Anxiety and insomnia.
- Mood swings, irritability.
- Intolerance to heat: feeling stifled, excessive perspiration, etc.
- Hair loss.
- Muscular weakness.
- Weight loss.
- Tiredness.
- Increased appetite.
- Intestinal complaints.
- High blood pressure.

What is a goiter?

- A goiter is an enlargement of the thyroid gland that is not associated with tumors or an inflammation. It usually appears when the thyroid gland is no longer able to produce thyroid hormones in a sufficient quantity to satisfy the body's demands. The thyroid gland enlarges to compensate for this situation, which is usually all it needs to do to correct minor thyroid-hormone deficiencies.
- Hyperthyroidism requires treatment only if it is producing symptoms. Enlargement of the thyroid can be treated using radioactive iodine to shrink the gland or through the surgical removal of part or all of the gland (thyroidectomy). Administering small doses of iodine can help when the goiter is due to iodine deficiency in a person's diet.
- Hyperthyroidism is usually treatable and is rarely fatal. It is very important for people suf-

Ultrasound techniques

An ultrasound thyroid scan is a diagnostic technique that uses high-frequency sound waves to generate an image of the gland. It is used to diagnose thyroid tumors, cysts, or goiters and is a risk-free, painless procedure.

fering hyperthyroidism to follow their physician's instructions to the letter.

- When being treated for a medical condition in which the metabolism is being accelerated—just as for the cardiovascular system—an individual may feel tired and can easily undergo minor crises. A person suffering from hyperthyroidism must get proper rest, avoid highly emotional or physical situations, and must not take medications that might accelerate the metabolism or cardiovascular system even more (nasal decongestants, certain types of anesthetic, stimulants, medication to reduce weight, etc.).

2. Hypothyroidism

- Hypothryroidism is caused when the thyroid gland releases very little thyroid hormone. This can lead to a wide range of symptoms and affect all of the body's functions.
- The most common cause of hypothyroidism is Hashimoto's disease, in which the body's own immune system attacks the thyroid.
- Another less common cause is failure of the pituitary gland, in which the gland fails to secrete the TSH hormones that stimulate the thyroid (secondary hypothyroidism).
- Other causes of hypothyroidism include congenital defects, thyroid surgery, radioiodine therapy, and inflammation.
- The body's metabolic processes slow down as the levels of thyroid hormone in the blood diminish, affecting a person both physically and mentally.
- In older people, the symptoms of hypothyroidism can be easily confused with the effects of aging, psychiatric illnesses, or dementia. Consequently, older people should have regular, routine thyroid function tests.

- In the most common cases of hypothyroidism—i.e. in primary hypothyroidism—a diagnosis is made by taking a blood sample for analysis. Hypothyroidism is confirmed if the sample shows very high concentrations of the hormone TSH.
- Analysis of T3 and T4 levels is not useful in the initial stages of the disease, as they may show no difference. Some types of medication and certain illnesses unrelated to the thyroid gland can affect these hormone levels, invalidating the test. Therefore, it is advised in most cases to quantify only TSH hormone levels, and if T3 and T4 hormones need to be quantified, they should be evaluated in their free form (concentrations of free T3 and free T4).
- Treatment for hypothyroidism relies on administering a substitute for the patient's thyroid hormone deficiency, usually taken in the form of tablets. A patient will have to take them for life, but it is important to evaluate the dose at least twice a year by means of checkups and blood sample analysis.
- Dosage varies from patient to patient and can range from very low doses to relatively high doses (300 micrograms a day). Nevertheless, a dose of between 50 and 150 micrograms a day is sufficient in most cases.
- Once a patient's treatment has been adjusted, thyroid hormone levels should return to normal, and the symptoms of hypothyroidism should disappear.

◾ Symptoms of hypothyroidism

- Tiredness.
- Depression.
- Intolerance to cold.
- Dry skin.
- Brittle nails.
- Hair loss.
- Memory problems.
- Constipation.
- Water retention (edema).
- Muscular aches.
- Weight gain.

mumps (parotitis)

Mumps, a form of parotitis, is a highly contagious, acute viral infection that affects both the parotid or salivary glands located between the ear and the jaw and, to a lesser extent, the testicles. There are no complications if the person infected is a prepubescent boy; however, if the testicles have already started to develop, there is a risk that the infected testicle will stop producing sperm, thus causing sterility. The mumps virus is transmitted from person to person through saliva or direct contact with objects contaminated with the virus.

- Mumps normally affects children from the age of 2 to 12, although it can occur at any age.
- In adults, it not only affects the salivary glands but can also affect other organs, such as the testicles, central nervous system, and the pancreas.
- The incubation time for this infection is generally 12 to 24 days. Its main symptoms include:
- Facial aching.
- Inflammation of the salivary glands.
- Fever.
- Headaches.
- Sore throat.
- Swellings around the temples or jaw (temporomandibular joint area).
- Men may also experience:
- Testicular pain.
- Lumps on the testicles.
- Inflammation of the scrotum.
- Mumps is diagnosed through a physical examination to confirm inflammation of the glands. If necessary, a saliva or urine sample may be taken for analysis to confirm the diagnosis.

Apart from a physical examination and a patient's complete medical history, it may be necessary to take either a saliva or urine sample, or both, to grow a culture and confirm the diagnosis.

- There is no specific treatment for mumps. The symptoms improve by applying a cold compress to the affected area and by taking medication to relieve pain and discomfort. Gargling with lukewarm, salt water, eating soft food, and drinking a lot of liquids can also help alleviate the symptoms.

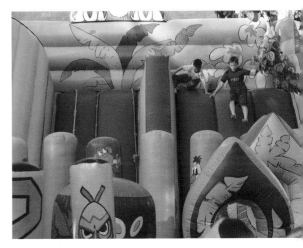

The mumps virus can be passed on 48 hours before the first symptoms appear and for up to 6 days afterward. The incubation period is between 14 and 24 days after first contact.

- The prognosis is usually good without complications arising, even if other organs are involved; and after the illness has passed, the patient has immunity to mumps for life.
- Mumps can usually be overcome without any specific treatment or bed rest. It is advisable to see your physician if you start to suffer an acute headache, persistent insomnia, vomiting and diarrhea, abdominal pain, bloodshot eyes, testicular pain, or lumps in the scrotum and on the testicles.
- The best way to prevent mumps is by vaccination. According to the US National Immunization Program, the first dose of the MMR vaccine that protects against mumps, measles, and rubella (German measles)

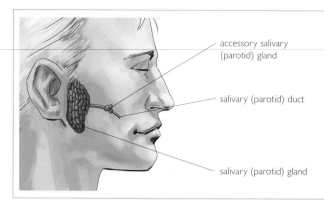

accessory salivary
(parotid) gland

salivary (parotid) duct

salivary (parotid) gland

The salivary (parotid) glands are situated between the ear and the jaw. In a case of mumps (parotitis), these glands become inflamed, causing discomfort and pain.

should be given to children between 12 and 17 months old. A repeat vaccination is issued to children between 4 and 6 years old or between the ages of 11 and 12 if they have not already received the MMR vaccine.

If a boy who has not yet reached puberty contracts mumps, there are no ensuing complications. However, there is a risk of complications if his testicles have already started to develop. The testicles become infected in 20 percent of all mumps cases. The condition usually affects only one testicle; only in rare circumstances does it affect both. Spermatogonia (immature

sperm) cells die as a result of the infection, leaving the infected testicle unable to produce sperm and leading in the long term to sterility. Once the infection is over, the size of the affected testicle or testicles may be reduced.

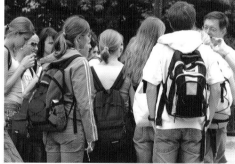

The most common viral cause of orchitis is mumps. Approximately 30 percent of all males who contract mumps after puberty will develop orchitis during the course of the illness. It is more commone among adolescent boys (only very rarely occurring before the age of 10), and generally appears 4 to 6 days after the viral process gets under way. Testicular atrophy (shrinkage of the testicles) occurs in a third of adolescents who develop orchitis as a result of mumps.

Mumps is most common among children between the ages of 2 and 12, although approximately 10 percent of adults are also likely to contract it.

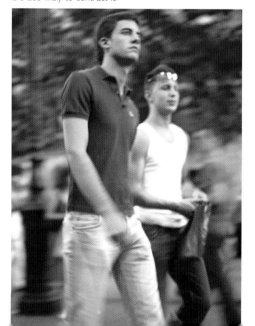

It has been proven beyond any doubt that immunization against mumps provides protection against the disease itself and its associated complication in males, orchitis, thus preventing the risk of sterility that mumps brings with it.

phimosis and circumcision

Phimosis refers to a condition in which it is either difficult or impossible to retract the foreskin, i.e. the skin that covers the end of the penis or glans in uncircumcised males. Phimosis can cause pain when an attempt is made to pull back the foreskin or when urinating and it is classed as a functional disorder, as it makes it impossible to have satisfactory sexual intercourse. In terms of personal hygiene, makes it difficult to keep the glans clean. Correction of the problem requires surgery, either circumcision or a technique known as prepucioplasty.

Phimosis describes a situation in which the foreskin is made up of a fibrous ring of tissue that prevents it from being retracted and thus uncovering the glans or head of the penis.

Phimosis may be a birth defect, but in many cases it is treated as an acquired condition due to repeatedly forced, traumatic retractions of the foreskin's delicate tissue during the first years of life (see below).

There is also another condition known as "paraphimosis" in which it is difficult to retract the foreskin over the glans as a result of inflammation of the foreskin.

Phimosis should not be confused with adherence of the foreskin to the glans of the penis, which is very common among boys under the age of three. For some boys, this adherence is accompanied by a narrowness of the foreskin, which causes inflammation and intense pain if any attempt is made to retract it. These adherences usually disappear of their own accord by the time a boy is out of diapers, and no attempt should be made to force back a foreskin, as it

In adult males, if the foreskin can be pulled back freely and there is no sense of tightening during erection, phimosis is not at issue. A longer than average foreskin is not an example of phimosis.

Balanitis

- This is an inflammation of the glans that may be bacterial, fungal, or viral in origin, or which may be due to the use of caustic soaps or not rinsing soap from the penis when washing.

- It usually involves irritation of the foreskin or the glans, rashes on the glans, a fetid odor, and pain affecting the foreskin and glans.

- It is usually diagnosed by means of a physical examination and the patient's medical history, although it may be necessary to grow a culture from the foreskin to investigate the organism responsible for the infection. In certain balanitis cases of unknown origin, it may be appropriate to take a biopsy of some of the skin from the penis.

- Depending on the cause of the balanitis, treatment may involve antibiotics, anti-inflammatories, skin therapies, and, in the most severe cases, circumcision.

- If not treated properly, balanitis can lead to phimosis or paraphimosis.

- Preventing balanitis depends on maintaining good personal hygiene.

Uncircumcised penis

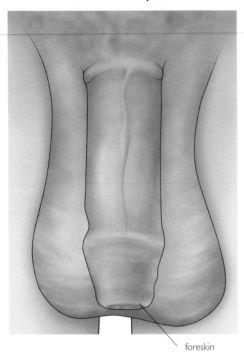

foreskin

Circumcised penis

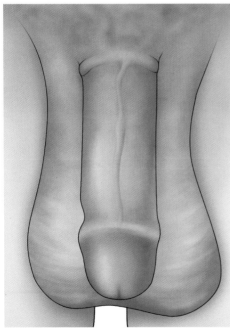

Circumcision involves the complete removal of the foreskin—the skin that covers the end of the penis (the glans).

Advice following a circumcision operation

- Avoid energetic exercise while healing.
- If the wound bleeds during the first 24 hours after the operation, you should dress the area to stop the bleeding.
- An ice pack or cold compress can be applied to the area during the first 24 hours after the operation to reduce inflammation and pain (except in the case of newborns).
- The wound should be washed using mild, non-perfumed soap.
- The dressing should be changed at least once a day, applying an antibiotic ointment each time. If the dressing becomes damp, it should be changed more frequently.
- Painkillers and anti-inflammatory medications can be taken to alleviate pain and discomfort. However, they will no longer be necessary after a week.
- You should try to avoid getting an erection.
- Sexual activity is not recommended until all the stitches have disappeared.
- You should see your physician if: moderate bleeding ensues, if the penis is very inflamed, if pus appears, if the pain is very intense, or if the pain and the healing process last longer than expected.

poses the risk of creating minor lesions, and the scar tissue that subsequently forms can become a cause of phimosis in itself.

Phimosis poses both a functional problem, since it makes it impossible to perform sexual intercourse properly, and a hygiene problem, since it becomes impossible to clean the glans—a fundamentally important issue for boys. The inability to clean the glans results in the buildup of a bodily secretion between the foreskin and glans referred to as "smegma," which often leads to painful local infections, frequently accompanied by the presence of pus (balanitis).

Phimosis can be corrected surgically by two methods: circumcision, which involves removing the entire foreskin, leaving the glans uncovered;

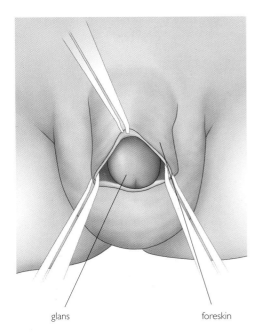

glans   foreskin

Circumcision is considered to be a safe procedure both for newborns and for adults. However, circumcision is usually avoided until a child is one year old to minimize the risk posed by anesthesia—except in the case of babies suffering repeated infections or in cases in which circumcision is practiced for cultural reasons, as occurs among Jews and Muslims, for example, where newborns are traditionally circumcised as a part of their religious customs.

or prepucioplasty, which involves dilating the narrowed section of the foreskin that prevents it from being retracted.

The choice of one technique or the other depends on the personal characteristics of each individual—although, in general, the recovery period following a circumcision involves more discomfort and the result is less aesthetic than in the case of prepucioplasty. Circumcision is recommended in cases of local infections or repeated urinary infections.

Before a circumcision is performed, the patient is injected with an anesthetic to numb the penis and reduce the pain. A ring-shaped clamp is placed around the foreskin, which it grips like a tourniquet to reduce bleeding, and

In some religions, such as Judaism or Islam, circumcision is part of a religious ceremony and is practiced on all newborn boys. However, in other cultures and areas of the world, including Europe, Asia, and Latin America, the circumcision of healthy males is very rare and is performed only if a medical imperative exists.

then the foreskin is cut below the clamp. Sometimes a disposable plastic device that, falls off by itself, after a week, is used once the area has started to heal. In newborns, scar tissue starts to form after approximately one week. Vaseline should be applied to the baby after changing his diaper in order to protect the wound. At first, it is normal for there to be some inflammation, and a yellow scab will form around the incision.

Complications do not usually arise after a circumcision, and recovery is usually swift—from eight to ten days. The only minor difficulties are maintaining hygiene and erections, which can cause minor bleeding and affect the stitches.

Although there are not usually any complications, consequential risks from this operation include minor bleeding, infection, localized irritation, and minor injuries to the penis.

■ Circumcision: the pros and cons

Great controversy exists about the practice of circumcising healthy males. Opinions differ, and many people believe that it is better to keep the foreskin intact, as it makes the experience of sex more natural during adult life. However, some studies insist that uncircumcised babies are at a greater risk of developing urinary tract infections. Other studies show that there is some increase in risk for uncircumcised men of penile cancer, some sexually transmitted diseases, penile infections, and the incidence of phimosis. In reality, the correlation between the risk of suffering from these conditions and being uncircumcised is relatively small. The results are not entirely conclusive, and the best way of preventing these conditions is to maintain good personal hygiene and behave safely and responsibly toward sex.